Understanding Hepatitis

Understanding Hepatitis

Editor: Terry May

AMERICAN
MEDICAL PUBLISHERS
www.americanmedicalpublishers.com

AMERICAN
MEDICAL PUBLISHERS
www.americanmedicalpublishers.com

Cataloging-in-Publication Data

Understanding hepatitis / edited by Terry May.
p. cm.
Includes bibliographical references and index.
ISBN 978-1-63927-199-3
1. Hepatitis. 2. Liver--Diseases. 3. Hepatitis, Viral. 4. Hepatitis viruses. 5. Inflammation. I. May, Terry.
RC848.H42 U53 2022
616.362 3--dc23

American Medical Publishers,
41 Flatbush Avenue,
1st Floor, New York,
NY 11217, USA

ISBN 978-1-63927-199-3 (Hardback)

Contents

Preface

The inflammation of the liver tissues is known as hepatitis. The most common symptoms of hepatitis include poor appetite, vomiting, diarrhea, abdominal pain, tiredness and yellow discoloration of the skin. There are five main kinds of hepatitis- type A, B, C, D and E. Contaminated food and water spread Hepatitis A and E. Hepatitis B and C are transmitted through needle sharing by intravenous drug users. Hepatitis D infects people who are previously infected by Hepatitis B. Hepatitis is majorly caused by viruses. Heavy intake of alcohol, certain medications and toxins can also cause hepatitis. Acute hepatitis resolves on its own while the chronic form of hepatitis causes liver failure, liver cancer and scarring of the liver. This book contains some path-breaking studies. It presents researches and studies performed by experts across the globe. For all readers who are interested in hepatitis, the case studies included in this book will serve as an excellent guide to develop a comprehensive understanding.

All of the data presented henceforth, was collaborated in the wake of recent advancements in the field. The aim of this book is to present the diversified developments from across the globe in a comprehensible manner. The opinions expressed in each chapter belong solely to the contributing authors. Their interpretations of the topics are the integral part of this book, which I have carefully compiled for a better understanding of the readers.

At the end, I would like to thank all those who dedicated their time and efforts for the successful completion of this book. I also wish to convey my gratitude towards my friends and family who supported me at every step.

Editor

1

Hepatitis E virus seroprevalence among the general population in a livestock-dense area in the Netherlands

Arianne B. van Gageldonk-Lafeber[1*], Wim van der Hoek[1], Floor Borlée[2,3], Dick J. J. Heederik[2], Sofie H. Mooi[1], Catharina B. M. Maassen[1], C. Joris Yzermans[3], Barry Rockx[1], Lidwien A. M. Smit[2] and Johan H. J. Reimerink[1]

Abstract

Background: Recent serological studies indicate that hepatitis E virus (HEV) is endemic in industrialised countries. The increasing trend in the number of autochthonous cases of HEV genotype 3 in Western European countries, stresses the importance to get insight in the exact routes of exposure. Pigs are the main animal reservoir, and zoonotic food-borne transmission of HEV is proven. However, infected pigs can excrete large amounts of virus via their faeces enabling environmental transmission of HEV to humans. This might pose a risk for of neighbouring residents of livestock farming.

Methods: Within a large study on the health of people living in the vicinity of livestock farming we performed a cross-sectional population-based serological survey among 2,494 non-farming adults from the general population in a livestock-dense area in the south of the Netherlands. Participants completed risk factor questionnaires and blood samples of 2,422 subjects (median age 58 years, range 20–72) were tested for anti-HEV IgG using an enzyme immune assay (Wantai). The aim of this study was to determine the HEV seroprevalence and to assess whether seropositivity in adults was associated with living in the vicinity of pig farms.

Results: The average seroprevalence of HEV was 28.7% (95% CI: 26.9–30.5). Determinants associated with an increased risk for HEV seropositivity were male gender and low level of education. There was a clear trend of increasing prevalence with increasing age (Chi-square test for linear trend, $X^2 = 83.1$; $p < 0.001$). A high number of pigs within 1,000 m of the residential address was not a risk factor for seropositivity.

Conclusions: This study confirmed the high HEV seroprevalence (29%) in the general population of the Netherlands, but presence of antibodies was not associated with residential proximity to pig farms. The prevalence increased with age from 10% in adolescents to 33% among those aged 50 and above, supporting the assumption of a cumulative lifetime exposure to HEV in the Netherlands as well a higher infection pressure in the past. Our findings cannot refute the assumption that transmission is primarily food-borne.

Keywords: Hepatitis E virus, Environmental exposure, Livestock, Seroprevalence, Zoonoses

* Correspondence: rianne.van.gageldonk@rivm.nl
[1]National Institute for Public Health and the Environment (RIVM), Bilthoven, The Netherlands
Full list of author information is available at the end of the article

Background

Hepatitis E virus (HEV) is a major cause of enterically transmitted hepatitis, especially in developing countries. However, recent studies show that autochthonous HEV infections are an increasing public health concern in industrialised countries [1–12].

The most common clinical presentation of HEV infection is acute hepatitis. Usually this is a self-limiting disease, with jaundice as the most common symptom [4, 13–15]. In patients with pre-existing liver disease and immunosuppressed patients, the clinical course of disease is often more severe and in developing countries excess mortality is seen in pregnant women [8, 10, 14–16]. However, most HEV infections in industrialised countries are either unrecognised or asymptomatic [1, 14, 16, 17]. This is supported by recent serological studies in several European countries, showing that the anti-HEV IgG seroprevalence in healthy blood donors varied between 7 and 52%, depending on both geographical area and the antibody assay used [17–22].

HEV is a non-enveloped single-stranded RNA virus belonging to the *Hepeviridae* family [16, 17, 23]. Four major genotypes, within species *Orthohepevirus A*, can infect humans [10, 15, 23, 24]. The genotypes 1 and 2 are restricted to human beings, and the genotypes 3 and 4 can infect both human beings and mammals. HEV-1 and HEV-2 are endemic in developing countries, leading to sporadic cases as well as large outbreaks. HEV-3 and HEV-4 are responsible for an increasing number of autochthonous hepatitis E infections worldwide [4, 10, 16, 17, 25]. The more recently discovered HEV genotypes 5 and 6 are so far only detected in animals, while genotype 7 is also described in humans [10, 26–29].

In contrast to HEV-1 and HEV-2, for which the faecal-oral transmission route via contaminated water has been confirmed, the transmission routes of HEV-3 and HEV-4 are largely unclear and the exact source of infection remains unknown for the majority of patients [4, 17, 27, 28]. The increasing trend in the number of autochthonous cases in Western European countries stresses the importance to get insight in the route of infection, enabling the implementation of control measures against human HEV infections [27, 28, 30].

It is hypothesized that HEV-3 and HEV-4 have a zoonotic origin, supported by the high prevalence of HEV-3 and HEV-4 among domestic pigs and wild boars [23, 26, 31]. In the Netherlands, the prevalence rate of HEV-3 in the domestic pig population is estimated at 55%, and domestic pigs may therefore be an important reservoir for human HEV infections [28, 32]. Furthermore, the frequent detection of HEV in pork products and the high similarity between porcine and human HEV sequences suggest zoonotic transmission of HEV-3 and HEV-4 worldwide [33–36]. Zoonotic food-borne transmission has been proven by the identification of identical nucleotide sequences in autochthonous HEV patients and in leftover portions of consumed contaminated food [37–40]. But zoonotic HEV transmission might also occur through exposure to contaminated environments. Infected pigs, which are generally asymptomatic, can excrete large amounts of virus via their faeces in the environment. This may lead to human infections [26–28, 41]. The high anti-HEV serum antibody rates in humans with occupational contact with pigs, like farmers and veterinarians, provide indirect evidence for this route of transmission [42–47]. However, environmental exposure to HEV might also pose a risk for of neighbouring residents of livestock farming, as was the case during the major Dutch Q-fever outbreak in 2007–2010 [48].

In the Netherlands there is an ongoing debate on the environmental health risks as a result of (intensive) livestock farming in areas highly populated with both livestock and people. At a surface of approximately 34.000 km^2 almost 17 million people are living together with 75 million chickens, 7 million pigs, 4 million cattle and 1.5 million goats and sheep. Within a large study on the health of people living in the vicinity of livestock farming, we performed a serological survey in order to assess the HEV seroprevalence among non-farming adults from the general population in a livestock-dense area in the south of the Netherlands. Furthermore, we investigated whether living close to pig farms is a risk factor for HEV seropositivity, focusing on the role of environmental transmission of HEV from pig farms to residents living in the vicinity of these farms.

Methods

In 2014 the Livestock Farming and Neighbouring Residents' Health study (Dutch acronym: VGO) started, aiming to assess the relationship between livestock farming and a number of health outcomes in people living in the eastern part of the province of Noord-Brabant and the northern part of the province of Limburg. This part of the Netherlands is a relatively highly populated rural area with a high density of livestock farms. Within the VGO study a cross-sectional health study was performed, investigating three categories of health effects: 1) respiratory health effects, 2) livestock-associated infections, and 3) carriage of resistant microorganisms. Furthermore, air sampling was conducted in order to assess to what extent residents living in the vicinity of livestock farms were exposed to emissions of these farms, including endotoxin amount, PM10 and DNA of *Staphylococcus aureus* and *E. coli*. Participants of the cross-sectional health study provided blood samples in order to assess (previous) exposure to several livestock-farming associated pathogens, including HEV.

Study population

The study population was selected in a two-step procedure. First, a questionnaire survey was conducted among 14,163 unrelated adults from the general population (aged 18–70 years) living in the study area. Participants were recruited via their general practitioner (GP). In the Netherlands each individual is registered with just one general practice, mostly close to residential address. Predefined inclusion criteria have been described previously by Borlée et al. [49]. Second, questionnaire participants who gave consent to be contacted for further studies, and who were not working or living on a farm, were eligible for the serological survey ($n = 8,714$) [50]. Based on their home addresses, twelve temporary study centres were established. Figure 1 shows the location of the temporary study centres, and pig density in the Netherlands in 2014. All participants living within a distance of approximately 10 km of a temporary study centre ($n = 7,180$) were invited to the nearest centre for a medical examination, including blood sampling for serological analyses against livestock-associated pathogens. Furthermore, they were asked to fill in a questionnaire comprising items on symptoms and diseases, home characteristics, smoking habits, education, profession, leisure activities, dietary habits (including the consumption of pork meat), and animal contact, including exposure to animal farm environment during childhood. Data were collected between 10 March 2014 and 27 February 2015. Patients' privacy was ensured as described earlier [49–51]. In short, medical information and address records were kept separated at all times by using a Trusted Third Party (Stichting Informatie Voorziening Zorg, Houten). The VGO study protocol was approved by the Medical Ethical Committee of the University Medical Centre Utrecht. All participants signed informed consent.

Exposure from livestock farms

Based on the home address of each participant, several exposure variables were computed, including distance to the nearest pig farm with more than 25 pigs and the total number of pigs within 1,000 m [52]. Information on farm characteristics in the study area was derived from the provincial database of mandatory environmental licenses for keeping livestock for 2012. This database contains amongst others data on number and type of animals and geographic coordinates of farms (specific for type of livestock).

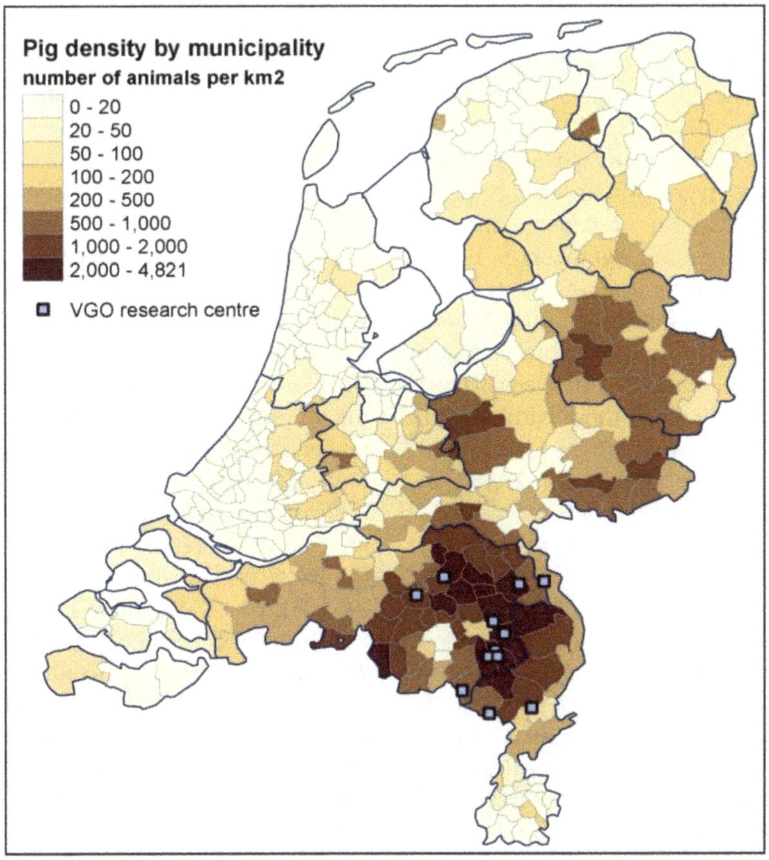

Fig. 1 Location of temporary study centres in relation to pig density in the Netherlands in 2014 (Source: Statistics Netherlands)

Serological analyses

Sera were analysed at the National Institute for Public Health and the Environment (RIVM) for the presence of IgG antibodies against HEV, using a commercial anti-HEV IgG enzyme immune assay (Wantai Biological Pharmacy Enterprise Co,. Ltd., Beijing, China). The test was performed according to the instructions of the manufacturer. Samples with anti-HEV IgG ratio <0.90 were considered negative, those with ratio > =0.90 but <1.10 were defined as borderline, and samples with ratio > =1.10 were considered as positive.

Statistical analyses

Seroprevalence, defined as the percentage of participants with borderline or positive anti-HEV IgG ratio, and 95% confidence intervals (CI) were calculated for the overall study population, per age group and per study centre.

Logistic regression analysis was performed to study potential determinants for HEV seropositivity. The following variables were included in the univariate analysis: age, gender, educational level, country of birth, consumption of pork meat, smoking status, spending childhood in the study region or on a (pig) farm, performing jobs on a farm during childhood, contact with animals during work or study, keeping farm animals and/or pigs for a hobby in the last 5 years, spending time abroad during the last 12 months, visiting a farm in the last 12 months (with or without contact with pigs during that visit) and the numbers of pigs within 1.000 m of the residential address of the participants. All variables with a *P*-value < =0.2 in the univariate analyses were included in the multivariate logistic regression model. Adjusted odds ratios (ORs) and 95% CIs were calculated and a *P*-value <0.05 was used to determine significance. T rend in seroprevalence with increasing age was tested with the Mantel-Haenszel chi square for linear trend.

Median distance from home address to nearest farm with more than 25 pigs was compared between participants with positive or borderline and those with negative anti-HEV IgG ratio using Mann-Whitney U test. This analysis was stratified by six age groups: 20–29, 30–39, 40–49, 50–59, 60–69 and 70 years and older.

The random forest method *(46)* was used to determine the ability of the potential risk factors to predict the anti-HEV IgG ratio or the infection status. Unlike regression, the random forest requires no underlying assumptions about the functional form of the model or distribution of the data and provides a reliable assessment of the contribution of the predictor variables to generate predictions of an outcome. The algorithm predicts the outcome (e.g. anti-HEV IgG ratio) of an individual based upon the individual's predictor variables, quantifies the prediction accuracy by means of estimates such as the mean square error (or proportion of correct classifications/statuses when predicting the status of an individual) and proportion of explained variance, and ranks the predictor variables according to their relative importance. Relative importance of a predictor variable is calculated by randomly permuting the data for that variable (leaving all other data unchanged) and comparing the prediction accuracy obtained with the 'shuffled' data set with that of the original data set. If the variable has little bearing on prediction, the mean square error will remain about the same after shuffling, while if the variable is useful for prediction the mean square error will deteriorate. The increase in mean square error that results from the shuffling is then a measure of variable importance which is used to rank the predictor variables.

Analyses were performed using SAS 9.3 and R version 3.1.0 (Random forest).

Results

A total of 2,494 of the 7,180 invited persons participated in the cross sectional serological survey, (response rate = 34.7%). Serum samples were available for 2,422 participants (97.1%). The primary reason for missing serum-samples was failure to collect enough blood for analysis. The median age of the participants, from whom a sample was available, was 58 years (range: 20–72 years) and 45.6% was male (Table 1). Although there were some differences between responders and non-responders, a non-response analysis within the initial questionnaire survey comparing the electronical medical records of the subjects recruited via GPs, showed that these differences do not affect the relationship between health and the presence of livestock [53]. A total of 2,163 of the 2,422 participants (89.3%) resided in the province of Brabant and Limburg during childhood, of which 1,816 (84.0%) lived in the specific study region. On average, the participants have lived at their current residential address for 20 years (standard deviation 13.5 years). The number of pigs within 1,000 m of the residential address varied between 0 and 79,057 (median = 2,701; interquartile range: 336–9,035) and the distance to the nearest pig farm with more than 25 pigs ranged from 11 to 2500 m (median = 687 m; interquartile range: 462–932).

Positive and borderline positive anti-HEV IgG ratio was found for respectively 666 (27.5%) and 29 (1.2%) of the 2,422 participants. Overall seroprevalence was 28.7% (95% CI: 26.9–30.5; Table 1), ranging between study centres from 16.7% (95% CI: 8.1–25.3) to 35.7% (95% CI: 25.5–46.0). Seroprevalence increased with age (Fig. 2).

Multivariate logistic regression analysis showed an increased risk for HEV seropositivity in participants aged 50 years or older, male participants and participants who reported a low level of education (Table 2). There was a clear trend of increasing prevalence with increasing age (Chi-square test for linear trend, $X^2 = 83.1$; $p < 0.001$). A high number of pigs within 1,000 m of residential address

Table 1 Density of pigs, details of study population and hepatitis E virus seroprevalence by study centre

Study centre	Density of pigs[a]	Number of participants	Median age (years)	Range (years)	Male participants (%)	Seroprevalence[b] (%)	[95% CI][c]
Afferden	717	49	59.2	[33.5–71.1]	57.5	25.5	[13.1–38.0]
Asten[d]	3,535	291	61.4	[20.4–71.4]	45.8	34.0	[28.6–39.5]
Bakel	3,756	315	59.3	[21.5–71.7]	47.1	29.2	[24.1–34.3]
Boxtel	988	170	59.3	[24.8–71.6]	45.0	27.2	[20.5–33.9]
Budel	1,080	200	61.4	[21.4–71.6]	49.5	32.6	[25.8–39.4]
Deurne	3,882	132	60.5	[29.0–71.7]	50.0	18.6	[11.7–25.4]
Heeswijk-Dinther	3,812	375	57.5	[20.1–71.4]	37.1	30.1	[25.5–34.8]
Heusden[d]	3,535	72	58.9	[24.2–71.4]	55.6	16.7	[8.1–25.3]
Horn	1,268	85	57.1	[24.0–71.7]	45.2	35.7	[25.5–46.0]
Someren	3,447	170	57.9	[28.6–71.2]	48.2	29.4	[22.6–36.3]
St. Anthonis	4,460	399	57.0	[22.6–71.8]	44.5	26.9	[22.4–31.4]
Stramproy	878	236	57.4	[21.3–72.0]	46.3	26.6	[20.9–32.4]
Total	2,506	2,494	58.6	[20.1–72.0]	45.6	28.7	[26.9–30.5]

[a]Number of pigs per km^2 by municipality, based on the provincial databases of mandatory environmental licenses for keeping livestock for 2012
[b]Anti-HEV IgG ratio > = 0.90
[c]95% Confidence Interval
[d]Asten and Heusden are both situated in the municipality Asten, and therefore have the same pig density

was not a risk factor. Other variables for exposure to pigs (e.g. number of pig farms or the presence of at least one pig farm within 1,000 m of residential address) gave similar results in both univariate and multivariate logistic regression analyses as number of pigs within 1,000 m of residential address (data not shown). Participants who reported to follow a diet without pork meat ($n = 47$) did not have a significantly lower risk for HEV seropositivity. Exclusion of the 29 samples with borderline positive anti-HEV IgG ratio did not affect the results of the of univariate and multivariate logistic regression analyses. This also holds when the borderline samples were considered as negative anti-HEV IgG ratio (data not shown).

Generally, seronegative participants lived closer to pig farms than seropositive participants. This difference was statistically significant for the overall group and for the age group 60–70 years (Table 3).

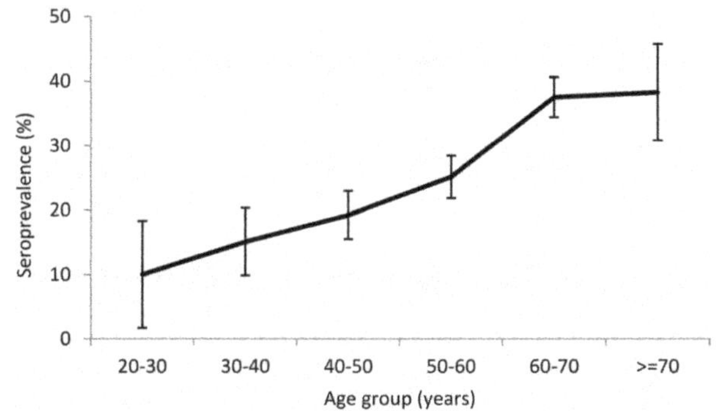

Fig. 2 Seroprevalence of antibodies against hepatitis E virus by age group

Despite the associations detected and reported above, the random forest method showed that the potential risk factors considered in this study are not at all able to predict anti-HEV IgG ratio nor disease status (results are omitted). Indeed, the proportion of explained variance was practically zero in our prediction analysis, which in particular prevents us from ranking the risk factors.

Discussion

The present population-based serological survey confirms the high HEV seroprevalence (29%) in the general population of the Netherlands, but provides no evidence for environmental transmission from pig farms to humans living in the vicinity of these farms.

Comparison of the seroprevalence found in this study with results from other European countries is difficult because of considerable differences in the studied populations, as well as the used assay for HEV antibody testing [54–56]. Recent studies using sensitive assays (like the Wantai assay we used) reported HEV seroprevalence varying between 16% and 52% [18, 57–61]. Our seroprevalence (29.7%) corresponds well with the 27% prevalence found in a large serological screening of Dutch blood donors [18]. Both studies used the Wantai assay to measure HEV specific IgG antibodies. In contrast, a population-based seroprevalence study in the general population in the Netherlands in 2006–2007, using a less sensitive assay for detection of prolonged IgG antibodies (MP Diagnostics, France), found a seroprevalence of only 3% [62]. Comparative studies suggest that the Wantai assay gives the most reliable estimate of the HEV seroprevalence, because it is more sensitive, it is positive

Table 2 Hepatitis E virus seroprevalence in the general population and potential determinants for HEV seropositivity

Determinants	N	Seroprevalence (%)[a]	Crude OR[b]	[95% CI][c]	Adjusted OR[b,d,e]	[95% CI][c]
Age (years)						
20–30	50	10.0	Ref.		Ref.	
30–40	179	15.1	1.60	[0.58–4.39]	1.49	[0.54–4.13]
40–50	432	19.2	2.14	[0.82–5.55]	2.01	[0.77–5.26]
50–60	661	25.1	3.02	[1.18–7.72]	2.58	[1.00–6.70]
60–70	938	37.5	5.40	[2.13–13.73]	4.22	[1.63–10.91]
> =70	162	38.3	5.58	[2.10–14.80]	4.15	[1.53–11.24]
Gender						
Female	1,318	25.6	Ref.		Ref.	
Male	1,104	32.3	1.39	[1.16–1.65]	1.21	[1.00–1.47]
Educational level						
High	733	24.8	Ref.		Ref.	
Medium	1,080	26.9	1.12	[0.90–1.38]	1.10	[0.87–1.38]
Low	609	36.5	1.74	[1.37–2.20]	1.36	[1.04–1.76]
Diet without pork meat						
No	2,360	28.8	Ref.		Ref.	
Yes	47	19.2	0.59	[0.28–1.22]	0.72	[0.33–1.59]
Missing	*15*					
Ever smoked						
No	1,034	26.5	Ref.		Ref.	
Yes	1,388	30.3	1.21	[1.01–1.45]	0.96	[0.79–1.17]
Childhood in study region						
No	580	32.2	Ref.		Ref.	
Yes	1,816	27.4	0.79	[0.65–0.97]	0.85	[0.68–1.07]
Missing	*26*					
Childhood on pig farm						
No	1,928	27.6	Ref.		Ref.	
Yes	468	32.5	1.26	[1.02–1.57]	1.21	[0.94–1.55]
Missing	*26*					
Performed jobs on farm during childhood						
No	1,090	26.9	Ref.	-	Ref.	
Yes	1,220	29.7	1.15	[0.96–1.38]	1.02	[0.83–1.27]
Missing	*112*					
Number of pigs within 1000 m of residential address (tertiles)						
Low[f]	807	32.1	Ref.		Ref.	
Intermediate[g]	808	26.9	0.78	[0.63–0.96]	0.79	[0.63–0.99]
High[h]	807	27.1	0.79	[0.64–0.98]	0.83	[0.66–1.04]

[a]Including both positive and borderline samples (anti-HEV IgG ratio > = 0.90)
[b]Odds Ratio
[c]95% Confidence Interval
[d]ORs are adjusted for age, gender, educational level, diet without pork meat, ever smoked, childhood in study region, childhood on pig farm, jobs on farm during childhood and number of pigs within 1000 m of residential address
[e]Adjusted ORs and 95% CIs were calculated for cases without missing answers (*N* = 2,301)
[f]Number of pigs within 1000 m < = 1,003
[g]Number of pigs within 1000 m > 1,003 and < = 5,771
[h]Number of pigs within 1000 m > 5,771

Table 3 Median distance from home address to nearest pig farm by anti-hepatitis E virus IgG ratio

	Positive or borderline anti-HEV IgG ratio[a]			Negative anti-HEV IgG ratio[b]			
Age group (years)	n	Median distance (m)	Range in distance (m)[c]	n	Median distance (m)	Range in distance (m)[c]	*P*-value
20–30	5	689	[469–850]	45	652	[489–843]	1.00
30–40	27	751	[373–1102]	152	581	[440–872]	0.16
40–50	83	702	[416–965]	349	665	[441–900]	0.68
50–60	166	701	[498–955]	495	674	[455–901]	0.28
60–70	352	748	[517–970]	586	686	[430–938]	0.02
> = 70	62	794	[539–1041]	100	672	[528–1004]	0.36
Total	695	730	[509–969]	1727	663	[447–916]	0.001

[a]Anti-HEV IgG ratio > =0.90
[b]Anti-HEV IgG ratio <0.90
[c]Range from the 25th to the 75th percentile of the distance from home address to nearest pig farm

in a higher proportion of proven infections and it remains positive for longer period post infection compared with the MP assay [56, 58, 59, 63].

In line with other serological studies, we found statistically significant higher seroprevalence in participants aged 50 years and older compared to 20–30 year olds [18, 44, 57, 62, 64]. This higher seroprevalence in older persons might be a result of age-dependent cumulative exposure, but can also be indicative of an age-cohort because of higher pressure of infection in the past. This age-cohort effect is also demonstrated in Denmark, the United Kingdom and the United States [60, 61, 65]. The HEV seroprevalence in blood donors as well as the high number of HEV RNA-positive donors found in serological screenings suggest an increasing HEV incidence in recent years in the Netherlands [18, 66, 67].

Proximity to pig farms and number of animals close to the home were used as proxy of potential environmental exposure to HEV. The lack of a positive association suggests that airborne spread of HEV is unlikely. Other environmental transmission routes cannot be excluded, for example through manure that may be transported to distant places or through surface water. In the Netherlands, HEV RNA has been detected in surface water samples [68]. Furthermore, a recent cross-sectional study suggests that consumption of tap water in France might be a risk factor for HEV infection [69]. Occupational exposure to pigs, which is a potential risk factor for seropositivity, was not investigated in our study since persons living or working on a farm were excluded [44, 47, 70]. Moreover, the present study was not designed to investigate the role of food-borne transmission. Presence of IgG antibodies is an indicator for HEV infection in the past and therefore suited to study exposure to HEV through the environment. Although we found no decreased risk for HEV seropositivity in participants who did not consume pork meat, this finding must be interpreted with caution because of the small numbers of participants on a diet without pork meat ($n = 47$, 2.0%). Moreover, some of these participants might have consumed pork meat in the past. A case-control study focussing mainly on food-borne transmission among patients with acute hepatitis E infection in the Netherlands is ongoing (study period: 2015–2017).

Conclusions

In conclusion, our study showed that the HEV seroprevalence in the general population in a livestock-dense area in the south of the Netherlands was not associated with living in proximity to pig farms. The higher seroprevalence among older participants supports the assumption of cumulative lifetime exposure to hepatitis E virus in the Netherlands, as well as an age-cohort because of higher pressure of infection in the past. Although it seems plausible that transmission is primarily food-borne, further research is needed to elucidate the exact sources and routes of infection.

Abbreviations

CI: Confidence interval; GP: General practitioner; HEV: Hepatitis E virus; OR: Odds ratio; RIVM: National Institute for Public Health and the Environment (Dutch acronym); VGO: Livestock farming and neighbouring residents' health study (Dutch acronym)

Acknowledgements

The authors would like to thank Najima Lamkaraf for performing the serological analyses, Ilse Zutt and Ngoc Hoa Roosen-Chung for technical assistance, José Ferreira for statistical advice, and Agnetha Hofhuis for critically reading the manuscript.

Funding

The Livestock Farming and Neighbouring Residents' Health (VGO) study was funded by the Ministry of Health, Welfare and Sports and the Ministry of Economic Affairs of The Netherlands, and supported by a grant from the Lung Foundation Netherlands (Grant number: 3.2.11.022).

Authors' contribution

AG, WH, FB, DH, CM, CY, LS and JR participated in the design and coordination of the study; BR and JR were responsible for the virological assays; AG, WH, FB, SM, and LS were involved in the statistical analyses; AG, WH, FB, DH, SM, CM, CY, BR, LS and JR participated in the interpretation of data and in drafting and reviewing the Manuscript. All authors read and approved the final manuscript.

Competing interests
The authors declare that they have no competing interests.

Consent for publication
Not applicable.

Author details
[1]National Institute for Public Health and the Environment (RIVM), Bilthoven, The Netherlands. [2]Institute for Risk Assessment Sciences, IRAS, Utrecht University, Utrecht, The Netherlands. [3]Netherlands Institute for Health Services Research (NIVEL), Utrecht, The Netherlands.

References

1. Lewis HC, Boisson S, Ijaz S, Hewitt K, Ngui SL, Boxall E, Teo CG, Morgan D. Hepatitis E in England and Wales. Emerg Infect Dis. 2008;14(1):165–7.
2. Kantala T, Maunula L, von Bonsdorff CH, Peltomaa J, Lappalainen M. Hepatitis E virus in patients with unexplained hepatitis in Finland. J Clin Virol. 2009;45(2):109–13.
3. Mansuy JM, Abravanel F, Miedouge M, Mengelle C, Merviel C, Dubois M, Kamar N, Rostaing L, Alric L, Moreau J, et al. Acute hepatitis E in south-west France over a 5-year period. J Clin Virol. 2009;44(1):74–7.
4. Perez-Gracia MT, Mateos Lindemann ML, Caridad Montalvo Villalba M. Hepatitis E: current status. Rev Med Virol. 2013;23(6):384–98.
5. Stroffolini T, Rapicetta M, Chionne P, Esvan R, Madonna E, Lombardo F, Toccaceli F, Pisani G, Ciccaglione A, Bortolotti F. Evidence for the presence of autochthonous (locally acquired) cases of acute hepatitis E virus infections in Italy since the 80s. Eur J Intern Med. 2015;26(5):348–50.
6. Tohme RA, Drobeniuc J, Sanchez R, Heseltine G, Alsip B, Kamili S, Hu DJ, Guerra F, Teshale EH. Acute hepatitis associated with autochthonous hepatitis E virus infection–San Antonio, Texas, 2009. Clin Infect Dis. 2011;53(8):793–6.
7. Ruggeri FM, Di Bartolo I, Ponterio E, Angeloni G, Trevisani M, Ostanello F. Zoonotic transmission of hepatitis E virus in industrialized countries. New Microbiol. 2013;36(4):331–44.
8. Echevarria JM. Autochthonous Hepatitis E virus infection in Europe: a matter of concern for public health? J Clin Transl Hepatol. 2014;2(1):7–14.
9. Aggarwal R, Naik S. Epidemiology of hepatitis E: current status. J Gastroenterol Hepatol. 2009;24(9):1484–93.
10. Khuroo MS, Khuroo MS. Hepatitis E: an emerging global disease - from discovery towards control and cure. J Viral Hepat. 2015;23(2):68–79.
11. Koot H, Hogema BM, Koot M, Molier M, Zaaijer HL. Frequent hepatitis E in the Netherlands without traveling or immunosuppression. J Clin Virol. 2015;62:38–40.
12. Lucarelli C1, Spada E, Taliani G, Chionne P, Madonna E, Marcantonio C, Pezzotti P, Bruni R, La Rosa G, Pisani G, Dell'Orso L, Ragone K, Tomei C, Ciccaglione AR. High prevalence of anti-hepatitis E virus antibodies among blood donors in central Italy, February to March 2014. Euro Surveill. 2016; 21(30). doi:10.2807/1560-7917.ES.2016.21.30.30299.
13. Turner J, Godkin A, Neville P, Kingham J, Ch'ng CL. Clinical characteristics of hepatitis E in a "Non-Endemic" population. J Med Virol. 2010;82(11):1899–902.
14. Arends JE, Ghisetti V, Irving W, Dalton HR, Izopet J, Hoepelman AI, Salmon D. Hepatitis E: An emerging infection in high income countries. J Clin Virol. 2014;59(2):81–8.
15. Kamar N, Dalton HR, Abravanel F, Izopet J. Hepatitis E virus infection. Clin Microbiol Rev. 2014;27(1):116–38.
16. Kamar N, Bendall R, Legrand-Abravanel F, Xia NS, Ijaz S, Izopet J, Dalton HR. Hepatitis E. Lancet. 2012;379(9835):2477–88.
17. Dalton HR, Bendall R, Ijaz S, Banks M. Hepatitis E: an emerging infection in developed countries. Lancet Infect Dis. 2008;8(11):698–709.
18. Slot E, Hogema BM, Riezebos-Brilman A, Kok TM, Molier M, Zaaijer HL. Silent hepatitis E virus infection in Dutch blood donors, 2011 to 2012. Euro Surveill. 2013;18(31).
19. Juhl D, Baylis SA, Blumel J, Gorg S, Hennig H. Seroprevalence and incidence of hepatitis E virus infection in German blood donors. Transfusion. 2014;54(1):49–56.
20. Fischer C, Hofmann M, Danzer M, Hofer K, Kaar J, Gabriel C. Seroprevalence and Incidence of hepatitis E in blood donors in Upper Austria. PLoS One. 2015;10(3):e0119576.
21. Mansuy JM, Saune K, Rech H, Abravanel F, Mengelle C, LH S, Destruel F, Kamar N, Izopet J. Seroprevalence in blood donors reveals widespread, multi-source exposure to hepatitis E virus, southern France, October 2011. Euro Surveill. 2015;20(19):27–34.
22. Hartl J, Otto B, Madden RG, Webb G, Woolson KL, Kriston L, Vettorazzi E, Lohse AW, Dalton HR, Pischke S. Hepatitis E Seroprevalence in Europe: A Meta-Analysis. Viruses. 2016;8(8). doi:10.3390/v8080211.
23. Perez-Gracia MT, Garcia M, Suay B, Mateos-Lindemann ML. Current knowledge on hepatitis E. J Clin Transl Hepatol. 2015;3(2):117–26.
24. Smith DB, Simmonds P, Jameel S, Emerson SU, Harrison TJ, Meng XJ, Okamoto H, Van der Poel WH, Purdy MA. Consensus proposals for classification of the family Hepeviridae. J Gen Virol. 2014;95(Pt 10):2223–32.
25. Khuroo MS. Discovery of hepatitis E: the epidemic non-A, non-B hepatitis 30 years down the memory lane. Virus Res. 2011;161(1):3–14.
26. Dalton HR, Hunter JG, Bendall RP. Hepatitis E. Curr Opin Infect Dis. 2013;26(5):471–8.
27. Pavio N, Meng XJ, Doceul V. Zoonotic origin of hepatitis E. Curr Opin Virol. 2015;10:34–41.
28. Van der Poel WH. Food and environmental routes of Hepatitis E virus transmission. Curr Opin Virol. 2014;4:91–6.
29. Lee GH, Tan BH, Teo EC, Lim SG, Dan YY, Wee A, Aw PP, Zhu Y, Hibberd ML, Tan CK, et al. Chronic infection with camelid hepatitis E virus in a liver transplant recipient who regularly consumes camel meat and milk. Gastroenterology. 2016;150(2):355–7. e353.
30. Adlhoch C, Avellon A, Baylis SA, Ciccaglione AR, Couturier E, de Sousa R, Epstein J, Ethelberg S, Faber M, Feher A, et al. Hepatitis E virus: Assessment of the epidemiological situation in humans in Europe, 2014/15. J Clin Virol. 2016;82:9–16.
31. Bouwknegt M, Rutjes SA, Reusken CB, Stockhofe-Zurwieden N, Frankena K, de Jong MC, de Roda Husman AM, Poel WH. The course of hepatitis E virus infection in pigs after contact-infection and intravenous inoculation. BMC Vet Res. 2009;5:7.
32. Rutjes SA, Lodder WJ, Bouwknegt M, de Roda Husman AM. Increased hepatitis E virus prevalence on Dutch pig farms from 33 to 55% by using appropriate internal quality controls for RT-PCR. J Virol Methods. 2007;143(1):112–6.
33. Bouwknegt M, Lodder-Verschoor F, van der Poel WH, Rutjes SA, de Roda Husman AM. Hepatitis E virus RNA in commercial porcine livers in The Netherlands. J Food Prot. 2007;70(12):2889–95.
34. Berto A, Martelli F, Grierson S, Banks M. Hepatitis E virus in pork food chain, United Kingdom, 2009-2010. Emerg Infect Dis. 2012;18(8):1358–60.
35. Di Bartolo I, Diez-Valcarce M, Vasickova P, Kralik P, Hernandez M, Angeloni G, Ostanello F, Bouwknegt M, Rodriguez-Lazaro D, Pavlik I, et al. Hepatitis E virus in pork production chain in Czech Republic, Italy, and Spain, 2010. Emerg Infect Dis. 2012;18(8):1282–9.
36. Berto A, Grierson S, Hakze-van der Honing R, Martelli F, Johne R, Reetz J, Ulrich RG, Pavio N, Van der Poel WH, Banks M. Hepatitis E virus in pork liver sausage, France. Emerg Infect Dis. 2013;19(2):264–6.
37. Li TC, Chijiwa K, Sera N, Ishibashi T, Etoh Y, Shinohara Y, Kurata Y, Ishida M, Sakamoto S, Takeda N, et al. Hepatitis E virus transmission from wild boar meat. Emerg Infect Dis. 2005;11(12):1958–60.
38. Tei S, Kitajima N, Takahashi K, Mishiro S. Zoonotic transmission of hepatitis E virus from deer to human beings. Lancet. 2003;362(9381):371–3.
39. Renou C, Roque-Afonso AM, Pavio N. Foodborne transmission of hepatitis E virus from raw pork liver sausage, France. Emerg Infect Dis. 2014;20(11):1945–7.
40. Riveiro-Barciela M, Minguez B, Girones R, Rodriguez-Frias F, Quer J, Buti M. Phylogenetic demonstration of hepatitis E infection transmitted by pork meat ingestion. J Clin Gastroenterol. 2015;49(2):165–8.
41. Pavio N, Meng XJ, Renou C. Zoonotic hepatitis E: animal reservoirs and emerging risks. Vet Res. 2010;41(6):46.

42. Withers MR, Correa MT, Morrow M, Stebbins ME, Seriwatana J, Webster WD, Boak MB, Vaughn DW. Antibody levels to hepatitis E virus in North Carolina swine workers, non-swine workers, swine, and murids. AmJTrop Med Hyg. 2002;66(4):384–8.
43. Aggarwal R, Jameel S. Hepatitis E. Hepatology. 2011;54(6):2218–26.
44. Drobeniuc J, Favorov MO, Shapiro CN, Bell BP, Mast EE, Dadu A, Culver D, Iarovoi P, Robertson BH, Margolis HS. Hepatitis E virus antibody prevalence among persons who work with swine. J Infect Dis. 2001;184(12):1594–7.
45. Bouwknegt M, Engel B, Herremans MM, Widdowson MA, Worm HC, Koopmans MP, Frankena K, de Roda Husman AM, De Jong MC, Van Der Poel WH. Bayesian estimation of hepatitis E virus seroprevalence for populations with different exposure levels to swine in The Netherlands. Epidemiol Infect. 2008;136(4):567–76.
46. Chaussade H, Rigaud E, Allix A, Carpentier A, Touze A, Delzescaux D, Choutet P, Garcia-Bonnet N, Coursaget P. Hepatitis E virus seroprevalence and risk factors for individuals in working contact with animals. J Clin Virol. 2013;58(3):504–8.
47. Krumbholz A, Joel S, Dremsek P, Neubert A, Johne R, Durrwald R, Walther M, Muller TH, Kuhnel D, Lange J, et al. Seroprevalence of hepatitis E virus (HEV) in humans living in high pig density areas of Germany. Med Microbiol Immunol. 2014;203(4):273–82.
48. van der Hoek W, Morroy G, Renders NH, Wever PC, Hermans MH, Leenders AC, Schneeberger PM. Epidemic Q fever in humans in the Netherlands. Adv Exp Med Biol. 2012;984:329–64.
49. Borlee F, Yzermans CJ, van Dijk CE, Heederik D, Smit LA. Increased respiratory symptoms in COPD patients living in the vicinity of livestock farms. Eur Respir J. 2015;46(6):1605–14.
50. Borlee F, Yzermans J, Krop E, Aalders B, Zock JP, Van Dijk C, Maassen K, Schellevis F, Heederik D, Smit LAM. Assessment of asthma and COPD prevalence: a comparison between three different data sources. In: American Thoracic Society, editor. B48 asthma: insights from the bench, genetics, and epidemiology. 2016. p. A3694.
51. Smit LA, Hooiveld M, van der Sman-de Beer F, Opstal-van Winden AW, Beekhuizen J, Wouters IM, Yzermans CJ, Heederik D. Air pollution from livestock farms, and asthma, allergic rhinitis and COPD among neighbouring residents. Occup Environ Med. 2014;71(2):134–40.
52. Smit LA, van der Sman-de Beer F, Opstal-van Winden AW, Hooiveld M, Beekhuizen J, Wouters IM, Yzermans J, Heederik D. Q fever and pneumonia in an area with a high livestock density: a large population-based study. PLoS One. 2012;7(6):e38843.
53. Maassen K, Heederik D, IJzermans J, Hagenaars T, van der Hoek W. Livestock Farming and Neighbouring Residents' Health [in Dutch]. Bilthoven: National Institute for Public Health and the Environment; 2016.
54. Lapa D, Capobianchi MR, Garbuglia AR. Epidemiology of Hepatitis E Virus in European Countries. Int J Mol Sci. 2015;16(10):25711–43.
55. Wenzel JJ, Preiss J, Schemmerer M, Huber B, Jilg W. Test performance characteristics of Anti-HEV IgG assays strongly influence hepatitis E seroprevalence estimates. J Infect Dis. 2013;207(3):497–500.
56. Schnegg A, Burgisser P, Andre C, Kenfak-Foguena A, Canellini G, Moradpour D, Abravanel F, Izopet J, Cavassini M, Darling KE. An analysis of the benefit of using HEV genotype 3 antigens in detecting anti-HEV IgG in a European population. PLoS One. 2013;8(5):e62980.
57. Faber MS, Wenzel JJ, Jilg W, Thamm M, Hohle M, Stark K. Hepatitis E virus seroprevalence among adults, Germany. Emerg Infect Dis. 2012;18(10):1654–7.
58. Bendall R, Ellis V, Ijaz S, Ali R, Dalton H. A comparison of two commercially available anti-HEV IgG kits and a re-evaluation of anti-HEV IgG seroprevalence data in developed countries. J Med Virol. 2010;82(5):799–805.
59. Mansuy JM, Bendall R, Legrand-Abravanel F, Saune K, Miedouge M, Ellis V, Rech H, Destruel F, Kamar N, Dalton HR, et al. Hepatitis E virus antibodies in blood donors, France. Emerg Infect Dis. 2011;17(12):2309–12.
60. Xu C, Wang RY, Schechterly CA, Ge S, Shih JW, Xia NS, Luban NL, Alter HJ. An assessment of hepatitis E virus (HEV) in US blood donors and recipients: no detectable HEV RNA in 1939 donors tested and no evidence for HEV transmission to 362 prospectively followed recipients. Transfusion. 2013;53:2505–11.
61. Christensen PB, Engle RE, Hjort C, Homburg KM, Vach W, Georgsen J, Purcell RH. Time trend of the prevalence of hepatitis E antibodies among farmers and blood donors: a potential zoonosis in Denmark. Clin Infect Dis. 2008;47(8):1026–31.
62. Verhoef L, Koopmans M, Duizer E, Bakker J, Reimerink J, Van Pelt W. Seroprevalence of hepatitis E antibodies and risk profile of HEV seropositivity in The Netherlands, 2006-2007. Epidemiol Infect. 2012;140(10):1838–47.
63. Avellon A, Morago L, Garcia-Galera del Carmen M, Munoz M, Echevarria JM. Comparative sensitivity of commercial tests for hepatitis E genotype 3 virus antibody detection. J Med Virol. 2015;87(11):1934–9.
64. Lagler H, Poeppl W, Winkler H, Herkner H, Faas A, Mooseder G, Burgmann H. Hepatitis E virus seroprevalence in Austrian adults: a nationwide cross-sectional study among civilians and military professionals. PLoS One. 2014;9(2):e87669.
65. Ijaz S, Vyse AJ, Morgan D, Pebody RG, Tedder RS, Brown D. Indigenous hepatitis E virus infection in England: more common than it seems. J Clin Virol. 2009;44(4):272–6.
66. Hogema BM, Molier M, Slot E, Zaaijer HL. Past and present of hepatitis E in the Netherlands. Transfusion. 2014;54(12):3092–6.
67. Hogema BM, Molier M, Sjerps M, de Waal M, van Swieten P, van de Laar T, Molenaar-de Backer M, Zaaijer HL. Incidence and duration of hepatitis E virus infection in Dutch blood donors. Transfusion. 2016;56(3):722–8.
68. Rutjes SA, Lodder WJ, Lodder-Verschoor F, van den Berg HH, Vennema H, Duizer E, Koopmans M, de Roda Husman AM. Sources of hepatitis E virus genotype 3 in The Netherlands. Emerg Infect Dis. 2009;15(3):381–7.
69. Mansuy JM, Gallian P, Dimeglio C, Saune K, Arnaud C, Pelletier B, Morel P, Legrand D, Tiberghien P, Izopet J. A nationwide survey of hepatitis E viral infection in French blood donors. Hepatology. 2016;63(4):1145–54.
70. Galiana C, Fernandez-Barredo S, Garcia A, Gomez MT, Perez-Gracia MT. Occupational exposure to hepatitis E virus (HEV) in swine workers. AmJTrop Med Hyg. 2008;78(6):1012–5.

2

Hepatitis B virus infection in hilly/mountainous regions of southeastern China: a locality-dependent epidemiology

Ping Chen[1,2], Qinfen Xie[1], Ting Chen[3], Jiawei Wu[3], Jie Wu[2], Bing Ruan[2], Zhiqin Zhang[4], Hainv Gao[1] and Lanjuan Li[2*]

Abstract

Background: The overall prevalence of hepatitis B virus (HBV) infection in China is declining. The purpose of this study was to use a community-based epidemiological study to update the infection status of hepatitis B virus (HBV) in mountainous regions of China, and to evaluate the impact of the Expanded Program of Immunization (EPI) on HBV transmission.

Methods: In total, 10,383 participants were selected by multi-stage stratified random cluster sampling in two mountainous regions, Xianju and Anji, in Zhejiang province, China.

Results: The positive rates of hepatitis B virus surface antigen (HBsAg), anti-HBV core antigen (anti-HBc), and anti-HBV surface antigen (anti-HBs) were 9.5%, 33.9%, and 51.0%, respectively. Positive HBV markers were more frequently detected in males than in females ($P < 0.01$). The alanine aminotransferase (ALT) levels were elevated (>38 IU/L) in 15. 3% of the HBsAg-positive and 6.3% of the HBsAg-negative subjects. The α-fetoprotein (AFP) level was elevated in 0.8% of the HBsAg-positive participants who were older than 30 years old.

Conclusions: The epidemiology of HBV infection is location dependent. The prevalence of HBV infection in the mountainous regions is higher than the national levels. Moreover, HBV infection in women of childbearing age is up to 10%, which represents a main factor for continuous HBV transmission.

Keywords: Hepatitis B virus, Community-based epidemiological study, Expanded program of immunization, Continuous HBV transmission

Background

Hepatitis B virus (HBV) infection is one of the most common viral infections [1]. Globally, almost two billion people have been exposed to HBV infection at some stage of their lives, and an estimated 240 million people are chronically infected. Approximately 780,000 patients die from advanced liver diseases caused by chronic HBV infection each year [2–4].

China has a high prevalence of chronic HBV infection. However, there is a significant difference in the HBV infection rate among different regions in China. Generally speaking, the prevalence of HBV infection in eastern, coastal, or rural areas is higher than that in western, inland, or urban regions [5]. In 1992, China released the first national hepatitis seroepidemiological survey, which showed that the prevalence of hepatitis B virus surface antigen (HBsAg) in the general population aged 1–59 years old was 9.75% [6]. The vertical infection of HBV from a HBV-positive mother to her infant is a major route for HBV transmission. To control HBV transmission, the Expanded Program of Immunization (EPI) for newborns was established in China in 1992. This program has been a great success and has resulted in a decline in the prevalence of chronic HBV infection, from 9.75% in 1992 to 7.18% in 2006 [7]. The overall prevalence of chronic HBV carriers in Zhejiang province was approximately 8.79% in 2006, a decline from 11.61% in 1992 [8].

* Correspondence: ljli@zju.edu.cn
[2]State Key Laboratory for Diagnosis and Treatment of Infectious Diseases, Collaborative Innovation Center for Diagnosis and Treatment of Infectious Diseases, The First Affiliated Hospital, College of Medicine, Zhejiang University, 79 Qing-Chun Road, Hangzhou 310003, China
Full list of author information is available at the end of the article

In hilly/mountainous areas of China, the prevalence of chronic HBV infection in the general population was 15.94% in 1993, [9, 10]. Mountains and hills account for 70.4% of the total land area of Zhejiang province, which is the largest of all Chinese provinces. An epidemiological study conducted in 2007 found that the prevalence of chronic HBV infection was 10.19% in the mountainous areas of Zhejiang province [11], which had declined from 15.94%, but it was still much higher than the provincial rate of 6.75% in Zhejiang province [12].

HBV seroepidemiological studies in the hilly/mountainous areas of China are relatively rare. The current status of chronic HBV infection and the related risk factors in those areas need to be assessed. The hilly/mountainous area in Xianju and Anji accounts for 80% and 70% of the territory, respectively. Geographically, the two counties are separately located. The economic development level also differs between the two counties. Therefore, we conducted a community-based epidemiological study in two representative hilly/mountainous areas in southeastern China to determine the current chronic HBV infection rate in the general population, to study the risk factors, and to evaluate the impact of the EPI on HBV transmission.

Methods

Study population

Under the sponsorship of the Mega-Project for National Science and Technology Development for the "12th Five-Year Plan of China" and the Department of Health of Zhejiang province, we initiated this HBV infection epidemiological study in two major hilly counties of Zhejiang province. This study was conducted between October 2012 and March 2014.

Sample size

Based on the previous HBV epidemiological studies, we assumed that the incidence of HBV infection in hilly/mountainous regions would be about 5–10%. Sample size was estimated with the following formula:

$$n = \frac{Z_{\alpha}^{2}P(1\text{-}P)}{\delta^{2}}$$

The calculated sample size is 8760 when we assume 80% power, 95% confidence level, and the incidence of HBV is set at 5%. In our analysis, we also take into account 20% possible attrition of subjects, and the final sample size is 9855.

Sampling strategy

Our study populations were chosen by multi-stage stratified random cluster sampling. First, Xianju and Anji were selected as two representative mountainous counties, because the hilly/mountainous region in Xianju and Anji accounts for 80% and 70% of the territory, respectively. Next, towns in each county were ranked into three tiers using the economic development index, one town was randomly selected at each tier. Lastly, three villages, each of which represented one of three income tiers, were selected from the selected three towns. A total of 18 villages were randomly selected from two included counties. All residents in each selected village mandated to complete yearly physical check-up at local health centers, which is organized by local health department. This annual physical check-up is part of public health service that aims to identify any diseases at early stage. The records indicate that approximately 90% of residents participate in this annual physical check-up. Our staff invited all of those who presented themselves for physical check-up to participate in our study at the time our study conducted. Approximately 80% of population (9855/11898) in all the selected villages were enrolled.

A panel of 360 physicians from 18 primary care hospitals in the two selected counties were invited by the Department of Health, Zhejiang province, to conduct medical examinations, interviews, and laboratory tests on subjects who volunteered for this project. All local citizens and migrant workers who had settled in these cities for at least 3 months (i.e., a documented residence before July 1, 2012) were eligible for screening. The collected information consisted of demographics (sex, age, occupation, and nationality), residency status, medical history (e.g., blood transfusion, hepatitis B, allergies), and laboratory tests (HBsAg, anti-HBV surface antigen (anti-HBs), anti-HBV core antigen (anti-HBc), α-fetoprotein (AFP), alanine aminotransferase (ALT) assays, and liver ultrasound). This study was performed in accordance with the guidelines and regulations for the use of human subjects and was approved by the Ethics Committee of the First Affiliated Hospital of Zhejiang University College of Medicine. All adult participants provided informed consent, or informed consent was obtained from the legal guardian of the children. The data were handled anonymously.

Serological testing

A 5-mL venous blood sample was collected from each participant, in accordance with strict hygiene and safety guidelines. The demographic information of the participants, including name, sex, age, and district, was recorded. Blood samples were kept in cool containers (4–10 °C) and delivered to Adicon Clinical Laboratories (Hangzhou, China), where sample processing and serological examinationwere performed on the same days. The HBV serological kits (ELISA) were purchased from Acon Biotech Co. (Hangzhou, China) for detection of HBsAg, HBsAb, and anti-HBc. In order to verify the test results, all samples were tested twice using the same kits. Only samples that were positive in both tests were considered positive. For the purpose of this analysis, HBsAg positivity was a marker for current HBV infection. Anti-HBc was indicative of previous exposure to HBV. Anti-HBs positivity without other HBV markers marked successful HBV vaccination. Individuals who tested negative for all HBV serological markers were categorized as having HBV exposure.

Testing ALT and AFP levels

The serum ALT level was determined within 2 h of sample arrival by an Architect C8000 automated biochemical analyzer (Abbott Laboratories, Abbott Park, IL, USA). An abnormal ALT level was defined as greater than 38 IU/L, representing 2.25 standard deviations (SD) above the mean established for normal subjects. An elevated ALT level was verified by retesting the samples using the same kits. If a sample was positive in both tests, it was considered positive [13]. Community-based preliminary screening of hepatocellular carcinoma (HCC) was performed for HBsAg-positive subjects who were older than 30 years old. Both AFP (AFP EIA Test Kit, BoSai, Zhengzhou, China) and ultrasonography were used for HCC screening. Liver ultrasonography was conducted by technicians from the Imaging Department of each community health center. Based on a positive AFP test and a focal mass indicated by ultrasonography, a tentative diagnosis of HCC was suggested.

Data analysis

The data were analyzed using SPSS software, version 21.0 (SPSS, Inc., Chicago, IL, USA). For categorical variables, the chi-squared test was used to determine group differences. Statistical significance was indicated when $P < 0.01$. The HBsAg, HBs-Ab, and HBc-Ab carrier rates were standardized by sex and age.

By referencing the 2010 Zhejiang population data [14], 95% confidence intervals (CIs) were calculated for percentages of HBsAg-positive individuals in the whole population and subgroups stratified by age and gender.

Results

Characteristics of the study group

A total of 10,383 serum samples were tested. However, 528 participants (5.1%) were excluded because of no age or sex data. Thus, 9855 samples were included for final analyses (Fig. 1). The prevalence of HBV infection was standardized according to the age and sex distribution of all participants to allow direct comparisons of the studied populations. The demographic characteristics of the participant populations are shown in Table 1.

Prevalence of HBV infection by age and sex

In total, 1056 individuals were HBsAg positive (Table 2). The prevalence of HBsAg positivity, a marker of current infection, in this group was 9.5% (95% CI: 8.6–10.4). The HBV infection rate gradually increased from 3.23% in those <20 years old to a peak of 12.40% in those 50–59 years old, but then it declined to 6.6% in the group older than 70 years old. There was a significant difference in the prevalence of HBsAg between male (11.9%) and female participants (9.8%) ($P < 0.01$). Alarmingly, HBV infection in women of childbearing age remains high (5.56% in those <20 years old, 7.67% in those 20–29 years old, and 10% in those 30–39 years old) (Fig. 2).

The prevalence of anti-HBc, a marker of HBV exposure, was 35.1% (95% CI: 33.4–36.8), and no significant variation was noted between genders. HBV exposure increased with age in both sexes, and it reached a peak in the group older than 70 years old, indicating that exposure to HBV had occurred in every age group (Fig. 3). The prevalence of anti-HBs increased from 39.9% to

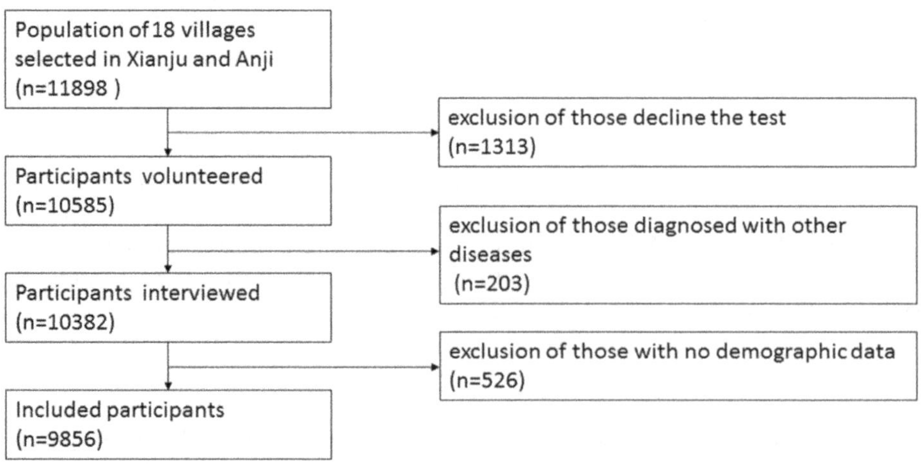

Fig. 1 Flow chart of the selection process in the study populations

Table 1 Demographic data of the study populations

Region	Population	Participants interviewed	Included participants	Percentage of males (%)	Mean Age ± SD (years)
Xianju	342,700	6362	5844	43.9	53.8 ± 17.5
Anji	466,552	4021	4011	39.8	41.4 ± 8.2
Total	809,252	10,383	9855	42.2	49.0 ± 15.9

57.7% in those aged 20–59 years old and to more than 60% among those >60 years old (Fig. 4). Having only anti-HBs positivity without other HBV markers was found in approximately 33.9% of the participants (95% CI: 31.5–36.3) (Table 2).

Difference in prevalence of HBV infection between the two mountainous regions

As shown in Table 3, the prevalence of HBV infection was calculated according to gender in each region. The total prevalence was calculated through normalization with the urban population in addition to the sex ratio. The prevalence of HBsAg was significantly higher ($P > 0.01$) in the Xianju region (12.6%; 95% CI: 10.9–13.8) than in the Anji area (8.6%; 95% CI: 5.1–9.1). The HBsAg prevalence was higher in males than in females ($P < 0.01$) in both locations. The anti-HBc prevalence in Xianju (45.7%) was significantly higher than that in Anji (35.9%; $P < 0.01$), but there was no significant difference in anti-HBc positivity between males and females in either region. The anti-HBs prevalence differed significantly between Xianju (61.2%) and Anji (41.8%). The prevalence of vaccination-induced immunity (only anti-HBs positivity) was also significantly higher (P < 0.01) in Xianju (Table 3).

HCC screening in the HBsAg-positive group and ALT levels

Eight HBsAg-positive participants (6 men and 2 women, 0.11%), who were >40 years old, were AFP positive. However, no liver tumors were detected by ultrasonography. The mean (± SD) ALT level was 18.8 ± 7.4 IU/L, and the proportion of participants with an elevated ALT level (>38 IU/L) was 6.8%. The proportion of patients with an abnormal ALT level was much higher in the HBsAg-positive group (15.3%), compared with the HBsAg-negative group (6.3%) ($P \leq 0.01$) (Table 4). The HBsAg-positive group had a significantly higher ALT level (25.32 ± 23.67 IU/L), compared with the HBsAg-negative group (18.05 ± 13.06 IU/L). Among all participants, the percentage of participants with an abnormal ALT level was significantly higher in males (9.55%) than in females (6.61%) ($P \leq 0.01$). The average ALT level in males (21.40 ± 16.67 IU/L) was higher than that in females (16.95 ± 12.84 IU/L). Additionally, the proportion of patients with an abnormal ALT level markedly decreased with age, from 7.67% in the group aged 30–39 years old to 3.45% in the group of subjects >70 years old ($P \leq 0.01$) (Fig. 5).

Discussion

We conducted a new epidemiological study of HBV infection in two mountainous regions of Zhejiang province and provided a fresh and interesting peek into the current status of HBV infection in China. We found that HBsAg positivity in the general population of the two study regions remains considerably high and that it increased with age. We also found that HBV infection in women of childbearing age is still at a high level (up to 10%). Finally, we found that the prevalence of HBV infection depends on the location, despite a similar landscape of the two areas.

The positive HBsAg rate in the mountainous areas of Zhejiang province decreased to 10.19% in 2011, from 15.94% in 1993 [9, 11]. The current study shows a chronic HBV infection rate of 9.5% in two mountainous areas of Zhejiang, which is lower than that reported previously but still higher than average national or provincial levels.

Maternal-neonatal HBV transmission is the main route for the spread of HBV infection in China. In

Table 2 Prevalence of hepatitis B virus markers, stratified by age group

Age	Only anti-HBs		HBsAg		Anti-HBc		Anti-HBs	
	No. positive/no. tested	Percent	No. positive/no. tested	Percent	No. positive/no. tested	Percent	No. positive/no. tested	Percent
<20	75/155	48.4	5/155	3.2	22/155	14.2	85/155	54.8
20–29	131/562	23.3	51/562	9.1	180/562	32.0	224/562	39.9
30–39	406/1551	26.2	180/1551	11.6	641/1551	41.3	738/1551	47.6
40–49	1047/3385	30.9	374/3385	11.0	1340/3385	39.6	1671/3385	49.4
50–59	670/1839	36.4	228/1839	12.4	814/1839	44.3	1062/1839	57.7
60–69	437/1147	38.1	138/1147	12.0	531/1147	46.3	702/1147	61.2
>70	455/1216	37.4	80/1216	6.6	568/1216	46.7	773/1216	63.6
total	3221/9855	33.9	1056/9855	9.5	4096/9855	35.1	5255/9855	51.0

The positive percentages were standardized by age

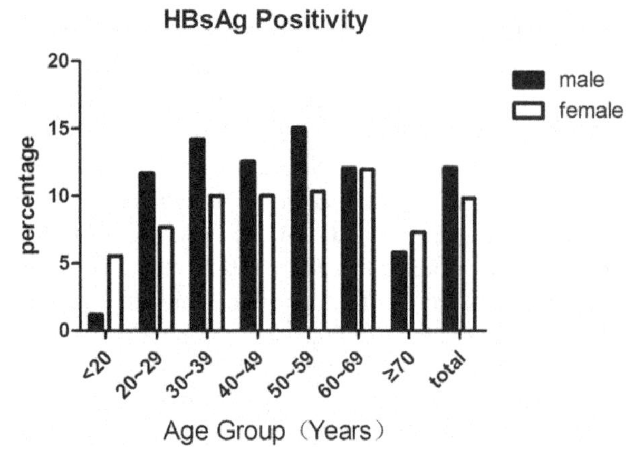

Fig. 2 Age-specific prevalence of hepatitis B virus surface antigen (HBsAg)

Zhejiang province, the EPI vaccination program is considered a success. Since the program was initiated in 1992, HBV infection in the participants who were younger than 20 years old was reduced to 3.2%, compared to a HBV infection rate of 9.5% in the total studied population. The success of universal HBV immunization of infants directly contributes to the decline in the HBV infection prevalence in China. However, the achieved success is not good enough because a portion of participants younger than 20 years old are infected with HBV. There are two possible reasons for the incomplete blockade of HBV transmission. One is HBV immunization coverage. Chen Xuejun et al. have reported that the average HBV vaccination coverage rate in Zhejiang was more than 95%, but not 100% [14]. A gap in the coverage can partially explain the data. The other reason could be related to the response rate to HBV immunization. As shown by our data, only anti-HBs positivity in the group younger than 20 years old was only around 50%. Assuming that 95% of them were immunized with the HBV vaccine, nearly 40% of immunized participants did not have detectable anti-HBs antibody, suggesting that the detectable anti-HBs antibody level has waned out or the response of the anti-HBs antibody to the HBV vaccine is unexpectedly lower than the reported 95% [14]. In a recent study, nearly 22% of HBV-vaccinated infants were negative for HBV-neutralizing antibody when they were tested at the age of one year (6 months after the last vaccine injection), and they had to be revaccinated, suggesting that the HBV-neutralizing antibody levels quickly declined or were initially lower than 10 mIU/mL [15]. Our results raise a serious question about the effectiveness of the current HBV vaccine and vaccination schedule. Clearly, our findings need to be verified in larger populations across different geographic locations.

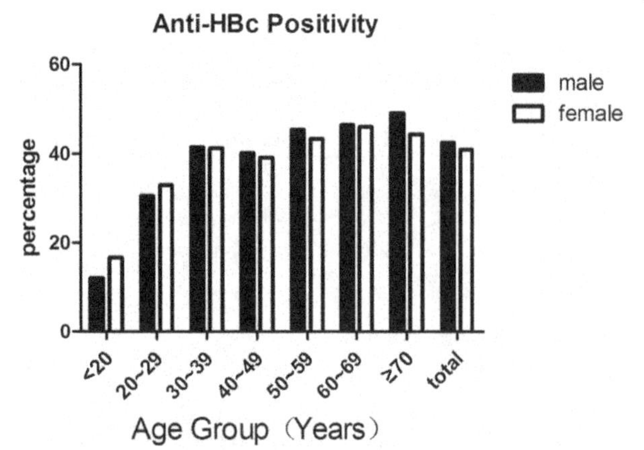

Fig. 3 Age-specific prevalence of anti-HBV core antibody (anti-HBc)

Another finding that surprises us is that chronic HBV infection in women younger than 20 years old was more than 5%. This result could be statistically skewed because of the relatively smaller number of participants in the group younger than 20 years old. In other age groups, the detected HBsAg positivity in females was generally lower than that in males. Despite relatively lower HBsAg positivity in females, the prevalence of chronic HBV infection among women of reproductive age (20–40 years old) is 9.36%, which is still a very high level. Chronic HBV-infected women of reproductive age represent an important source for HBV transmission. It has been reported that the HBV vaccination rate in mountainous regions was significantly lower than that in plains areas [16]. Incomplete coverage of HBV immunization and a lower response rate of anti-HBs antibody in immunized children will contribute to perinatal HBV infection, the majority of whom will become chronically infected. Our results reflect a severe challenge that we are facing in completely blocking the vertical transmission of HBV. Government agencies ought to expand HBV immunization coverage and strengthen the screening test for HBsAg among pregnant women to increase the HBV interruption rate of perinatal transmission [17–19]. Additional HBV immunization drugs that are more effective than the currently available hepatitis B immunoglobulin and HBV vaccine are needed to completely block the vertical transmission of HBV.

Several reasons have been suggested for the relatively high chronic HBV infection in the hilly region: first, the economy in the mountainous region is at a lower level compared to other regions that are easily accessible by transportation. Sun et al. have found that the positive rate of HBsAg in less-developed regions was significantly higher than that in developed areas [20]; second, the population living in the mountainous villages may not have sufficient awareness of HBV infection and lack protection against HBV transmission in daily life, which may have caused the spread of hepatitis B infection [21, 22]; third, poor hygiene in the hilly region is also a risk factor

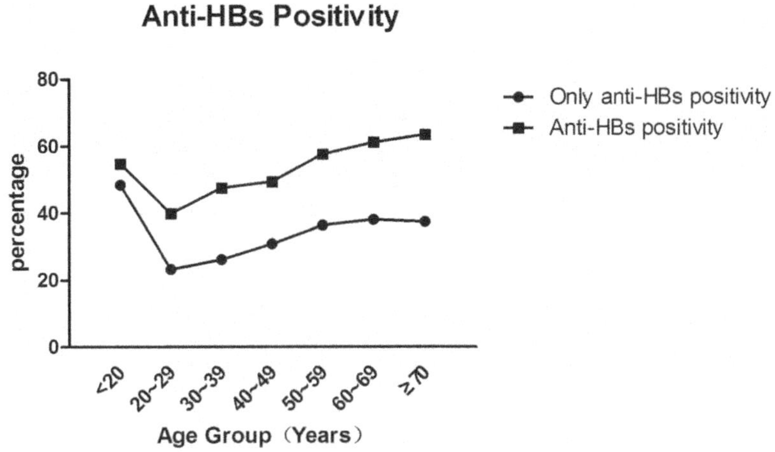

Fig. 4 Age-specific prevalence of anti-hepatitis B surface antigen (anti-HBs) antibody positivity with or without other HBV markers

for HBV infection B [23]; finally, the primitive lifestyle of those who live in hilly regions makes HBV spread easily [24].

The results of this study showed that the HBcAb-positive rate increased with age, which is consistent with the results of an earlier survey [25]. Thus, horizontal HBV transmission may occur more frequently than realized previously.

Interestingly, the distribution of anti-HBc by age was not different between the two genders (Fig. 2), while the distribution of HBsAg by age did not follow the same pattern (Fig. 1): The HBs-Ag positive frequency in male adults was much greater than that of female adults. This finding indicates that while exposure to HBV transmission among male and female subjects was similar, a higher portion of the HBV-exposed male adults became chronically infected in this cohort. This observation was consistent with the pattern described by a long-term study of HBV infection in Fujian [26].

The current survey showed that the positivity rates of HBsAg and anti-HBc in the Xianju area were significantly higher than those in the Anji region (Table 3). Anji is located in the Yangtze River delta and has a more developed economy than Xianju. In addition, the prosperous tourist industry in Xianju may have facilitated the spread of HBV infection [27]. Though both areas were included in the EPI in 1992, which initially only covered infants, Xianju started implementing free HBV immunization for all residents including infants and adults in 2010 to expand immunization. These facts may explain the difference in the prevalence of only anti-HBs detection between the two regions.

The association between abnormal ALT levels and HBsAg status was also indicated in the current study. The HBsAg-positive group had higher levels of ALT, compared with the HBsAg-negative group. Furthermore, abnormal ALT levels were significantly more frequent among HBsAg carriers than those who were not carriers.

HCC is the fifth most common malignancy and the third leading cause of cancer-related deaths worldwide. Approximately 85% of HCC cases are borne in developing countries, especially in East and Southeast Asia and sub-Saharan Africa, where a major risk factor is chronic HBV infection [28, 29]. The prevalence of abnormal AFP levels among HBsAg-positive individuals aged >30 years old was 0.8% in this group, greater than the recently reported 0.13% found in the general population of the same age range in Zhejiang province [30]. Although no HCC cases were identified among the AFP-

Table 3 Prevalence of hepatitis B virus markers, stratified by region

Region	Sex	Anti-HBs		HBsAg		Anti-HBc		Only anti-HBs	
		No. positive/total	Percent	No. positive/total	Percent	No. positive/total	Percent	No. positive/total	Percent
Xianju	Male	1583/2585	61.2	352/2585	13.6	1205/2585	46.6	1010/2585	39.1
	Female	2019/3301	61.2	383/3301	11.6	1475/3301	44.7	1227/3301	37.2
	Total	3602/5886	61.2	735/5886	12.6	2680/5886	45.7	2237/5886	38.1
Anji	Male	673/1595	42.2	154/1595	9.7	572/1595	35.9	422/1595	26.5
	Female	1002/2416	41.5	180/2416	7.5	867/2416	35.9	573/2416	23.7
	Total	1675/4011	41.8	334/4011	8.6	1439/4011	35.9	995/4011	25.1

Percentages of HBV markers were standardized by gender

Table 4 Percentages of elevated ALT in HBsAg-positive and HBsAg-negative groups

	HBsAg-positive						HBsAg-negative					
	<38 UI/L			>38 UI/L			<38 UI/L			>38 UI/L		
Serum ALT	No. positive/no. test	Mean ALT ± SD	%	No. positive/no. test	Mean ALT ± SD	%	No. positive/no. test	Mean ALT ± SD	%	No. positive/no. test	Mean ALT ± SD	%
Male	398/499	20.19 7.50	79.8	101/499	65.62 50.84	20.2	3364/3660	17.34 7.66	91.9	296/3660	54.63 20.41	8.1
Female	501/557	17.65 7.06	89.9	56/557	57.86 20.02	10.1	4920/5139	14.59 6.34	95.7	219/5139	57.85 30.78	4.3
Total	899/1056	18.76 7.35	84.7	157/1056	62.85 42.57	15.3	8284/8799	16.69 6.79	93.7	515/8799	56.00 25.37	6.3

positive individuals by the ultrasound examination, an elevated APF level warrants close monitoring.

We acknowledge several limitations in this study. First, as a community-based epidemiology study, we did not collect information on genotype, IgM antibody, and participants' vaccine history, which may better inform the HBV epidemiological characteristics in study areas. Second, the exclusion of those who missed the information of age and gender from our analysis may have potential impact on overall prevalence estimate. Moreover, the exclusion of those who were diagnosed with hepatitis C, hepatitis D, other liver diseases, HIV, immune-suppression disorders, or those who were undergoing antiviral therapy may have underestimated the HBV prevalence because they were probably at greater risk of being infected with hepatitis B. Finally, we did not collect data on risk factors of these populations, including homosexual activity, intravenous drug use, transfusion, and shared medical equipment (e.g., dialysis and dental procedures).

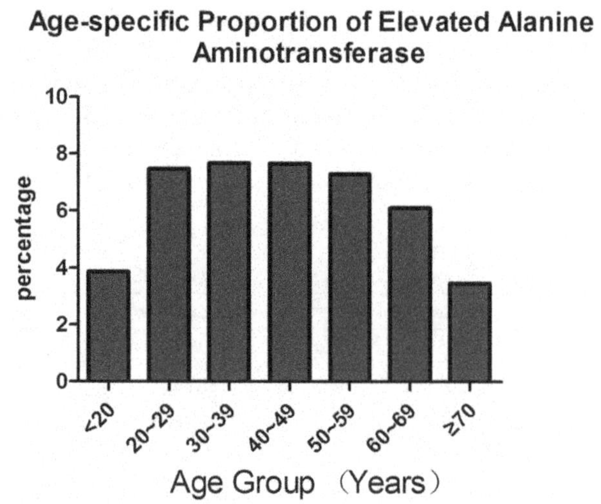

Fig. 5 Age-specific percentages of elevated alanine aminotransferase (ALT) levels

Conclusions

In conclusion, this community-based study of HBV infection in hilly/mountainous regions in China describes the current status of HBV infection in China. We found that after more than 20 years of the EPI, HBsAg positivity in the general population of the two study regions remains considerably high at 9.5%, which is significantly higher than the national level. We also found that HBV infection in women of childbearing age is still at a high level (up to 10%). Finally, we found that the prevalence of HBV infection depends on the location, despite a similar mountainous landscape of the two areas. Our data serve as a reminder that it is a long journey to block HBV transmission completely through HBV vaccination alone in China and that a more effective treatment that can clear chronic HBV infection is required to lower the prevalence of HBV infection in China.

Abbreviations

AFP: α-fetoprotein; ALT: Aminotransferase; anti-HBc: Anti-HBV core antigen; anti-HBs: Anti-HBV surface antigen; HBsAg: Hepatitis B virus surface antigen; HBV: Hepatitis B virus

Acknowledgements

Not applicable

Funding

This study was supported by grants from the Mega-Project for National Science and Technology Development under the "12th Five-Year Plan of China" (2013ZX10004904 and 2014ZX10004008), the opening foundation of the State Key Laboratory for Diagnosis and Treatment of Infectious Diseases and Collaborative Innovation Center for Diagnosis and Treatment of Infectious Diseases, The First Affiliated Hospital of Medical College, Zhejiang University (grant No. 2017KF10) and the Medical & Health Technology Program of Zhejiang Province (grant No. 2016KYA079).

Authors' contributions

PC, TC and JWW designed the study. BR and ZQZ collected and analyzed the data. HNG, ZQZ, and LJL contributed to sample collection and provided intellectual input. PC, QFX and LJL drafted and wrote the manuscript. PC, TC, and JW revised the manuscript critically for intellectual content. All authors gave intellectual input to the study and approved the final version of the manuscript.

Consent for publication
Not applicable

Competing interests
The authors declare that they have no competing interests.

Author details
[1]Shulan (Hangzhou) Hospital, Zhejiang University International Hospital, Hangzhou 310012, China. [2]State Key Laboratory for Diagnosis and Treatment of Infectious Diseases, Collaborative Innovation Center for Diagnosis and Treatment of Infectious Diseases, The First Affiliated Hospital, College of Medicine, Zhejiang University, 79 Qing-Chun Road, Hangzhou 310003, China. [3]College of Medicine, Zhejiang University, Hangzhou 310058, China. [4]Xianju Hospital of Traditional Chinese Medicine, Zhenjiang, Xianju 317300, China.

References

1. Trepo C, Chan HL, Lok A. Hepatitis B virus infection. Lancet. 2014;384:2053–63.
2. WHO. Guidelines for the prevention, care and treatment of persons with chronic hepatitis B infection. http://www.who.int/hepatitis/publications/hepatitis-b-guidelines/en.
3. Marcellin P, Gane E, Buti M, Afdhal N, Sievert W, Jacobson IM, Washington MK, Germanidis G, Flaherty JF, Aguilar Schall R, Bornstein JD, Kitrinos KM, Subramanian GM, McHutchison JG, Heathcote EJ. Regression of cirrhosis during treatment with tenofovir disoproxil fumarate for chronic hepatitis B: a 5-year open-label follow-up study. Lancet. 2013;381:468–75.
4. El-Serag HB. Epidemiology of viral hepatitis and hepatocellular carcinoma. Gastroenterology. 2012;142:1264–73. e1
5. Chen YS, Li L, Cui FQ, Xing WG, Wang L, Jia ZY, Zhou MG, Gong XH, Wang FZ, Zheng H, Luo HM, Bi SL, Wang N, Yang WZ, Liang XF. A sero-epidemiological study on hepatitis C in China. Zhonghua Liu Xing Bing Xue Za Zhi. 2011;32:888–91.
6. Liang X, Bi S, Yang W, Wang L, Cui G, Cui F, Zhang Y, Liu J, Gong X, Chen Y, Wang F, Zheng H, Wang F, Guo J, Jia Z, Ma J, Wang H, Luo H, Li L, Jin S, Hadler SC, Wang Y. Reprint of: epidemiological serosurvey of hepatitis B in China–declining HBV prevalence due to hepatitis B vaccination. Vaccine. 2013;31(Suppl 9):J21–8.
7. Ding Y, Sheng Q, Ma L, Dou X. Chronic HBV infection among pregnant women and their infants in Shenyang. China Virol J. 2013;10:17.
8. Yang SG, Wang B, Chen P, Yu CB, Deng M, Yao J, Zhu CX, Ren JJ, Wu W, Ju B, Shen JF, Chen Y, Li MD, Ruan B, Li L. Effectiveness of HBV vaccination in infants and prediction of HBV prevalence trend under new vaccination plan: findings of a large-scale investigation. PLoS One. 2012;7:e47808.
9. Xu WJ. Seroepidemiological survey of hepatitis B virus infection in normal population. Chin J Public Health. 1993;9:346.
10. Zhou ST. Analysis of hepatitis B virus infection of different occupation groups in a city. In: The third National Academic Symposium on epidemic worker epidemiology of infectious diseases; 2005. p. 82–3.
11. Zhang DY, Wei-Ling HE, Zhang HF, Zhou YY. Study on hepatitis B virus infection status and risk factors among populations in Lishui city Zhejiang province. Dis Surveill. 2009;24:238–41.
12. Chen YP. Exploring the influence of health education on the prevention of hepatitis B knowledge popularization rate. China Health Care & Nutrition. 2013;23:2676–7.
13. Chen P, Yu C, Ruan B, Yang S, Ren J, Xu W, Luo Z, Li L. Prevalence of hepatitis B in insular regions of southeast China: a community-based study. PLoS One. 2013;8:e56444.
14. Lu ZY, Shan FX, Wang WX. Analysis on hepatitis B surface antibody level and effect of blocking HBV maternal-infant transmission in Shenzhen. Practical Prev Med. 2013;1:017.
15. Evans AA, Cohen C, Huang P, Qian L, London WT, Block JM, Chen G. Prevention of perinatal hepatitis B transmission in Haimen City, China: results of a community public health initiative. Vaccine. 2015;33:3010–5.
16. Yao J, Yang JZ, Mo SH. Investigation on Immunization Coverage Rate and Immune Effect of Hepatitis B Vaccine among Newborns in Zhejiang Province. Zhejiang Prev Med. 2000;04:3–5.
17. Chen XJ, Pan YX, Cheng YZ. Detection and distribution characteristics of serological markers of hepatitis B in neonates, infants and preschool children in Zhejiang province. Chinese J Lab Med. 2011;34:200–5.
18. Wang FZ, Gong XH, Liu LR. Analysis on infection of hepatitis B virus among pregnant women in Beijing. Chin J Vaccines Immunization. 2007;1:009.
19. Wang HX, Liu L, Wu D, Wang SY. Analysis of the effect of maternal and child block in 200 cases of hepatitis B surface antigen positive pregnant women. World Latest Medicine Information. 2015;15:184.
20. Sun LY, Zeng ZZ, Chen HY, Fu ZW, Chen SM, Yan XJ, Deng HY, Pan ZF. Seroepidemiological survey of hepatitis B virus infection in Hainan Province. China Trop Med. 2007;7:182–9.
21. Li KQ, Wu GC, Xu H, Zou K. Hepatitis B virus infection in a mountainous area. Modern Preventive Medicine. 2007;34:2557–8.
22. Dan DU, Wang R. KAP survey on hepatitis B among hepatitis B patients and their families in Lanzhou City. Chinese Journal of Disease Control & Prevention. 2011;04:323–6.
23. Zhang HL, He LX, Zhang QJ, Ma XY. Investigation of HBV infection and nosocomial infection control in hospitalized patients with pulmonary tuberculosis. Modern Journal of Integrated Traditional Chinese and Western Medicine. 2002;11:2266–7.
24. Qu MWN, Zhuo XM, Lu YC. The exploration of the development of the county area of the poor mountainous areas of the Yi nationality in the poor mountainous areas: Xide Liangshan County as an example. Communist Party Committee of the Provincial Party School in Suchuan Journal. 2013;2:98–101.
25. Chen P. Seroepidemiological and molecular epidemiological studies of viral hepatitis B after 20 years from the Inroduction of hepatitis B vaccine in insular regions of Southeast China. Hangzhou: Zhejiang University; 2013.
26. Lin CL, Kao JH. Risk stratification for hepatitis B virus related hepatocellular carcinoma. J Gastroenterol Hepatol. 2013;28:10–7.
27. Zhang YB, Cheng JQ, Hao YT, Chen WH, Ma ZC, Liao YX, Zhang R. Comparisons and analysis of the hepatitis B infection status of transient population and registered residents in Shenzhen City. Chinese Journal of Disease Control & Prevention. 2012;16:424–7.
28. Li C, Zhang Z, Zhang P, Liu J. Diagnostic accuracy of des-gamma-carboxy prothrombin versus alpha-fetoprotein for hepatocellular carcinoma: a systematic review. Hepatol Res. 2014;44:E11–25.
29. Li G, Cai G, Li D, Yin W. MicroRNAs and liver disease: viral hepatitis, liver fibrosis and hepatocellular carcinoma. Postgrad Med J. 2014;90:106–12.
30. Zou LL, Hu MZ, Tang HZ. Analysis of the detection results of serum AFP, CEA, CA125, CA19-9 in health examination population. Zhejiang Medical Journal. 2013;13:1298–300.

3

Genotypes of hepatitis a virus in Turkey: first report and clinical profile of children infected with sub-genotypes IA and IIIA

Huseyin Yilmaz[1*], Asiye Karakullukcu[2], Nuri Turan[1], Utku Y. Cizmecigil[1], Aysun Yilmaz[1], Ayse A. Ozkul[3], Ozge Aydin[1], Alper Gunduz[4], Mahmut Mete[5], Fadile Y. Zeyrek[6], Taner T. Kirazoglu[2], Juergen A. Richt[7] and Bekir Kocazeybek[2]

Abstract

Background: Hepatitis A virus (HAV) is a food and water-borne virus causing clinical (mainly hepatitis) and subclinical disease in humans. It is important to characterize circulating strains of HAV in order to prevent HAV infections using efficacious vaccines. The aim of this study was the detection and characterization of the circulating strains of HAV in Turkey by performing serology, RT-PCR, sequencing and phylogenetic analysis.

Methods: In this study, 355 HAV suspected cases were analysed by ELISA for the presence of antibodies to HAV. RNA was extracted from 54 HAV IgM positive human sera. None of the suspect cases were vaccinated against HAV and they never received blood transfusions. Samples found positive by RT-PCR using primers targeting the VP1/VP2A junction and VP1/VP3 capsid region of HAV, were subjected to sequencing and phylogenetic analyses.

Results: IgM type antibodies to HAV were detected in 54 patients. Twenty one of them were students. The age of IgM positive cases was between 3 and 60 years. IgM positivity differed in age groups and was higher in the age group 3 to 10 years. Phylogenetic analysis showed that the majority of HAV strains detected in this study belong to the "HAV 1B" cluster. In addition, the HAV sub-genotypes IA (KT874461.1) and IIIA (KT222963.1) were found in 2 children. These sub-genotypes were not previously reported in Turkey. The child who carried sub-genotype IIIA travelled to Afghanistan and presented with abdominal pain, icterus and vomitus. He was positive for anti-HAV IgM and IgG but negative for hepatitis B and C. Liver enzymes like aspartate aminotransferase, alanine aminotransferase, alkaline phosphatase, gamma-glutamyl transferase and lactate dehydrogenase were severely elevated. Bilirubin levels were also increased. White blood cells, neutrophils and hemoglobin were decreased while lymphocytes and monocytes were increased. Similar clinical signs and laboratory findings were reported for the child infected with sub-genotype IA but aspartate aminotransferase and alanine aminotransferase were not severely elevated.

Conclusions: The results indicate that molecular studies determining the HAV genotype variation in Turkey are timely and warranted. The majority of IgM positive cases in 3–10 year old patients indicate that childhood vaccination is important. Sub-genotype IB is the most prevalant genotype in Turkey. Surprisingly, sub-genotype IA and IIIA are also present in Turkey; future diagnostic efforts need to include diagnostic methods which can identify this emerging HAV genotypes. Our results also show that one important risk factor for contracting hepatitis A virus is international travel since genotype IIIA was detected in a child who had travelled to Afghanistan.

Keywords: Hepatitis a virus sequencing, Phylogenetic, VP1/VP2A, VP1/VP3, Turkey

* Correspondence: hyilmaz@istanbul.edu.tr
[1]Department of Virology, Veterinary Faculty, University of Istanbul, Avcilar, Istanbul, Turkey
Full list of author information is available at the end of the article

Background

Hepatitis A virus (HAV) infections occur worldwide with approximately 1.4 million new cases reported each year with 11–22% of the cases being hospitalized [1]. The severity and symptoms of HAV infections are strongly associated with age. HAV infections are asymptomatic in childhood while symptoms like jaundice and acute liver failure are more prominent in older people with mortality rates up to 1.8%, depending on the region and vaccination policy [2, 3].

Hepatitis A virus is a non-enveloped RNA virus with positive polarity and the only member of genus *Hepatovirus* in the family *Picornaviridae*. The viral genome is about 7.5 kb and contains 5′ and 3′ untranslated regions and one open reading frame (ORF) [4]. The open reading frame of HAV RNA encodes a large polyprotein (P0) with 2227 amino acid residues. Protease cleavage of the HAV polyprotein yields four major proteins which are VP1- VP4. It has 3 regions as P1, P2 and P3. The P1 region encodes capsid or structural proteins, 1A (VP4), 1B (VP2), 1C (VP3) and 1D (VP1). The P2 and P3 regions encode non-structural proteins, 2A, 2B and 2C, and 3A, 3B, 3C and 3D, respectively [5–7].

Complete genome sequence analysis have shown that HAV can be divided into 7 genotypes [7, 8]. Genotypes I, II, III and VII have been associated with hepatitis in humans. Most of the HAV strains detected in humans belong to genotypes I and III with 80% of them being genotype I. Genotypes I and III are divided in to sub-genotypes A, B and C. Genotypes IV, V and VI are found in simians and have been also recovered from pigs [7, 8].

HAV is transmitted by the feco-oral route mainly through contaminated food (sandwiches, fruits, salads and shellfish) and water and to a lesser extend from person to person or via blood transfussion [9–12]. Hepatitis A virus is endemic mainly in the Middle East, Asia and in North African countries [3] but outbreaks have also been reported in Europe [13, 14], especially in tourists returning from HAV endemic countries. Incidence rates of HAV are strongly associated with socioeconomic factors correlating with poor hygienic conditions, which affects the hygiene of food and water [2]. However, with improvement of food safety, HAV incidence in endemic countries decreased in young children but increased in adolescents and adults [3]. Since mainly children are vaccinated in many countries, elderly people are more affected by HAV in recent years because of the decrease in vaccine immunity to HAV.

In order to prevent HAV infections, it is important to know the HAV strains circulating in an endemic area in order to establish effective vaccination strategies. Several regions of the HAV genome have been used for genotyping to investigate molecular variants of HAV. These are the entire VP1 region, the N terminus of the VP1 region, the VP1–2A junction region, the VP1–2B region, the VP3-2B region, the C terminus of the VP3 region and the 5'UTR region [7, 15–18]. The aim of this study was detection and investigation of the circulating strains of HAV in Turkey by performing serology, RT-PCR, sequencing and phylogenetic analysis.

Methods

Patients and diagnosis of hepatitis A

The study population consisted of 355 patients who showed one or two clinical symptoms of hepatitis (abdominal pain, diarrhea, vomiting and/or icterus) and were admitted to the clinical department at the Cerrahpasa Medical School Hospital in Istanbul, Turkey, between 2012 and 2015 as well as the Sisli Research Hospital, Dicle University, Izmir University and Harran University. The clinical symptoms, age, gender, occupation, travel history and vaccination status were recorded. Sera were collected for serological and molecular analyses in the first week after the onset of clinical symptoms. Samples were transported to the research laboratory using cold storage (4°–8 °C). In order to confirm hepatitis A diagnosis, all sera were analysed by an ELISA for the presence of IgM antibodies to HAV as described in detail by the manufacturer (HEPAVASE MA-96, TMB; General Biologicals Corporation, Germany).

RNA extraction and cDNA synthesis

For the extraction of viral RNA, QIAamp Viral RNA mini kit (Qiagen, Germany) was used to extract RNA from 54 sera which were found to be IgM positive to HAV. Extraction procedures were carried out according to the instructions described by the manufacturer (Qiagen, Germany). The amount of RNA in the extracted material was measured using a NanoDrop spectrophotometer (NanoDrop 1000c, Thermo Scientific). Approximately 500–600 ng/µl RNA was used for reverse transcription (RT). RT was performed in 2 steps. For the first step, 9 µl of RNA template (about 400 ng) was mixed with 1 µl random hexamers (Promega) and incubated at 70 °C for 5 min, followed by a cooling step to 4 °C using a thermal cycler (Biorad Chromo4). For the second step, a total volume of 20 µl reaction mixture was prepared consisting of 10 µl RNA/primer mixture from the first step, 4 µl 5X RT buffer, 2.4 µl 25 mM $MgCl_2$, 1 µl 10 mM dNTPs, 1.6 µl nuclease-free water, and 1 µl reverse transcriptase (Improm II, Promega). The mixture was returned to the thermal cycler and incubated at 20 °C for 5 min, 42 °C for 30 min and 70 °C for 15 min before being cooled to 4 °C. After completion of the RT reaction, 30 µl of nuclease-free water was added to each cDNA sample and the samples were kept at −80 °C until required.

Sequencing and phylogenetic analyses

Samples (n = 54) found positive by IgM ELISA were subjected to RT-PCR, sequencing and phylogenetic analyses. Commercially synthesized primers were used in these analyses (DNA Technology, Denmark). Two different PCR reactions were set up using primers targeting the VP1/VP2A junction region and the VP1/VP3 region (Table 1). The primers and method used to amplify the VP1/VP3 region were the same as described previously [16]. However, in order to amplify the VP1/VP2A junction region, a modification of the previous method was used [15]. For this purpose, a nested PCR was performed. For the first amplification step, the newly designed primers (HAV-OtF and HAV-Ot-R) were used (Table 1). Briefly, a total volume of 25 μl reaction mixture was prepared for an optimized PCR consisting of 12.5 μl Maxima Hot Start PCR Master Mix (Thermo Scientific), 1 μl HAV-OtF primer (2.5 pmol/μl), 1 μl HAV-OtR primer (2.5 pmol/μl), 0.5 μl $MgCl_2$ (25 mM), 5 μl nuclease free water and 5 μl cDNA. The mixture was placed in a thermal cycler (Stratagene mx3000p). Cycling conditions were as follows: 95 °C for 4 min then 40 cycles of 94 °C for 40 s, 54 °C for 1 min, 72 °C for 1 min and final incubation at 72 °C for 7 min. For the second nested amplification step, primers (HAV BR5F and HAV newRT) (Table 1) and a method described by Reuter and others (2006) were used. Briefly, a total volume of 50 μl reaction mixture was prepared for an optimized PCR consisting of 25 μl Maxima Hot Start PCR Master Mix (Thermo Scientific), 1 μl BR5F primer (20 pmol/μl), 1 μl newRT primer (20 pmol/μl), 21 μl nuclease free water and 2 μl first step product. The mixture was placed in a thermal cycler (Stratagene mx3000p). Cycling conditions were as follows: 95 °C for 4 min then 40 cycles of 94 °C for 1 min, 58 °C for 1.5 min, 72 °C for 1 min and final incubation at 72 °C for 7 min. After PCR, a HAV-specific 360 bp product was visualized by 1.5% agarose gel electrophoresis.

For all RT-PCR reactions, nuclease free water was used as negative control in place of a template. Positive controls were obtained from sera samples submitted to Cerrahpasa Hospital laboratory, which were previously confirmed to be HAV positive by RT-PCR and sequencing. Products obtained by PCR using the primers specific for the VP1/VP2A and VP1/VP3 regions were sequenced by a commercial company (MedSanTek, Istanbul, Turkey; REFGEN, Ankara, Turkey). Multiple alignments of VP1/VP2A and VP1/VP3 region sequences were made using the Mega 7 software. Phylogenetic analyses were carried out using the criterion of neighbour-joining trees based on genetic distance model by Tamura-Nei [19]. After the generation of phylogenetic trees, the sequences were analyzed for the presence of possible recombination event or recombinant HAV strains.

Results

Clinical findings and demography of HAV IgM positive cases

HAV-specific IgM antibodies were detected in 54 patients. All patients with IgM type antibodies to HAV were suffering from one or two of the following clinical signs: abdominal pain, diarrhea, vomitus and/or icterus. None of these patients were vaccinated against HAV or received a blood transfusion. Twenty one (n = 21) of them were students.. Fourty three (n = 43) cases were from Istanbul, 8 cases from the east of Turkey and 3 cases from the west of Turkey. Two (n = 2) patients have recently travelled to Afghanistan. Thirty four (n = 34) of them were male and 20 were female. The ages of IgM positive cases were between 3 and 60 years old. IgM positivity differed in age groups and was higher in ages between 3 to10 years (Table 2). Various characteristics of the HAV IgM positive patients and some factors like age, occupation, eating habit, sea food consumption and presence of icterus in patients are summarized in Table 2.

Sequencing and phylogenetic analyses

VP1/VP2A region

Amplification of a 360 bp product of the VP1/VP2A region of HAV was successful with 23 out of 54 IgM positive sera. The partial VP1/VP2A sequences detected in 22 sera (Fig. 1) were closely related to HAV sub-genotype IB strains detected in Netherlands (KM261588.1), Hungary (DQ163904.2), France (GU646039.1), Italy (AY294047), Bulgaria (KX859023.1) and Egypt (KX228692.1). In addition, HAV sub-genotype IA (KT874462.1) was

Table 1 Primers and their sequences used in this study

Primers	Sequences 5'-3'	Product size	Target gene	Target Sequences	References
HAV-ot-VP1-2- 2848 F	GAGCACTGGATGGTTTGGGW	466 bp	VP1/VP2A junction	2848–2867	Designed in this study
HAV-ot-VP1-2- 3314 R	WGCAGTCACWCCTCTCCAAG			3314-3295[a]	
HAV BR5F	TTGTCTGTCACAGAACAATCA	360 bp	VP1/VP2A junction	2952–2973	Reuter et al., 2006
HAV newRT	AGC AGT CAC TCC TCT CCA G			3294–3311[b]	
HA2F	GTTTTGCTCCTCTTTATCATGCTATG	247 bp	VP1-VP3 capsid	2165–2191	Namsai et al., 2011
HA1R	GGAAATGTCTCAGGTACTTTCTTTG			2411–2387[c]	

[a]M20273; [b]M14707 and [c]KP879217 indicates the sequences derived from the GenBank accession numbers

Table 2 Characteristics and some factors associated with HAV IgM positive patients by age groups

	Age Groups (Year)					
	3–10	11–20	21–30	31–40	41–50	51–60
Sex (%)						
Male	15 (68)	6 (50)	9 (75)	2 (66.6)	2 (66.6)	0 (0)
Female	7 (32)	6 (50)	3 (25)	1 (33.4)	1 (33.4)	2 (100)
Job (%)						
Student	12 (54.5)	12 (100)	3 (25)	0 (0)	0 (0)	0 (0)
Waiter	0 (0)	0 (0)	1 (8.3)	0 (0)	0 (0)	0 (0)
Sailor	0 (0)	0 (0)	1 (8.3)	0 (0)	0 (0)	0 (0)
Others	0 (0)	0 (0)	1 (8.3)	3 (100)	3 (100)	1 (50)
Non-working	10 (45.5)	0 (0)	6 (50)	0 (0)	0 (0)	1 (50)
City of residence (%)						
Istanbul	14 (63.6)	11 (91.6)	10 (83.3)	3 (100)	3 (100)	2 (100)
Other cities	8 (36.4)	1(8.4)	2 (16.7)	0 (0)	0 (0)	0 (0)
Eating habit (%)						
Homemade	19 (86.3)	4 (33.3)	9 (75)	3 (100)	3 (100)	2 (100)
Fast food	3 (13.7)	8 (66.7)	3 (25)	0 (0)	0 (0)	0 (0)
Consumption of seafood (%)						
Fish	1 (4.5)	0 (0)	3 (25)	0 (0)	1 (33.4)	1 (50)
Mussels	1 (4.5)	1(8.4)	0 (0)	0 (0)	0 (0)	0 (0)
No seafood	20 (91)	11 (91.6)	9 (75)	3 (100)	2 (66.6)	1 (50)
Presence of symptoms (%)						
Icterus	9 (41)	7 (58.3)	1 (8.4)	1 (33.4)	2 (66.6)	1 (50)
Others[a]	13 (59)	5 (41.7)	11 (91.6)	2 (66.6)	1 (33.4)	1 (50)

None of the patients received blood transfusion. [a]Presence of vomitus and/or abdominal pain and/or diarrhea

detected in one serum and was closely related to HAV sub-genotype IA strains previously reported in China (KP177965.1) and Japan (AB258550.1), but slightly different than those reported in United States of America (K02990.1), Russia (EU251188.1), Germany (X75215.1) and Italy (AJ505572.1) (Fig. 1). No recombination or circulating recombinant forms were present amongst the strains detected when analyzing the HAV VP1/VP2 junction region.

VP1/VP3 region

Amplification of a 247 bp product of the VP1/VP3 region of HAV was successful with 16 out of 54 IgM positive sera. The partial VP1/VP3 sequences detected in 14 sera (Fig. 2) were similar to HAV sub-genotype IB strains detected in Hungary (EF190998.2), Spain (HQ401242.1), Italy (AY294046.1), Egypt (KX228694.1) but different from HAV genotypes IA, IIA, IIB, IIIA and IIIB (Fig. 2). In addition, HAV sub-genotype IA was found in one serum and sub-genotype IIIA in another serum; these 2 sub-genotypes were not previously detected in Turkey. The HAV sub-genotype IA (KT874461.1) detected in this study is closely related to IA strains previously reported in China (KP177965.1) and Japan (HQ822089.1) but slightly different than those reported in Hungary (AY956357.2), Russia (EU251188.1), and Germany (X75215.1) (Fig. 2). The HAV sub-genotype IIIA (KT222963.1) detected in this study is closely related to HAV sub-genotype IIIA strains previously reported in Iran (KC669701), Netherlands (AY343856.1) and South Korea (GU908279.1) but slightly different than those reported in Japan (AB279732.1) and India (DQ991030.1). No recombination or circulating recombinant forms were present amongst the strains detected when analyzing the HAV VP1/VP3 region.

Clinical signs and laboratory findings of children infected with HAV sub-genotype IA and IIIA

The child which was found positive for HAV sub-genotype IIIA (KT222963.1) had abdominal pain, icterus, vomitus and a travel history to Afghanistan. He was positive for anti-HAV IgM and IgG but negative for hepatitis B and C. He had elevated levels of total IgM, IgG and IgE. Liver enzymes like aspartate aminotransferase, alanine aminotransferase, alkaline phosphatase, gamma-glutamyl transferase and lactate dehydrogenase were very high. Bilirubin levels were also increased.

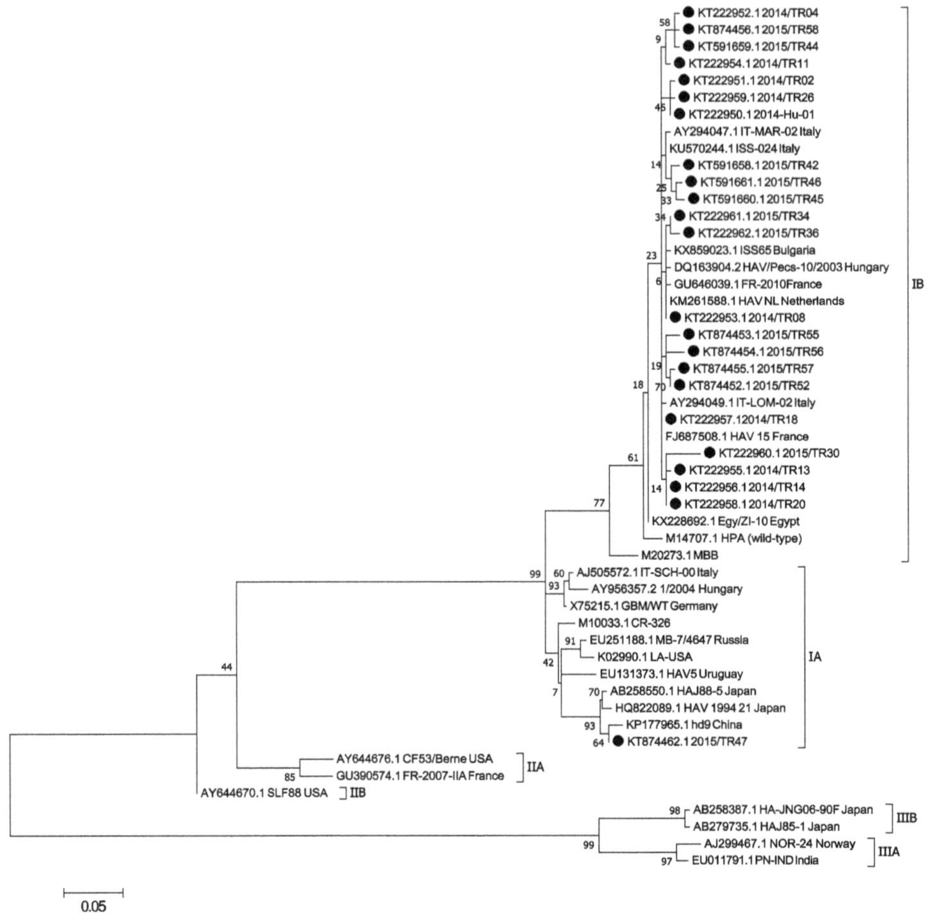

Fig. 1 Phylogenetic tree generated by using the sequences obtained from the VP1/VP2A junction. Phylogenetic tree, using Neighbour Joining and Bootstrap analysis, was generated following alignment of the sequences, by Mega 7, and compared with partial VP1/VP2A junction sequences of HAV strains deposited in GenBank from other investigators in Turkey and other countries

White blood cells, neutrophils and hemoglobin were decreased while lymphocytes and monocytes were increased (Table 3).

Similar clinical signs and laboratory findings were reported for the child infected with sub-genotype IA, but liver enzymes aspartate aminotransferase and alanine aminotransferase were not very high.

Discussion

Hepatitis A virus is an important human pathogen, reported worldwide including Turkey. Undercooked seafood, vegetables, fruits, ready-to –eat food and water are the main source of infection [9, 11, 20]. In order to prevent HAV infections ms, it is important to know the virus source, circulating genotypes and variants of HAV by performing molecular epidemiology. In many studies, the VP1–2A junction of HAV was choosen for analysis since this junction is the most variable region of the HAV genome [14, 18]. Results of previous studies have shown that genotype I is more prevalent in Europe and America than in other continents while genotype III is endemic in Asia [21–24]. However, genotype III has recently been reported in Spain [18]. Sub-genotype IA has been circulating mainly in Mediterranean countries like Greece, Italy and France whereas sub-genotype IB seems to be present in Spain, Jordan and Egypt [3, 18, 22]. Similar to previous studies from Turkey [17, 25]' sub-genotype IB was detected in the majority of patients when the VP1/VP2A junction and VP1/VP3 capsid region of HAV was amplified.

Sequencing and phylogenetic analyses of this study targeting the VP1/VP2A junction region revealed that 22 out of 23 HAVs clustered as sub-genotype IB. The IB sub-genotype was confirmed with 14 of those sera when the VP1/VP3 region was analyzed. The Turkish IB sub-genotype is similar to the one reported in Netherlands, Hungary, France, Italy, Bulgaria and Egypt (Fig. 1). In addition, sub-genotype IA and IIIA strains were found for the first time in Turkey; both sub-genotypes were detected in sera of children. Sub-genotype IIIA was detected by using the primers targeting the VP1/VP3 region but not the VP1/VP2A junction region (Fig. 2).

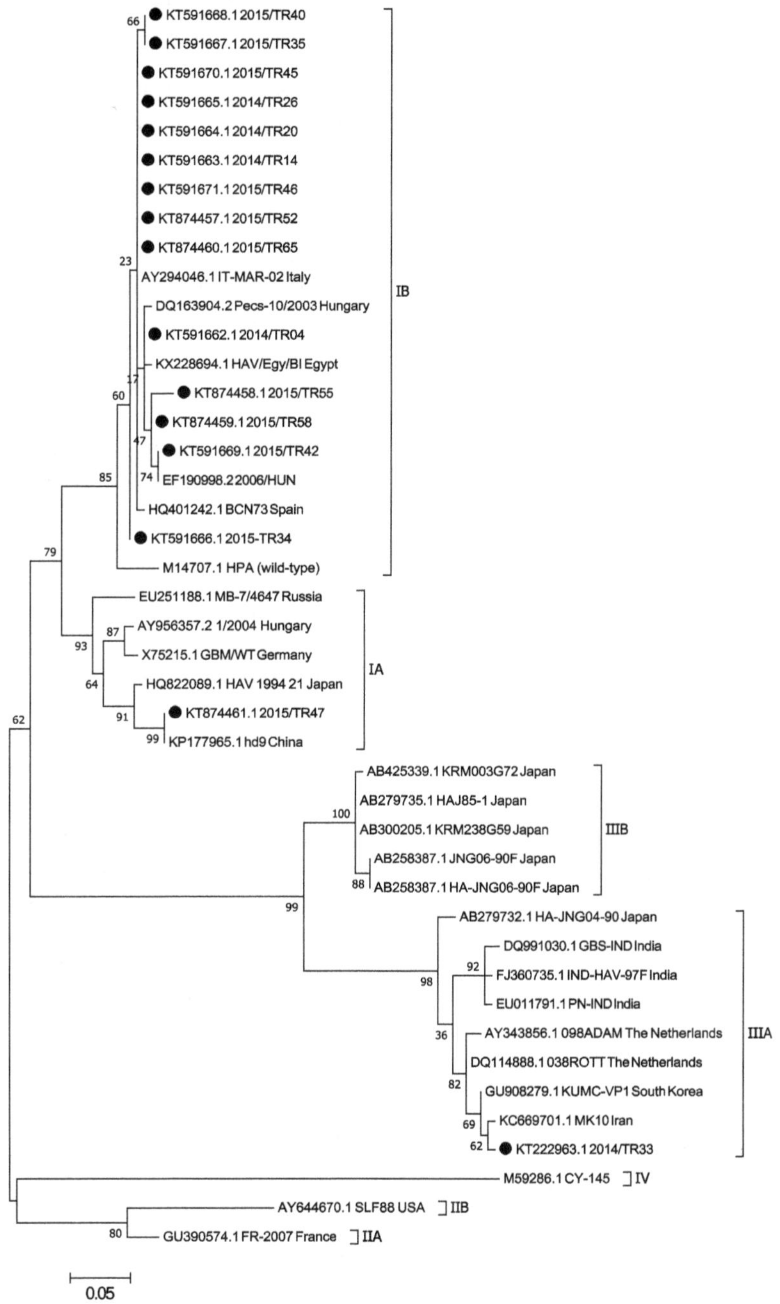

Fig. 2 Phylogenetic tree generated by using the sequences obtained from the VP1/VP3 capsid region. Phylogenetic tree, using Neighbour Joining and Bootstrap analysis, was generated following alignment of the sequences, by Mega 7, and compared with partial VP1/VP3 capsid sequences of HAV strains deposited in GenBank from other investigators in Turkey and other countries

This indicates the importance of targeting different regions of the HAV genome to detect different genotypes. Interestingly, the travel history of the child carrying sub-genotype IIIA indicated that the child had travelled to Afhganistan. The sub-genotype IIIA (KT222963.1) detected in this study, associated with rather severe clinical symptoms, was found to be similar to strains found in Iran, The Netherlands, South Korea, Japan and India (Fig. 2). These data indicate that the Turkish HAV sub-genotype IIIA detected might have originated from Iran or India, and made his way through Afghanistan to Turkey (Barde et al., 2014). The sub-genotype IA detected in this study was found to be similar to HAV sub-genotype IA reported in China, Japan, Russia, Hungary and Germany (Figs. 1 and 2). So far, these newly detected genotype IA and IIIA

Table 3 Serological, biochemical and heamatological test results of the child positive for HAVsub-genotype IIIA

Parameters	Results	Units	Reference Values
Total IgM	914,4[a]	mg/dl	40–320
Total IgA	153,9	mg/dl	34–305
Total IgG	1852[a]	mg/dl	700–1600
Total IgE	292[a]	IU/ml	<100
Anti-HBs	33	IU/ml	-
HBs Ag	Negative	-	Negative
Anti-HCV	Negative	-	Negative
Anti-HAV IgM	Positive	-	Negative
Anti-HAV IgM	Positive	-	Negative
AST	2555[a]	IU/L	0–40
ALT	2163[a]	IU/L	0–40
ALP	252[a]	IU/L	20–155
GGT	165[a]	IU/L	3–25
LDH	1066[a]	IU/L	<764
Total protein	5,6[a]	g/dl	6–8
Albumin	2,9[a]	gr/dl	3,2–5,4
CRP	0,5	mg/dl	0–0,5
Urea	8[a]	mg/dl	10–50
Uric acid	2,2	mg/dl	2–5,5
Creatinine	0,3	mg/dl	0,3–1,1
Total bilirubin	3,26[a]	mg/dl	0,3–1,2
Direct bilirubin	3,09[a]	mg/dl	0–0,2
WBC	4,1[a]	10^3mm^3	5,2–12,4
RBC	4,3	10^6mm^3	4–6,2
HGB	10,9[a]	g/dl	12–18
HCT	33[a]	%	37–52
PLT	574[a]	10^3mm^3	130–400
NEUT %	27[a]	%	40–74
LYMPH %	58,3[a]	%	19–48
MONO %	17,8[a]	%	3,4–9
EOS %	1,8	%	0–7
BASO %	0,3	%	0–1,5

AST aspartate aminotransferase, *ALT* alanine aminotransferase, *ALP* alkaline phosphatase, *GGT* gamma-glutamyl transferase, *LDH* lactate Dehydrogenase, *CRP* c-reactive protein, *WBC* white blood cell, *RBC* red blood cell, *HGB* hemoglobin, *NEUT* neutrophil, *LYMPH* lymphocyte, *MONO* monocyte, *EOS* eosinophil, *BASO* basophil; [a]Values below or above the reference range

were only found in 2 children, but more epidemiological studies are needed to understand the real distribution of HAV sub-genotypes IA and IIIA in Turkey. If these novel sub-genotypes are more widely spread, a new vaccination policy might need to be considered since these sub-genotypes seem to be causing severe disease in children [18, 26].

As it was reported previously, Turkey is considered to be an intermediate endemic region for HAV [17, 25]. In this study, age distribution of HAV positives was different with a higher incidence in children than in adults. This confirms the results reported in another studies [17, 25] performed in Turkey, indicating that childhood vaccination program should continue particularly in endemic areas in Turkey. In fact, until September 2012, a hepatitis A vaccine containing genotypes (A HM175, CR 326, GBM starin) was used in children as a voluntary immunization (Ministry of Health, Turkey). After September 2012, children are being routinely vaccinated at 18 and 24 months old age in Turkey (Ministry of Health, Turkey). These vaccination regime seems to provide lifelong protection against the currently circulating HAV strain sub-genotype IB [27]. However, further investigations are necessary to evaluate the current vaccines in protection against the newly identifed HAV genotypes IA and IIIA in Turkey.

Conclusion

The present study with the identification of novel HAV-subgenotypes indicates that molecular studies determining the HAV genotype variation in Turkey are warranted. The majority of IgM positive cases in 3–10 year old patients indicates that childhood vaccination in Turkey is important. Sub-genotype IB is the most prevalent genotype in Turkey. Surprisingly, sub-genotype IA and IIIA are also present in Turkey; therefore, future diagnostic efforts should include methods which can identify these emerging HAV genotypes. Our results also show that one important risk factor for contracting hepatitis A virus is travelling since genotype IIIA was detected in a child who had travelled to Afghanistan.

Abbreviations

cDNA: Complementary DNA; HAV: Hepatitis A virus; IgM: Immunoglobulin M; RT-PCR: Reverse transcriptase PCR; VP: Viral protein

Acknowledgements

We would like to thank to TUBITAK for financial support (Project No: 1130390).

Funding

Turkish Scientific and Technical Research Council (TUBITAK); Project No: 1130390.

Consent for publication

Authors consent was taken for publication.

Authors' contributions

HY, NT, AY, JAR, BK made substantial contributions to conception and design and have been involved in the interpretation of data and drafting of the manuscript AAO, OA, AK, AG, MM, FYZ, TTK, BK, AK, AY, UYC, HY, NT: made substantial contributions in acquisition, analysis, data input and interpretation of data. All authors read and approved the final manuscript.

Competing interests
The authors declare that they have no competing interests.

Author details
[1]Department of Virology, Veterinary Faculty, University of Istanbul, Avcilar, Istanbul, Turkey. [2]Department of Microbiology, Cerrahpasa Faculty of Medicine, University of Istanbul, Cerrahpasa, Istanbul, Turkey. [3]Department of Child Health and Diseases, Faculty of Medicine, University of Izmir, Karsiyaka, Izmir, Turkey. [4]Division of Infectious Diseases and Clinical Microbiology, Sisli Hamidiye Etfal Training and Research Hospital, Istanbul, Turkey. [5]Department of Microbiology, Faculty of Medicine, University of Dicle, Diyarbakir, Turkey. [6]Department of Microbiology, Faculty of Medicine, University of Harran, Urfa, Turkey. [7]Department of Diagnostic Medicine and Pathobiology, College of Veterinary Medicine, Kansas State University, Manhattan, USA.

References

1. Fiore AE, Wasley A, Bell BP. Advisory Committee on Immunization Practices (ACIP), Prevention of hepatitis A through active or passive immunization: recommendations of the Advisory Committee on Immunization Practices (ACIP). The MMWR Recommendations and Reports. 2006;55(RR-7):1–23.
2. Jacobsen KH, Wiersma ST. Hepatitis a virus seroprevalence by age and world region, 1990 and 2005. Vaccine. 2010;28(41):6653–7.
3. Melhem NM, Talhouk R, Rachidi H, Ramia S. Hepatitis a virus in the Middle East and North Africa region: a new challenge. J Viral Hepat. 2014;21(9):605–15.
4. Lauber C, Gorbalenya AE. Partitioning the genetic diversity of a virus family: approach and evaluation through a case study of picornaviruses. J Virol. 2012;86(7):3890–904.
5. Melnick JL. Properties and classification of hepatitis a virus. Vaccine. 1992; 10(1):24–6.
6. Totsuka A, Moritsugu Y. Hepatitis A virus proteins. Intervirology. 1999;42(2–3):63–8.
7. Yong HT, Son R. Hepatitis a virus – a general overview. Int Food Res J. 2009;16:455–67.
8. Arauz-Ruiz P, Sundqvist L, García Z, Taylor L, Visoná K, Norder H, Magnius LO. Presumed common source outbreaks of hepatitis a in an endemic area confirmed by limited sequencing within the VP1 region. J Med Virol. 2001;65(3):449–56.
9. Kokkinos P, Kozyra I, Lazic S, Bouwknegt M, Rutjes S, Willems K, Moloney R, de Roda Husman AM, Kaupke A, Legaki E, D'Agostino M, Cook N, Rzeżutka A, Petrovic T, Vantarakis A. Harmonised investigation of the occurrence of human enteric viruses in the leafy green vegetable supply chain in three European countries. Food Environ Virol. 2012;4(4):179–91.
10. Bellou M, Kokkinos P, Vantarakis A. Shellfish-borne viral outbreaks: a systematic review. Food Environ Virol. 2013;5(1):13–23.
11. Maunula L, Kaupke A, Vasickova P, Söderberg K, Kozyra I, Lazic S, van der Poel WH, Bouwknegt M, Rutjes S, Willems KA, Moloney R, D'Agostino M, de Roda Husman AM, von Bonsdorff CH, Rzeżutka A, Pavlik I, Petrovic T, Cook N. Tracing enteric viruses in the European berry fruit supply chain. Int J Food Microbiol. 2013;167(2):177–85.
12. Hughes JA, Fontaine MJ, Gonzalez CL, Layon AG, Goodnough LT, Galel SA. Case report of a transfusion-associated hepatitis a infection. Transfusion. 2014;54(9):2202–6.
13. MacDonald E, Steens A, Stene-Johansen K, Gillesberg Lassen S, Midgley S, Lawrence J, Crofts J, Ngui SL, Balogun K, Frank C, Faber M, Gertler M, Verhoef L, Koopmans M, Sane J, van Pelt W, Sundqvist L, Vold L. 2013. Increase in hepatitis A in tourists from Denmark, England, Germany, the Netherlands, Norway and Sweden returning from Egypt, November 2012 to March 2013. Euro Surveil. 2014;18(17):20468.
14. Petrignani M, Verhoef L, Vennema H, van Hunen R, Baas D, van Steenbergen JE, Koopmans MP. Underdiagnosis of foodborne hepatitis a, The Netherlands, 2008-2010 (1.). Emerg Infect Dis. 2014;20(4):596–602.
15. Reuter G, Juhász A, Kosztolányi L, Lefler E, Fekete Z. Co-circulation of genotype IA and new variant IB hepatitis a virus in outbreaks of acute hepatitis in Hungary–2003/2004. J Med Virol. 2006;78(11):1392–7.
16. Namsai A, Louisirirotchanakul S, Wongchinda N, Siripanyaphinyo U, Virulhakul P, Puthavathana P. Surveillance of hepatitis a and E viruses contamination in shellfish in Thailand. Lett Appl Microbiol. 2011;53(6): 608–13.
17. Dinc B, Koyuncu D, Karatayli SC, Berk E, Karatayli E, Parlak M, Çelık I, Akgüç M, Sertöz R, Berktaş M, Bozdayi G, Bozdayi AM. Molecular characterization of hepatitis a virus isolated from acute infections in Turkey. Turk J Gastroenterol. 2012;23(6):714–9.
18. D'Andrea L, Pérez-Rodríguez FJ, de Castellarnau M, Manzanares S, Lite J, Guix S, Bosch A, Pintó RM. Hepatitis a virus genotype distribution during a decade of universal vaccination of preadolescents. Int J Mol Sci. 2015; 16(4):6842–54.
19. Tamura K, Nei M. Estimation of the number of nucleotide substitutions in the control region of mitochondrial DNA in humans and chimpanzees. Mol Biol Evol. 1993;10(3):512–26.
20. Koopmans M, Duizer E. Foodborne viruses: An emerging problem. Int J Food Microbiol. 2004;90:23–41.
21. Robertson BH, Jansen RW, Khanna B, Totsuka A, Nainan OV, Siegl G, Widell A, Margolis HS, Isomura S, Ito K. Genetic relatedness of hepatitis a virus strains recovered from different geographical regions. J Gen Virol. 1992;73:1365–77.
22. Cristina J, Costa-Mattioli M. Genetic variability and molecular evolution of hepatitis a virus. Virus Res. 2007;127(2):151–7.
23. Lee H, Jeong H, Yun H, Kim K, Kim JH, Yang JM, Cheon DS. Genetic analysis of hepatitis a virus strains that induced epidemics in Korea during 2007-2009. J Clin Microbiol. 2012;50(4):1252–7.
24. Barde PV, Shukla MK, Pathak R, Kori BK, Bharti PK. Circulation of hepatitis a genotype IIIA virus in paediatric patients in central India. Indian J Med Res. 2014;139(6):940–4.
25. Normann A, Badur S, Onel D, Kilic A, Sidal M, Larouzé B, Massari V, Müller J, Flehmig B. Acute hepatitis a virus infection in Turkey. J Med Virol. 2008; 80(5):785–90.
26. Yoon YK, Yeon JE, Kim JH, Sim HS, Kim JY, Park DW, Sohn JW, Chun BC, Kim MJ. Comparative analysis of disease severity between genotypes IA and IIIA of hepatitis a virus. J Med Virol. 2011;83:1308–14.
27. FitzSimons D, Hendrickx G, Vorsters A, Van Damme P. Hepatitis a and E: update on prevention and epidemiology. Vaccine. 2010;28(3):583–8.

Prevalence and risk factors of hepatitis B infection among mothers and children with hepatitis B infected mother in upper Dolpa, Nepal

Purusotam Raj Shedain[1*], Madhu Dixit Devkota[2], Megha Raj Banjara[3], Huang Ling[4] and Subash Dhital[5]

Abstract

Background: Hepatitis B Virus (HBV) infection is a worldwide public health problem. In Nepal, the prevalence of HBV is found to be low (0.9%), although high prevalence (≥8%) of HBV infection is depicted among subgroup/ population in the mountain region by various studies. This study assessed the prevalence and the risk of HBV infection among mothers, as well as among the youngest child under 5 years old living with hepatitis B positive mothers in Dolpa, the most remote mountain district of Nepal.

Methods: The cross sectional study survey was conducted between June and July 2014. All mothers with their youngest child under 5 years old were invited to participate in the survey and tested for hepatitis B surface antigen (HBsAg). The HBsAg positive mothers were further tested by 5-panel HBV test card. Children living with HBsAg positive mothers were also tested for HBsAg.

Results: One hundred fifty-one mothers, comprising 37% of the total study population in the selected Village Development Committees (VDCs), were surveyed in the mobile health camps. The seroprevalence of HBsAg among mothers and their youngest child under 5 years old living with HBsAg positive mothers were 17% (95% CI, 11.01–22.99%) and 48% (95%CI, 28.42–67.58%) respectively.

The majority of HBV infected mothers were indigenous (84%) followed by Dalit (4%) and other castes (12%). Among HBV infected mothers, 40% were hepatitis B envelope antigen (HBeAg) positive. The prevalence of HBsAg was higher among children living with HBeAg positive mothers as compared to HBeAg negative (60% vs 40%) and male children compared to female (60% vs 33%). Thirty-six percent of children were vaccinated with a full course of the hepatitis B vaccine. Of these vaccinated children, 56% were HBsAg sero-positive.

Conclusions: The HBV infection rate is high among mothers and children living with HBsAg positive mothers in the indigenous population of the most remote mountain community of Nepal.

Keywords: Children, Hepatitis B infection, Mothers, Nepal, Upper Dolpa

* Correspondence: shedaindr@gmail.com
[1]Department of Community Medicine and Public Health, Institute of Medicine/Ministry of Health, RamshahPath, Kathmandu, Nepal
Full list of author information is available at the end of the article

Background

Hepatitis B Virus (HBV) infection is a worldwide public health problem. Two hundred and forty million people are estimated to be chronically infected, particularly in low and middle income countries [1–3].HBV poses a serious concern worldwide as the virus is the major cause of chronic hepatitis, cirrhosis, and eventually hepatocellular carcinoma (HCC). The prevalence of HBV is highest in Sub-Saharan Africa and East Asia where 5–10% of the general population is infected, while in the Indian Subcontinent prevalence is estimated to be 2–5% [3]. Although most of the infections are self-limiting, the remainder persist as chronic infections in carrier individuals [2]. Around 15–40% of HBV infected patients develop cirrhosis, liver failure, or HCC [4]. Approximately 500,000 to 1.2 million people die of complications related to HBV infection annually [5].

In Nepal, the prevalence of HBV in the general population is believed to be heterogeneous, though there is no representative study or survey to confirm the national prevalence among the adults [6–8]. Most of the studies have depicted low prevalence of hepatitis B surface antigen (HBsAg) seroprevalence among the general population and blood donors, ranging from 0.4–1.2% [9–11].

A serosurvey of children born before and after hepatitis B vaccine introduction revealed that the prevalence of infection in pre-vaccination (10–12 years) and post-vaccination (5–6 years) cohorts of children were 0.28 and 0.13% respectively [12]. However, the prevalence of HBV infection is not homogenous due to differences observed within regions as well as ethnic groups. The Sherpas and Gurung residing at northern border of the country have a higher prevalence. HBsAg seroprevalence was found to be 7.35% of healthy individuals in Manang and 3.5% of individuals in Gurung at Mt. Everest Base camp [13]. Similarly, many other studies have suggested that there is high prevalence (≥8%) of hepatitis B infection among subgroups in mountain region of Nepal, ranging from 21 to 38% [8, 14–16].

In endemic areas, most infections occur in infants and children as a result of maternal-neonatal transmission or close childhood contact [17]. Children who are not HBV infected at birth remain at risk from long-term interpersonal contact with their infected mothers [18]. The disease outcome is determined by the time of exposure as early neonatal exposure has high morbidity and mortality rates [19, 20].

The determining factor for progression of acute HBV infection to the chronic lifelong carrier stage is the patient's age at acquisition of the virus. Thus children acquiring infection perinatally or within 6 years of age are prone to develop chronic infection [21].

This study was conducted to determine the prevalence and identify the risk factors of hepatitis B infection among the children with a hepatitis B infected mother in upper part of Dolpa district, the most remote part of Nepal.

Methods

Study site

Dolpa is the most remote district of Nepal with 23 Village Development Committees (VDCs). Five VDCs (Chharka, Dho, Mukot, Saldhang and Tinje) of the upper part of the Dolpa were purposely selected for the study because these areas are home for the indigenous people that are highly mobile due to trade, seasonal migration, grazing cattle, and pilgrimage [14, 22].

Study design and participants

A cross-sectional survey was performed among the target population of mothers with their youngest child under 5 years old. The sample size was based on a population of 503 children under 5 years old given by the Department of Health Services (DOHS, fiscal year 2014/2015), and the proportion of mothers with children under 5 years old (0.804) as per the Nepal Demographic Health Survey (NDHS 2011). The estimated total population was 404 individuals. Given the parameters, $N = 404$, Level (α) = 0.05, Tolerance (δ) = 0.05, and Prevalence (ρ) = 0.19 (from various studies), the required sample size would be 150 individuals with simple random sampling. A significant portion of $N = 151$, which comprised 37% of the total population, participated in this study.

All mothers with their youngest child under 5 years old were invited to participate in the survey. Written/verbal consent was obtained prior to the survey from the mothers for themselves and their children.

Two to three camps were organized in each VDC to ensure access and coverage of the survey in their cluster settlements. Participants were informed about the camps through Female Community Health Volunteers (FCHV), Amchi (local traditional doctors), local health workers, and non-governmental organization (NGO) staff working in the areas.

The participants were counseled on HBV infection including how to protect themselves from the infection, how to maintain health if they were infected, ways to protect their children from transmission of infection, and where to get vaccines if they were not immunized or not fully immunized.

Sampling

Mothers with their youngest child under 5 years old and the youngest children of the HBsAg positive mothers who attended the camps were all enrolled in the study. The camps were organized in early June to late July 2014.

Inclusion and exclusion criteria

Mothers with their youngest child under 5 years old were eligible for the study. Respondents who were not able to donate blood samples due to history of bleeding disorders, such as hemophilia, and unable to consent due to severe mental illness were not included in the survey.

Data collection

Sociodemographic data collection

A structured questionnaire was administered to HBsAg seropositive mothers. Information on sociodemographic variables; history of antenatal care, delivery, and postnatal care services during the pregnancy of their youngest child; risk factors for hepatitis B infection; and vaccination history of mothers and children for hepatitis B virus were collected.

Blood specimen collection

A 3.5 ml blood sample was collected from mothers and a 1 ml blood sample was collected from children by venipuncture. Samples were centrifuged and serum from both mothers and children were tested for HBsAg at the sites with SD Bioline(Standard Diagnostic, Inc., Korean, Sensitivity 100%, 95% CI 96.5–100%, Specificity 100%, 95% CI 97.9–100%).Serum sample was transported to the Research Laboratory, Institute of Medicine, maintaining cold chain. Serum of HBsAg positive mothers were further tested with a 5panel HBV test card (Lumi-Quick) with accuracy for HBsAg99.6%, HBsAb97.9%, HBcAb97.4%, HBeAg99.6%, and HBeAb98.2%. The 5panel HBV test card is an immunochromatographic test involving antibody or antigen sandwich and competitive immunoassay. All positive samples and random selection of 10% of negative samples were tested by enzyme-linked immunosorbentassay [23] for an HBsAg at the National Public Health Laboratory (NPHL), Teku Kathmandu.The sensitivity and specificity of the HBsAg rapid test was similar when compared with enzyme-linked immunosorbent assay.

Data analysis

Data was entered in EpiData 3.1 and analyzed by SPSS 20 version. Descriptive analysis was performed.

Results

Description of the study population

One hundred fifty-one mothers attended the mobile health camp, which comprised 37% of the total study population. Among them, 125 mothers (83%) were HBsAg seronegative and the remaining 26 mothers (17%) were HBsAg seropositive. The proportion of HBsAg positive mothers was significantly lower than the proportion of HBsAg negative mothers in the population with the difference being greater than 2 standard error (SE).One child refused to give a blood sample, therefore only 25 mother-children pairs were included in the data analysis (Fig. 1).

Infected mothers by sociodemographic characteristics, condom use, and antenatal care services

The majority of HBsAg positive mothers (52%) were from two VDCs, Chharka and Dho. The median age of mothers was 32 years, ranging from 19 to 46 years. The majority of the mothers belonged to Janajati group (84%) followed by Dalit (4%) and other groups (12%). Most of the mothers (96%) had never attended school (Table 1).

More than half (60%) of the participants had heard about the infection; however, only 16 % were tested for the hepatitis B infection in the past, and about 12% were informed about the status of their hepatitis B infection. An overwhelming number of participants (92%) had never had vaccination against hepatitis B infection.

None of the mothers used condoms during their last episode of sexual intercourse. Less than one-third (28%) of mothers had utilized antenatal care (ANC) services

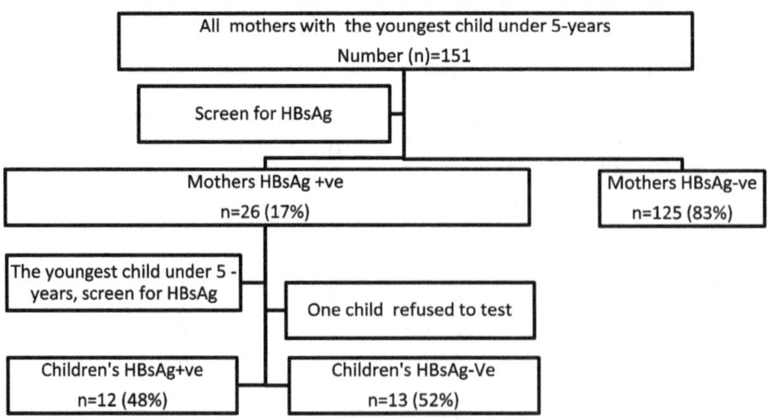

Fig. 1 Research participants

Table 1 The residence, age and caste/ethnicity of the HBsAg sero-positive mothers

Characteristics	Number (*N* = 25) and Percentage	
	n	%
Residence (VDCs)		
Chharka	5	20
Dho	8	32
Mukot	4	16
Saldang	4	16
Tinje	4	16
Age		
19–24 Years	2	8
25–29 Years	8	32
30–34 Years	7	28
35 Years and higher	8	32
Mean	32.04	
Range	19–46	
Cast/ethnicity		
Gurung/Lama (Indigenous)	21	84
Rokaya/Budha	3	12
BK	1	4

Table 2 ANC services and alcohol consumption during the last pregnancy

ANC services and alcohol consumption	N	%
ANC services		
Yes	7	28
No	18	72
De-worming		
Yes	4	16
No	21	84
Iron tab or syrup		
Yes	8	32
No	17	68
Drinks containing alcohol during the last pregnancy		
Yes	19	76
No	6	24
Regularity of alcohol consumption during pregnancy (among users)		
Every day	8	42
2–3 times a week	8	42
At least once a week	1	5
Less than once a week	2	11
Form of alcohol taken during the pregnancy (among users)		
Jand (raw local fermented alcohol)	4	21
Chhyang (filter local fermented alcohol)	12	63
Homemade alcohol	3	16

during the pregnancy of their youngest child. Some mothers (16%) had taken anthelminthic medication and nearly one-third (32%) had taken iron tablets or syrup during their most recent pregnancy (Table 2). Alcohol consumption was common among the participants (76%) with daily usage in a high proportion of the users (42%). The *Jand* and *Chhayang* (local fermented alcohols) were the most common (84%) form followed by homemade alcohol (16%). Only a few mothers (8%) consumed alcohol containing drinks less than once a week (Table 2).

Characteristics of the children by sex, size at birth, and newborn care

Birth weight was obtained by recall from mothers. Less than half (40%) children were average size at birth, one-fifth were smaller than average, and one-third were larger than average. All children were born at home without skilled birth attendants and most (64%) were not fed colostrum (Table 3). Unsterile knives and scissors (96%) were commonly used instruments for cord cutting.

Prevalence of hepatitis B infection

The seroprevalence of HBsAg among mothers and the youngest children living with HBsAg positive mothers was 17% (95% CI, 11.01–22.99%) and 48% (95% CI, 28.42–67.58%) respectively.

Characteristics of mothers and status of their children's HBsAg seroprevalence

The HBsAg seroprevalence was higher among children who lived with mothers having no ANC services (71.4%) compared to those having some ANC services (28.6%). The prevalence was higher among children with mothers that drank alcohol during pregnancy (57.9%) compared to those that did not (16.7%). The prevalence was higher among children with mothers that consumed alcohol daily (63%) (Table 4).

The prevalence of HBeAg and HBeAb seropositive mothers was 76% with 10 mothers (40%) HBeAg positive and 9 mothers (36%) HBeAb positive out of a total of 25 mothers. All mothers were HBcAb positive. The majority of children (60%) with HBeAg positive mothers were HBsAg positive, whereas less children (40%) were HBsAg positive with HBeAg negative mothers. Less children (11%) were HBsAg positive with HBeAb positive mothers, where as an overwhelming number of children (69%) were HBsAg positive with HBeAb negative mothers (Table 4).

Characteristics of children and HBsAg seroprevalence

A greater proportion of male children (61.5%) were HBsAg seropositive compared to female children (33.3%). Children with average or greater size at birth

Table 3 Sex, size at birth and newborn care of the children

Children's characteristics	Number	Percentage
Sex of baby		
Male	13	52.0
Female	12	48.0
Perceived Size of the child at birth		
Very large	2	8.0
Larger than average	7	28.0
Average	10	40.0
Smaller than average	5	20.0
Very small	1	4.0
Cord cutting instruments		
New/boiled blade	1	4.0
Knife/ Scissor	24	96.0
Colostrums feeding		
Yes	9	36.0
No	16	64.0

Table 4 Mother's socio-demographic, serological characteristics and HBsAg sero-prevalence of children

Mother's characteristics	Children's HBsAg sero-prevalence, n (%)		*P* value*
	Yes	No	
Age			
Below 30 years	6 (50)	6 (50)	.848
30 and highest	6 (46.2)	7 (53.8)	
Caste/ethnicity			
Janajati	10 (47.6)	11 (52.4)	.930
Others	2 (50)	2 (50)	
ANC visit			
Yes	2 (28.6)	5 (71.4)	.225
No	10 (55.6)	8 (44.4)	
De-worming			
Yes	2 (40)	3 (60)	.689
No	10 (50)	10 (50)	
Iron taken			
Yes	3 (37.5)	5 (62.5)	.471
No	9 (52.9)	8 (47.1)	
Drinks containing alcohol during pregnancy			
Yes	11 (57.9)	8 (42.1)	.078
No	1 (16.7)	5 (83.3)	
Regularity of alcohol consumption during pregnancy (among users) (*n* = 19)			
Every day	5 (62.5)	3 (37.5)	.729
2–3 times to less than once week	6 (54.5)	5 (45.5)	
Form of alcohol taken during the pregnancy (among users %))			
Jand/Chhyang	8 (50)	8 (50)	.107
Homemade alcohol	3 (100)	–	
Mother's HBeAg			
Positive	6 (60)	4 (40)	.327
Negative	6 (40)	9 (60)	
Mother's HBeAb			
Positive	1 (11.1)	8 (88.9)	.002
Negative	11 (68.8)	5 (31.2)	

*Calculated using chi-square test

were less frequently HBsAg seropositive (47.6%) compared to those that were smaller than average size at birth (50%). Children who were fed colostrum within 1 h after delivery were less HBsAg seropositive (44.4%) compared to no colostrum fed ones (50%) (Table 5).

Administration of the first dose of the hepatitis B vaccine was high (88%) among the children; however, only half of the children that had been vaccinated were HBsAg seronegative. Nearly two-thirds of children (68%) were vaccinated with the second dose, but nearly half of them (53%) were HBsAg seronegative. Only one-third (36%) of children were vaccinated with full series of the hepatitis B vaccine ($^{\text{HepB3}}$), although more than half of children (56%) were HBsAg seropositive (Table 5 and Fig. 2). Furthermore, the percentage of HBsAg seropositivity increased in older age groups with rates of 20, 50, and 72% respectively in age groups 0 to 12 months, 12 to 24 months, and 24 to 60 months (detailed data not shown).

Discussion

The prevalence of HBsAg, if equal or greater than 8% is considered as high endemic [1]. This study showed that the prevalence of hepatitis B infection is very high among the mothers, and the youngest children under 5-years living with HBsAg sero-positive mothers in the upper part of the district, whereas the national prevalence of the infection in the general population is considered low (0.9%) [6]. Hence, it can be described as an issue of health disparity affecting indigenous mothers and children in Nepal.

Among HBV infected mothers, 40% were carried HBeAg seroprevalence. The majority of the children living with HBeAg positive mothers were HBsAg positive. Obviously, in highly endemic areas with HBeAg positive mothers, HBV is most commonly spread from mother-to-child at birth or perinatal transmission (WHO, #1292;Li, 2015 #1200;WHO, 2017 #1424). But in this study the proportion of positivity has increased with age group, so it can be assumed that there was other horizontal mode of transmission along with vertical one, which calls for a further study to know the relationship.

In our study 60% of children living with HBeAg positive mothers were found to be HBsAg positive, which

Table 5 Children's characteristics and HBsAg sero-prevalence

Children's characteristics	HBsAg sero-prevalence, n (%)		*P* value*
	Yes	No	
Sex of baby			
Male	8 (61.5)	5 (38.5)	.159
Female	4 (33.3)	8 (66.7)	
Size of baby at birth			
Average and above	9 (47.4)	10 (52.6)	.910
Smaller than average	3 (50)	3 (50)	
Cord Cutting Instruments			
New/boiled blade	0 (0.0)	1 (100)	.327
Other (knife/sickle/khukuri/ scissor)	12 (50)	12 (50)	
Colostrums feeding			
Yes	4 (44.4)	5 (55.6)	.790
No	8 (50)	8 (50)	
Hepatitis B vaccination, n (%)			
Hep (1), 22 (88)	11 (50)	11 (50)	0.680
Hep (2), 17(68)	8 (47)	9 (53)	
Hep (3), 9 (36)	5 (56)	4 (44)	

*Calculated using chi-square test

was higher than sub-Sahara Africa (38.3%) between 3 and 12 months of age and lower than many other studies (70–90%) in Asia; whereas 40% of children living with HBeAg negative mothers were HBsAg positive, it is higher than sub-Saharan Africa (4.8%) [24] but in concordance with many other studies (< 10–40%), in the absence of post exposure immunoprophylaxis [25–27].

A significant proportion of children were HBsAg negative who were living with HBeAb positive mothers as in other studies [28]. It is due to the seroconversion from HBeAg to HBeAb, which usually indicates lower viral loads [29]. Further studies are required whether the seroconversion was due to spontaneous or local food or medicines as the "*Thikpa or Thigba*", a local name of disease which is characterized by loss of appetite, distension of abdomen, yellowish discoloration of the conjunctiva/skin, dark urine are extensively treated by the local Amchi (a traditional doctor) and Lama with a various local herbs [8]. They perform wide ranges of health care activities such as chanting mantras for well-being and prescribing local herbal pills to cure the diseases as per their own diagnosis criteria and disease classification system [8, 14]. The Amchis also provide various surgical interventions to cure *Thigba/Thikpa* to their community through sucking, cutting and letting the blood from the big veins of the body but they are still unaware of proper sterilization practices and procedures [8], the impact of intervention needs to be assessed whether it has risked the transmission or prevented the infection in the community.

In this study male children were more infected than female ones. The proper explanations are not known, but male child is prone to most of infections compared to female child [30, 31]. Some of the studies had identified behavioral differences between sexes as an influencing factor, while other hypothesized that double X chromosome in females and random activation is also a factor for antibody development which may have protected the female child [32]. The explanation behind the cause of disparity of the prevalence of hepatitis B among sexes is not known. However, the disparity could have an impact on public health as it is estimated that the lifetime risk of death from Chronic Hepatitis B Infection (CHB) was 40–50% in men, and about 15% in women [33].

Using condom in their last sexual intercourse was nil. Utilization of ANC services was poor. It could be due to lack of awareness, unavailability of health care services and a far-flung settlement from the health post and district hospital. Only few (4%) mothers used a new/boiled blade to cut their newborns' umbilical cord, majority of the mothers used old scissors and knives to cut the baby cord. There is a high chance of transmission of the infection while using the unsterilized

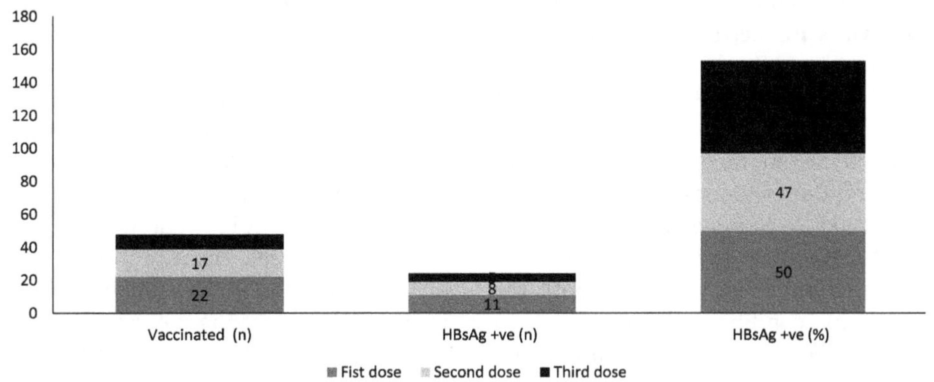

Fig. 2 Children's vaccination and HBsAg sero-prevalence

contaminated scissors and knives. Furthermore, the poor availability of indicated items for infection prevention (0.2%) at health facilities in the mountain ecological region [34] could be a contributor to the high prevalence of the infection.

The National Immunization Program (NIP) has administered hepatitis B vaccine starting at 6 weeks of age [35] considering the low prevalence of the infection and other feasibility issues. Mothers were not screened for the HBsAg, an overwhelming numbers of participants had never had vaccinated against the HBV. Newborns were neither administered hepatitis B vaccine at birth nor hepatitis B immunoglobulin by the NIP. In the high endemicity setting (HBsAg prevalence ≥ 8%), the infection is mainly transmitted at birth or during early childhood (< 5 years), the first vaccine dose at birth are recommended, which prevent transmission of the infection by more than 90% of cases [36].

Only one-third of the children were administered three dose of hepatitis vaccine, among them more than half children were infected. The proportion of infection among the children increased with an increase in age groups. It has suggested that there is a horizontal transmission of hepatitis B infection among the children in addition to perinatal transmission. However, the perinatal and early neonatal transmission could be effectively prevented by at birth vaccination and immunoglobulin [2, 37]. Likewise, the horizontal transmission could be prevented with effective vaccination, awareness and education program. The finding has raised questions on the coverage of the NIP, the timing of the vaccination and effectiveness of the program.

Alcohol consumption was very common among the women and the infection prevalence was high among the children living with mothers who consumed drinks containing alcohol during their pregnancy compared to non drinkers. Generally, an alcohol use is associated with sexual risk behavior [38], though it requires a research for culture-specific and context-specific ways of dealing with the problems. There is a need for an indepth understanding of the alcohol consumption that influences the risk behaviors for hepatitis B transmission and its consequences on them. Furthermore, both heavy alcohol consumption and hepatitis B are independent risk factors for the hepatocellular carcinoma [39, 40].

The majority of the infected mothers belonged to Janajati followed by Dalit and others. Janajati is Nepali word for indigenous people [41]. *Indigenous and Tribal Peoples Convention*, 1989 defines the indigenous people as the, tribal peoples in independent countries whose social, cultural and economic conditions distinguish them from other sections of the national community, and whose status is regulated wholly or partially by their own customs or traditions or by special laws or regulations." In Nepali history the Janajatis have been excluded from the mainstream and these people are living in abject poverty [41]. Likewise, these people have been excluded from the modern health care services as they live in the remotest areas from the hospitals, have poor access to other promotive and preventive health care services [8].

Limitations of the study

As far as we are aware, this is the first study ever done in the remotest hard-to-reach community of seminomadic population of upper Dolpa in Nepal. The geographically inaccessible setting; the silent nature of the infection; extremely mobile population; constraints of resources and the set objectives were the context.

The estimated target populations were 404. Given the parameters, $N = 404$, Level $(\alpha) = 0.05$, Tolerance $(\delta) = 0.05$ and Prevalence $(\rho) = 0.19$ (from a various studies), the required sample size would be 150 with the simple random sampling. A significant portion ($N = 151$, 37% of the total) of the population participated in this study. Camps were organized in each VDC to ensure access and coverage of the survey in their settlements. Participants were informed about the camps through FCHV, Amchi (local traditional doctors), local health workers, and non-governmental organization (NGO) staff working in the areas. We assume that there was no information bias as the target populations were informed through various social networks; there was no disease-bias as the chronic hepatitis B infection is often asymptomatic, even in advanced diseased stage; there was no selection bias as the all participants who attended the camps were enumerated; and researchers were bound to limit the methodology due to resources constraint.

Altogether, 151 participants attended the camps with their children, out of which (mothers) 26 were HBsAg positive and 125 were HBsAg negative. The prevalence of HBsAg in mother is 17%. The HBsAg positive prevalence proportion was significantly lower as compared to HBsAg negative mothers i.e. the difference between the proportion is greater than 2SE.

The sample size of interest of outcome (subset) is small (26 paired). One child refused to participate. Out of 25 children, 12 were HBsAg positive and 13 were HBsAg negative. Obviously the prevalence of HBsAg among children living with HBsAg positive mothers is higher than the WHO cutoff value (≥ 8). However, the difference between their proportions is not significant, i.e., < 2SE. On the basis, we can conclude that the prevalence of HBsAg among children living with HBsAg positive mothers is not significantly different from the HBsAg negative children living with HBsAg positive mothers. A further study with sufficient sample size is required to differentiate the discrepancy of the prevalence of the infection in the subset population.

Conclusion

This study revealed that the prevalence of HBsAg is high among mothers and children living with hepatitis B positive mothers in the indigenous community of the upper Dolpa. In this endemic setting, the infection is mainly transmitted at birth or during early childhood. The hepatitis B vaccine series with the first dose at birth prevents the transmission of the infection in greater than 90% of cases.

A comprehensive intervention on prevention, control, and treatment are required in endemic areas to address the current and future associated liver health problems considering the high prevalence of the infection and additional risk factors, such as alcohol abuse, lack of safe sexual practices, poor access to modern health care services, and harmful traditional health care practices.

Abbreviations

ANC: Antenatal care; CHB: Chronic hepatitis B infection; ELISA: Enzyme-linked immunosorbent assay; FCHV: Female Community Health Volunteers; HBcAb: Hepatitis B core antibody; HBeAb: Hepatitis B e antibody; HBeAg: Hepatitis B e antigen; HBsAg: Hepatitis B Surface Antigen; HBV: Hepatitis B Virus; HCC: Hepatocellular Carcinoma; IOM: Institute of Medicine; NGO: Non-Governmental Organization; NIP: National Immunization Program; NPHL: National Public Health Laboratory; TU: Tribhuvan University; VDC: Village Development Committees; WHO: World Health Organization

Acknowledgements

We would like to thank the Member of Parliament Mr. Dhana Bahadur Budha, Dr. Senendra Raj Upreti (Secretary, Ministry of Health), Dr. Dipendra Raman Singh (Director, NCASC), Dr. Baburarm Marasini (Director, EDCD), Dr. Yub Raj Pokharel (EDCD), Mr. Rana Lal Kula (DPHO, Dolpa), Mr. Khadga Shrestha (IOM, TU), Mr. Rajan Paudel(IOM, TU), Mr. Durga Pahari(IOM, TU), Mr. Ashok Bhurtayl(IOM/TU), Mr. Padam Dahal (Research Officer), Dr. Rajman Shrestha (Statistician), Mr.Santa Budha (Research Assistant), Mr. Harilal Khadka (Medical technologist), Mr. Hari Prasad Kattel (Medical technologist/Microbiologist), Ms.Pedol Gurung (Staff nurse) and Dr. med. Till Kinkel for their support during our study. We would also like to thank all the staff of District Health Office, Dolpa, for their support on providing the logistic transportation for the study. We would also like to thank Dr. Karen Hussein, Neonatal fellow at Robert Wood Johnson Medical School, Rutgers University, New Brunswick, New Jersey, and Mr. Ram Saran Sedhai, a freelance editor for their time and effort in editing the manuscript. Our special thanks go to the research participants from Dolpa district.

Funding

None.

Authors' contributions

PRS conceptualized the framework and designed the study. MDD and HL provided feedback on the framework. SD prepared the lab report. PRS and MRB analyzed the data. MDD and SD revised the analysis. PRS drafted the paper, all other contributors revised it. All are agreed to be accountable. All authors read and approved the final manuscript.

Authors' information

PRS was completing a PhD in public health while conducting the study at the DCMPH, at present he is working with the Ministry of Health in Nepal. MDD is a professor and head of the DCMPH. MRB is a professor at Central Department of Microbiology, Tribhuvan University, Nepal. HL was completing a PhD in public health at the DCMPH. SD is lab technologist at National Public Health Laboratory, Department of Health Services in Nepal.

Consent for publication

Not applicable.

Competing interests

The authors declare that they have no competing interests.

Author details

[1]Department of Community Medicine and Public Health, Institute of Medicine/Ministry of Health, RamshahPath, Kathmandu, Nepal. [2]Department of Community Medicine and Public Health, Institute of Medicine, Tribhuvan University, Kathmandu, Nepal. [3]Central Department of Microbiology, Tribhuvan University (TU), Kirtipur, Kathmandu, Nepal. [4]Department of Preventive Medicine, Medical College of CTGU/Department of Community Medicine and Public Health, Institute of Medicine, Kathmandu, Nepal. [5]National Public Health Laboratory, Department of Health Services, Teku, Kathmandu, Nepal.

References

1. WHO. Weekly epidemiological record, Hepatitis B vaccines, WHO position paper. 2009. http://www.who.int/wer/2009/wer8440.pdf.
2. WHO. Guidelines for the prevention, care and treatment of persons with chronic hepatitis B infection. 2015. http://apps.who.int/iris/bitstream/10665/155081/1/WHO_HIV_2015.5_eng.pdf?ua=1&ua=1.
3. Naghavi M, Wang H, Lozano R, et al. Global, regional, and national age–sex specific all-cause and cause-specific mortality for 240 causes of death, 1990–2013: a systematic analysis for the Global Burden of Disease Study 2013. Lancet. 2015;385(9963):117–71.
4. Anna SF, Lok MD. Chronic Hepatitis B. N Engl J Med. 2002;346:1682–83. doi: 10.1056/NEJM200205303462202.
5. Hou JLZ, Gu F. Epidemiology and prevention of hepatitis B virus infection. Int J Med Sci. 2005;2(1):50–7.
6. Shrestha SM. Chronic hepatitis B in Nepal: An Asian country with low prevalence of HBV Infection. Trop Gastroenterol. 2012;33(2):95–101.
7. Kinkel HT, Karmacharya D, Shakya J, Manandhar S, Panthi S, Karmacharya P, et al. Prevalence of HIV, Hepatitis B and C Infections and an Assessment of HCV-Genotypes and Two IL28B SNPs among People Who Inject Drugs in Three Regions of Nepal. PLoS One. 2015;10(8):e0134455.
8. Shedain PJA, Bhattarai KD. Himalayan Seasonal Migration and STI/HIV Infection: A Case Study among Seasonal Migrants in Kathmandu from Dolpa District, Nepal. J Nepal Health Res Counc. 2006;4:1.
9. Shrestha S, Shrestha SM. Seroepidemiology of Hepatitis B in Nepal. J Commun Dis. 1990;22(1):27–32.
10. Shrestha ACGP, Tiwari BR, Rajkarnikar M. Transfusion-transmissible infections among blood donors in Kathmandu, Nepal. J Infect Dev Ctries. 2009;3(10):794–7.
11. Tiwari BRGP, Kandel SR, Rajkarnikar M. Seroprevalence of HBV and HCV in blood donors: A study from regional blood transfusion services of Nepal. Asian J Transfusion Sci. 2010;4(2):91.
12. Upreti SR, Gurung S, Patel M, Dixit SM, Krause LK, Shakya G, et al. Prevalence of chronic hepatitis B virus infection before and after implementation of a hepatitis B vaccination program among children in Nepal. Vaccine. 2014;32(34):4304–9.
13. Shrestha SMSS. Chronic hepatitis B in Nepal: An Asian country with low prevalence of HBV infection. Trop Gastroenterol. 2012;33(2):95–101.
14. Shedain. Cultural Construct of HIV/STI; A case study from Dolpa. J Nepal Pub Health Stud Soc. 2005;6:200–6.
15. Foundation DTC. Dolpo Tulku Foundation 2012 Winterclinic Report 2012.
16. CharitableFoundation DT. Report of seventh Free Winterclinic 2014. 2014.
17. Li ZH, X.Cao, G. Is mother-to-infant transmission the most important factor for persistent HBV infection? Emerging Microbes Infections. 2015;4(5):e30.
18. CDC. A Comprehensive Immunization Strategy to Eliminate Transmission of Hepatitis B Virus Infection in the United States, Recommendations of the Advisory Committee on Immunization Practices (ACIP) Part 1: Immunization of Infants, Children, and Adolescents. 2005. https://www.ncbi.nlm.nih.gov/pubmed/16371945.
19. Shepard CW SE, Finelli L, Fiore AE, Bell BP. Hepatitis B virus infection: epidemiology and vaccination. https://www.ncbi.nlm.nih.gov/pmc/articles/PMC3435776/.

20. Han G-R. Management of chronic hepatitis B in pregnancy. World J Gastroenterol. 2012;18(33):4517.
21. JL. D. Hepatitis B virus infection. New England J Med 2008;359(14):1486–500.
22. Bhattachan KB. Indigenous Nationalities & Minorities of Nepal. 2003. https://madhesi.files.wordpress.com/2006/09/bhattachan_report.pdf.
23. Nayagam S, Thursz M, Sicuri E, Conteh L, Wiktor S, Low-Beer D, et al. Requirements for global elimination of hepatitis B: a modelling study. Lancet Infect Dis. 2016;16(12):1399–408.
24. Keane E, Funk AL, Shimakawa Y. Systematic review with meta-analysis: the risk of mother-to-child transmission of hepatitis B virus infection in sub-Saharan Africa. Aliment Pharmacol Ther. 2016;44(10):1005–17.
25. Kumar MST, Sinha S. Chronic hepatitis B virus infection and pregnancy. J Clin Exp Hepatol. 2012;2(4):366–81.
26. Piratvisuth T. Optimal management of HBV infection during pregnancy. Liver Int. 2013;33(Suppl 1):188–94.
27. Degli Esposti S SD. Hepatitis B in pregnancy: challenges and treatment. Gastroenterol Clin North Am. 2011;40(2):355–72.
28. Gussetti N PE, Largajolli G, D'Elia R. Vertical transmission of HBV from mothers HBsAg positive, anti-HBe positive. Dev Biol Stand. 1983;54:405–8. PMID: 6653895.
29. Fang ZL, Sabin CA, Dong BQ, Wei SC, Chen QY, Fang KX, et al. The association of HBV core promoter double mutations (A1762T and G1764A) with viral load differs between HBeAg positive and anti-HBe positive individuals: A longitudinal analysis(). J Hepatol. 2009;50(2):273–80.
30. Blumberg BS, Melartin L, Guint RA, Werner B. Family Studies of a Human Serum Isoantigen System (Australia Antigen). Am J Human Genetics. 1966; 18(6):594–608.
31. Blumberg BS. Sex differences in response to hepatitis B virus. I. History. Arthritis Rheum. 1979;22(11):1261–6.
32. BS B. Blumberg BS. Sex differences in response to hepatitis B virus. Arthritis Rheum. 1979;22(11):1261–6.
33. WHO/CDS/CSR/LYO/2002.2: Hepatitis B. WHO, Department of Communicable Diseases Surveillance and Response; 2002. http://www.who.int/emc. Accessed 4 Sept 2017.
34. MOH. Nepal Health Facility Survey 2015 In: Ministry of Health (MOH) NE, and Nepal Health Sector Support Program (NHSSP); and ICF, editor. 2017.
35. CHD. Comprehensive Multi-Year Plan 2068–2072 (2011–2016). 2011.
36. WHO. Hepatitis B vaccines, WHO position paper. 2009.
37. Behrouz Navabakhsh NM. Arezoo estakhri, Mehdi Mohamadnejad, Hossein Poustchi. Hepatitis B Virus Infection during Pregnancy: Transmission and Prevention. Middle East J Digestive Dis. 2011;3:2.
38. WHO. Alcohol use and sexual risk behaviour: a cross-cultural study in eight countries. Geneva: WHO; 2005.
39. Jee SH, Ohrr H, Sull JW, Samet JM. Cigarette smoking, alcohol drinking, hepatitis B, and risk for hepatocellular carcinoma in Korea. J Natl Cancer Inst. 2004;96(24):1851–6.
40. McMahon BJ. The Natural History of Chronic Hepatitis B Virus Infection. 2009.
41. UN. Janajatis in Nepal. UN Nepal Information Platform. 2004.

5

Hepatitis B vaccination coverage among healthcare workers at national hospital in Tanzania

Dotto Aaron[1†], Tumaini J. Nagu[1*†], John Rwegasha[2] and Ewaldo Komba[1]

Abstract

Background: Hepatitis B vaccination for healthcare workers (HCWs) is a key component of the WHO Hepatitis B Elimination Strategy 2016–2021. Data on current hepatitis B vaccine coverage among health care workers in Sub-Saharan Africa are scarce, but these data are vital for effective programming. We assessed the proportion of HCWs vaccinated for hepatitis B and the factors associated with adequate vaccination coverage at a national hospital in Tanzania.

Methods: A descriptive cross-sectional study was conducted among consenting healthcare workers between 30th July and 30th September 2015. Vaccination histories were obtained through self-administered questionnaires. Means and proportions were used to summarize the data. Student's t and chi-squared tests were used as appropriate. Logistic regression was used to determine the factors associated with vaccination.

Results: A total of 348 HCWs were interviewed, of whom 198 (56.9%) had received at least one dose of hepatitis B vaccination, while only 117 (33.6%) were fully vaccinated. About half of the 81 HCWs with partial vaccination (49.4%) had missed their subsequent vaccination appointments. Among unvaccinated HCWs, 14 (9.3%) had either HBV infection or antibodies against HBV infection upon pre-vaccination screening. However, the remaining participants were not vaccinated and did not know their immune status against HBV.

Nearly all respondents (347, 99.3%) had heard about the hepatitis B viral vaccine. The following reasons for non-vaccination were given: 98 (65.3%) reported that they had not been offered the vaccine; 70 (46.7%) observed standard precautions to ensure infection prevention and 60 (41.3%) blamed a low level of awareness regarding the availability of the hepatitis B vaccine.

Conclusion: The current vaccination coverage among practicing healthcare workers at Muhimbili National Hospital is low, despite a high level of awareness and the acceptance of the vaccine. Expedited and concerted efforts to scale vaccine uptake should include improved access to the vaccine, especially for newly recruited HCWs. The extension of the study to private healthcare settings and lower-level facilities would be useful.

Keywords: Vaccine, Hepatitis, HBV, Prevention, Liver cirrhosis, Hepatoma, SSA, Sub-Saharan Africa, Tanzania

* Correspondence: jtjoyce20@hotmail.com
†Equal contributors
[1]School of Medicine, Muhimbili University of Health and Allied Sciences, P.O. Box 65001, Dar es Salaam, Tanzania
Full list of author information is available at the end of the article

Background

Viral hepatitis infection was the seventh leading cause of global mortality and was responsible for 1.5 million deaths and 42 million disability-adjusted life years (DALYs) in 2013 [1]. Among the hepatitis viruses, Hepatitis B and C are responsible for more than 90% of the global burden of viral hepatitis [1]. It is estimated that about 240–257 million people have chronic HBV infections around the world [1]. The global prevalence of HBV infection is 1.3% and varies by geographical setting from as low as 0.2% in America to 3% in Africa [1]. More than two-thirds of hepatitis patients are in Sub-Saharan Africa and East Asia, where the prevalence is more than 8% [1–3]. The Hepatitis B vaccine has been available since 1981 and is considered a key strategy for preventing HBV infections.

HBV is endemic in East Africa, with an estimated HBsAg prevalence of 8% [1, 3]. In Tanzania, the HBV prevalence varies from one population to another, ranging between 8.8 and 11% among blood donors, [4–6] between 4 and 8% among pregnant women [7–10] and between 8 and 17% among HIV-infected individuals [11]. A study performed in Uganda showed that the seroprevalence of HBV infection in the general population was 10% [12], and in Kenya, a recent national survey reported an HBV prevalence of 2.1%, with some regions recording a prevalence of 7.5% [13]. Earlier studies in Kenya reported an HBV prevalence between 8 and 10% [14, 15].

Healthcare workers (HCWs) are exposed to the constant risk of HBV infection due to their occupational contact with blood, blood products and other body fluids, as well as the risk of needle-stick injuries. In East Africa, the prevalence of HBV among HCWs is estimated to be between 7 and 8% [16, 17]. In developing countries, 40–65% of HBV infections among healthcare workers are attributable to percutaneous occupational exposure, whereas the corresponding risk in developed countries is as low as 10% [18]. A safe and effective HBV vaccine is available and recommended by the world Health Organization (WHO) for the primary prevention of HBV among all healthcare workers [19]. The introduction of the Hepatitis B vaccine, along with health education, reduced HBV prevalence from 10% to 1% among healthcare workers in India [19–21].

In Tanzania, the Hepatitis B vaccine is offered without charge to all public healthcare workers. However, only one in five healthcare workers were found to have protective immunity resulting from vaccination in a tertiary referral hospital in Tanzania [17]. In such a setting, it is important to assess the facilitators of and hurdles to HBV protection among healthcare workers. This study therefore seeks to determine the proportion of HCWs vaccinated against HBV, as well as to un-cover the factors associated with vaccination status. The findings of this study will guide policy and interventions in similar settings, particularly in Sub-Saharan Africa (SSA), as the global community works toward the elimination of HBV.

Methods

Design, patients and study procedures

A descriptive cross-sectional study was conducted at Muhimbili National Hospital (MNH), Dar es Salaam, from 30th July to 30th September 2015. The study included healthcare providers working in all departments, including trained nurses, medical attendants, and clinicians – both surgical and medical-related specialties and laboratory technicians. The investigator approached healthcare workers through the hospital administration and the heads of the departments. A self-administered questionnaire was used to obtain information from the participants. The questionnaires were collected from the healthcare workers upon completion by appointment with the participant. The sample size was calculated using the following formula for cross-sectional studies: $N = \{Z^2P\ (1 - P)\}\ /D^2$, where N = minimum sample size required; Z = standard normal deviation, which was set at 1.96; P = estimated proportion of healthcare workers vaccinated for HBV, which was unknown during the planning of this research and was estimated at 50%, and D = type 1 error, which we set at 0.05. The required sample size was 384.

Definition of terms

HBV vaccination schedule

HBV vaccination is provided in the form of an intramuscular injection in three doses. The first dose is the baseline dose, and the second and third doses are provided one and 6 months after the first dose, respectively.

Complete HBV vaccination

Healthcare workers who had received three HBV vaccine doses according to the HBV schedule were considered to have complete HBV vaccination.

Incomplete but on schedule HBV vaccination

Healthcare workers who had received one or two HBV vaccine doses according to the schedule but were not due for their next dose were considered to have a vaccination level that was incomplete but on schedule.

Incomplete HBV vaccination

Healthcare workers who had not received a full vaccination course but who were otherwise 1 month or more post-appointment for their scheduled dose were considered to have incomplete vaccination.

Ineligible for HBV vaccination

Healthcare workers with HBV infection or immunity to HBV upon their vaccination screening visit were considered ineligible for HBV vaccination.

Statistical analysis

The information requested via the questionnaire included vaccination status, knowledge about the transmission of and protection against HBV, and attitudes toward the Hepatitis B vaccine. The questionnaires were initially prepared in English, translated into Kiswahili and then back-translated in English to ensure that there was no loss of meaning. Both questionnaires were pretested for clarity and adjusted accordingly. The data were analyzed using Statistical Software for the Social Sciences (SPSS) Version 20. The categorical variables were summarized using proportions, while means were used to summarize the continuous variables. The variable of interest was complete or on-schedule vaccination as per the hepatitis B vaccination schedule. The differences between participants with complete/on-schedule vaccination and those with incomplete or no vaccination were tested using student's t- and chi-squared tests as appropriate. Logistic regression was used to investigate the factors associated with complete and on-schedule vaccination. HCWs who were ineligible for HBV vaccination were removed from the comparative analyses.

Ethics, consent and permissions

Ethical clearance was sought from the Muhimbili University of Health and Allied Sciences (MUHAS) review board. Permission to conduct the study was sought from the MNH administration. Informed written consent was obtained from participants before recruitment into the study. Confidentiality and privacy were ensured, and the information provided was stored securely, with access being limited to the investigators. No individual information or data that could lead to identity disclosure are published in this manuscript.

Results

During the study, 348 healthcare workers (HCWs) were interviewed at the hospital, of whom 158 (45%) were males and 190 (54.5%) were females. Table 1 provides the demographic characteristics of the study participants. The mean age was 33 years, and half of the participants were 30 years old or younger. More than three-quarters of the participants had worked for 10 years or fewer. The nurse cadre was predominant in the study group, making up 124 (35.6%) of the participants. Specialist doctors were the least common, at 22 participants (6.3%). Details regarding these demographic characteristics are provided in Table 1.

Table 1 General characteristics of the Health Care Workers at Muhimbili National Hospital ($n = 348$)

Variable	Frequency (%)
Gender	
Male	158 (45.4)
Female	190 (54.6)
Age group (years)	
21–30	191 (54.9)
31–40	94 (27.0)
41–50	44 (12.6)
>50	19 (5.5)
Medical cadre	
Intern doctor	48 (13.8)
Registrar/resident	62 (17.8)
Specialist	22 (6.3)
Nurse	124 (35.6)
Hospital attendants	48 (13.8)
Laboratory technicians	44 (12.6)
Duration of employment (years)	
0–1	97 (27.9)
2–5	106 (30.5)
5–10	71 (20.4)
11–20	42 (12.1)
>20	32 (9.2)
Department	
Medical/pediatrics	96 (27.6)
Surgical and [a]OBGY	81 (23.3)
Theater/Laboratory	76 (21.3)
[b]EMD/[c]ICU/Mortuary	49 (14.1)
[d]OPD	46 (13.2)

[a]OBGY = Obstetrics and Gynecology
[b]EMD = Emergency department
[c]ICU = intensive care unit
[d]OPD = Outpatient department

Table 2 shows the vaccination status of the interviewed HCWs. Partial or full vaccination for the Hepatitis B virus was reported by 198 (56.9%) interviewees. However, only 117 (33.6%) were fully vaccinated, with three doses of the vaccine. Among HCWs with partial vaccination, 41 (50.6) were not yet due for their next dose according to the vaccination schedule. The remaining half, some 40 individuals (49.4%) with partial vaccination, had missed their scheduled vaccination visit for 1 month or more. Among unvaccinated HCWs, 14 (9.3%) had either HBV infection or antibodies against HBV infection upon pre-vaccination screening.

Table 3 provides an unadjusted comparison of vaccination coverage among the interviewed HCWs by department. Outpatient departments had the lowest proportion

Table 2 Hepatitis B Vaccination status among Health Care Workers at Muhimbili National Hospital ($n = 348$)

	n(%)
HB vaccination status	
Only one HB vaccine dose	30 (8.6)
Two HB vaccine doses	51 (14.7)
Full vaccination (3 doses)	117 (33.6)
Un-vaccinated	150 (43.1)
Vaccination status among HCW with Partial vaccination[a]	
Partial vaccination on schedule	41 (50.6)
Partial vaccination missed appointments	40 (49.4)

[a]Among those with partial vaccination

of vaccinated HCWs, at ten individuals (22.7%), while emergency departments, intensive care units (ICUs) and mortuary departments had the highest proportion of vaccinated individuals (76.6%) (Table 3). Healthcare workers (HCWs) who underwent partial or full-course vaccination had a mean employment duration 2.3 years, as compared to 2.5 years among those who were not vaccinated ($p = 0.72$).

Regarding knowledge of the transmission and prevention of HBV, the majority of the respondents, 342 individuals (98.3%), had heard about hepatitis B viral infection prior to the interview. A total of 337 (96.8%) HCWs correctly identified their work as increasing the risk of acquiring HBV infection.

Unvaccinated health workers provided the following reasons for non-vaccination: they had not been offered a chance for hepatitis B vaccination (98 individuals, 65.3%), or they were very careful and observed standard precautions while at work (70 individuals, 46.7%) (Table 4). Others reported that there was not enough awareness concerning access to hepatitis B vaccination (62 individuals, 41.3%) (Table 4).

Table 5 shows attitudes towards the hepatitis B vaccine. Among the respondents, 326 (93.7%) agreed that

Table 3 Comparison of vaccination status by department the participant worked at the time of interview ($n = 334$)[a]

Department**	Number (%)		
	Vaccinated $n = 198$	Unvaccinated $n = 136$	Total $n = 334$
Medical/Pediatrics	63 (67.0)	31 (33.0)	94
Surgical/[b]OBGY	48 (63.2)	28 (36.8)	76
Theater/laboratory	41 (56.2)	32 (43.8)	73
[c]EMD/[d]ICU/Mortuary	36 (76.6)	11 (23.4)	47
[e]OPD	10 (22.7)	34 (77.3)	44

[a]excluding HCW with HBV infection or HBV immunity at screening
**$P < 0.001$
[b]OBGY = Obstetrics and Gynecology
[c]EMD = Emergency department
[d]ICU = intensive care unit
[e]OPD = Outpatient department

Table 4 Reasons for non-vaccination status among health care personnel at Muhimbili National Hospital ($n = 150$)

Reasons	Frequency (%)
I have never heard about the vaccine before	7 (4.7)
The vaccine is not available at my working place	44 (29.3)
I have not been offered a chance for HBV vaccination	98 (65.3)
I have no time for hepatitis B vaccination, very busy schedule	27 (18.0)
I am very careful, I observe standard precautions when I work	70 (46.7)
There is no enough education concerning HBV vaccination	62 (41.3)
I can't afford the HBV vaccine	21 (14.0)
I was found infected on initial screening	8 (5.3)
I had HBsAb already on screening	10 (6.7)

the Hepatitis B vaccine was effective in preventing HBV infection, while a few either disagreed (seven individuals, 2.0%) or were unsure about the effectiveness of the hepatitis B vaccine (15 individuals, 4.3%). Similarly, to a large extent, HCWs reported having trust in the vaccine (312 individuals, 89.7%), while a few (15 individuals, 4.3%) did not trust hepatitis B vaccine or had doubts about it (21 individuals, 6%). When we enquired into whether the hepatitis B vaccine should be compulsory among HCWs in Tanzania, 333 (96.8%) of the respondents agreed, while seven (2%) disagreed and four (1.1%) were undecided about mandatory hepatitis B vaccination for HCWs.

Based on the multivariate logistic regression analysis, medical attendants (PR 6.6; 95% CI 2.0–21.7) and laboratory technicians (PR = 5.7; 95% CI 1.4–22.6) were more like likely to have incomplete or no vaccination compared to interns. Similarly, newly recruited HCWs were more likely to be associated with incomplete or non-vaccination status as compared to HCWs who had been working for more than 10 years (Table 6). It is worth noting that HCWs working in the outpatient department were significantly less likely to be vaccinated

Table 5 Attitude towards hepatitis B vaccine as reported by health care workers at Muhimbili National Hospital ($n = 348$)

	Agree n (%)	Disagree n (%)	Undecided n (%)
Effective for the disease prevention	326 (93.7)	7(2.0)	15 (4.3)
I trust hepatitis B vaccine	312 (89.7)	15 (4.3)	21 (6.0)
The vaccine is not safe	17 (4.9)	225 (73.3)	76 (21.8)
Should be compulsory for all health care workers	333 (96.8)	7 (2.0)	4 (1.1)

Table 6 Multivariate analysis of factors associated with incomplete or non-vaccination status among health care workers at Muhimbili National Hospital ($n = 334$)[a]

	PR[b]	95.0% C.I.		*P*
Male	1.23	0.717	2.11	0.453
Age (years)	1.433	0.877	2.34	0.151
Cadre				
Intern doctors	1			
Registered doctors/specialists	0.578	0.208	1.605	0.293
Nurses	1.972	0.81	4.797	0.135
Medical attendants	6.611	2.018	21.659	0.002
Laboratory technicians	5.707	1.442	22.583	0.013
Work duration (years)				
0 – 1	9.501	2.629	34.329	0.001
2 – 5	10.148	2.921	35.254	<0.0001
6 – 10	2.792	1.05	7.423	0.04
>10	1			
Work department				
Medical/Pediatrics	1			0
Surgical/ [c]OBGY	1.256	0.64	2.464	0.507
Theatre/Laboratory	0.776	0.285	2.108	0.618
[d]EMD/[e]ICU/Mortuary	0.472	0.2	1.114	0.087
[f]OPD	7.815	2.743	22.263	<0.0001

[a]excluding HCW with HBV infection or HBV immune at screening
[b]PR = Prevalence ratio
[c]OBGY = Obstetrics and gynecology
[d]EMD = Emergency department
[e]ICU = intensive care unit
[f]OPD = Outpatient department

as compared to HCWs from medical (internal medicine and pediatrics) departments (PR 7; 95% CI 2.0–21.7). The detailed multivariate analysis results are provided in Table 6.

Discussion

In this study, we have observed that only one in three HCWs at the national referral hospital had undergone full hepatitis B vaccination, despite high levels of awareness and the near complete acceptance of the vaccine. These rates are lower than those in Europe 50–90% [22–29] and North America 63.4% [30]. Hepatitis B vaccine coverage is even lower in the neighboring countries of Kenya (12%) [31] and Uganda (5%) [32]. These low vaccination rates are worrisome because accidental exposure to blood and body fluids is common among healthcare workers [32–34] and has been associated with occupational hepatitis B infections. Efforts must be made to increase coverage.

Addressing incomplete vaccination (81 individuals, 23%) is also important, particularly among those who have already missed their scheduled visit and are thus potential defaulters on the vaccination program (40 individuals, 11.4%). These HCWs are potentially at risk for infection should they be exposed to HBV. A full--course hepatitis B vaccine (three doses) is safe and tolerable and offers 95–100% protection for adults [35, 36]. The first and second HBV vaccine doses provide less protection, specifically up to 85% protection against HBV infection [35]. A significant proportion of the HCWs who received two doses and even more of those who received only one dose of the vaccine are at risk of contracting hepatitis B infection should they be exposed. This message must clearly delivered to HCWs because incomplete vaccination is largely attributed to carelessness or forgetfulness [31]. There should be no misconceptions regarding HCWs having full protection with less than three doses without demonstrated evidence of immunity through antibody level assessment.

Improving hepatitis B vaccination coverage among healthcare workers at MNH requires addressing various bottlenecks. Based on previous studies, as well as the findings from our study, hepatitis B knowledge [14, 23], access to hepatitis B vaccination [31] and a lack of publicity are the major stumbling blocks to increased coverage [31, 38, 39]. Our study revealed that 47% of unvaccinated HCWs thought that observing infection control precautions and being careful would be enough to prevent HBV infection at their workplace. Healthcare personnel who view their susceptibility to HBV infection as high are more likely to be vaccinated than their counterparts who view their susceptibility to infection as low [23]. In other studies, those who wore gloves all or most of the time when they cared for patients or instruments were more likely to be vaccinated [37]. Appropriate knowledge about the transmission and prevention of HBV infection is vital in this regard. Two out of the three unvaccinated HCWs who responded reported that they had not been offered hepatitis B vaccination. Increased publicity for the vaccine would empower HCWs to demand vaccine and know how to access the vaccine. Reports show that publicity campaigns regarding the vaccination of HCWs yielded nearly complete protection rates among HCWs [38, 39]. Given the high acceptance rates regarding the vaccine among the HCWs in our study (97%) and those in Uganda (98%) [32], publicity is important in improving vaccine coverage. Therefore, a vaccination program, when properly planned and guided with policies such as mandatory vaccination among HCWs, could be successful [29, 40]. In European countries, policies differ; some countries enforce the mandatory vaccination of HCWs [41].

Multivariate analysis demonstrated that, laboratory technicians and medical attendants were six and seven times more likely to be unvaccinated/incomplete vaccination as compared to intern doctors. This finding is worrisome because the risk of occupational injury and exposure to HBV is higher among nurses and intern doctors [22, 42–44]. In other places such as India, vaccination for HBV was highest among interns and lowest among nursing attendants [45]. Our data, suggest that the majority of HCWs who worked at the outpatient department, were less likely to be vaccinated. Previous reports have shown that higher vaccination coverage has been associated with surgical and laboratory departments, where the risk is high [44]. It is therefore important that these departments be sensitized to and educated about the risks and advantages of vaccination. The locations for vaccine administration, the conflicting schedules for vaccine administration vs. duty stations, and the varying workloads among departments should be considered when designing and implementing HCW vaccination programs at a given health facility. Similarly, there was an association between the probability of non-/incomplete vaccination and increased employment duration. Education must particularly target recent employed health personnel to reduce risk of new hepatitis infections.

This study has shown the level of awareness of HBV infection among HCWs. Through first-hand information gathered via self-administered questionnaires, we were able to assess HCWs' acceptance of the hepatitis B vaccine and address bottlenecks regarding increased uptake. Notwithstanding this important contribution, our study has certain weaknesses. Vaccination status was assessed through self-provided information, which is prone to recall bias. Given the fact that the participants were healthcare workers and recent national efforts to vaccinate healthcare workers in the country, we believe this bias to be very low. Vaccination does not always translate into immunity. Therefore, the use of a hospital database and coupling this study with an assessment of anti-HBsAb titres would have helped to inform policy change. Secondly, HCWs from all departments were approached through the administration, regardless of cadre and duration of employment. Purposeful selection would probably have increased the number specialist doctors included in the study.

Conclusion

Hepatitis B vaccination coverage at this national hospital in Tanzania is currently low, despite good knowledge of and positive attitudes towards the vaccine. More effective programming, including publicity, as well as increasing access to the vaccination, could improve hepatitis B vaccine coverage. Feasibility studies regarding mandatory vaccination as a pre-requisite for employment should be conducted. Similar studies at private and lower-level health facilities are also warranted.

Abbreviations

DALYs: Disability-adjusted life years; EMD: Emergency medicine department; HBsAb: Hepatitis B surface antibody; HBsAg: Hepatitis B surface antigen; HBV: Hepatitis B virus; HCW: Health care worker; ICU: Intensive care unit; IDU: Injection drug use; MNH: Muhimbili National Hospital; MUHAS: Muhimbili University of Health and Allied Sciences; OBGY: Obstetrics and gynecology; OPD: Outpatient department; PR: Prevalence ratio; SPSS: Statistical software for the social sciences; WHO: World Health Organization

Acknowledgements

The authors are grateful to the following: the Government of Tanzania, which provided funds to support this study; the Muhimbili University of Health and Allied Sciences for assisting with logistical issues; Muhimbili National Hospital authority for allowing the study to be performed and all staff who participated in the study.

Funding

Funding for this research was provided by the Government of Tanzania through the Ministry of Education as part of research training for medical doctors. The funder had no role in the design, data acquisition, data management, data analysis or the presentation of the findings.

Authors' contributions

The study was conceived and developed by DA and TJN. Data collection was performed by DA. Analysis and results interpretation was performed by DA, TJN, EK and JR. The manuscript was first drafted by TJN. All authors contributed to the draft, and finally, all authors approved the manuscript.

Consent for publication

Not applicable. There are no personal identifiers in the data we are presenting in this manuscript.

Competing interests

All authors declare that they have no any competing interests with regard to this publication.

Author details

[1]School of Medicine, Muhimbili University of Health and Allied Sciences, P.O. Box 65001, Dar es Salaam, Tanzania. [2]Muhimbili National Hospital, P.O. Box 65000, Dar es Salaam, Tanzania.

References

1. Stanaway JD, Flaxman AD, Naghavi M, Fitzmaurice C, Vos T, Abubakar I, et al. The global burden of viral hepatitis from 1990 to 2013: findings from the global burden of disease study 2013. Lancet. 2016;388(10049):1081–8.
2. Global Hepatitis Report 2017. Geneva: World Health Organization; 2017. Available at http://apps.who.int/iris/bitstream/10665/255016/1/9789241565455-eng.pdf?ua=1. Accessed 15 Dec 2017.
3. Schweitzer A, Horn J, Mikolajczyk RT, Krause G, Ott JJ. Estimations of worldwide prevalence of chronic hepatitis B virus infection: a systematic review of data published between 1965 and. Lancet. 2013;386:1546–55.
4. Hollinger FB, Liang TJ. Hepatitis B virus. In: Knipe DM, et al., editors. Field virology. 4th ed. Philadelphia: Lippincott Williams & Wilkins; 2001. p. 2971–3036.
5. Matee MI, Lyamuya EF, Mbena EC, et al. Prevalence of transfusion-associated viral infections and syphilis among blood donors in Muhimbili medical Centre in Dar es salaam, Tanzania. East Afr Med J. 1999;76:167–71.
6. Matee MN, Magesa PM, Lyamuya EF. Seroprevalence of human immunodeficiency virus, hepatitis B and C viruses and syphilis infections among blood donors at the Muhimbili National Hospital in Dar Es Salaam, Tanzania. BMC Public Health. 2006;6:21.

7. Rashid S, Kilewo C, Aboud S. Seroprevalence of hepatitis B virus infection among antenatal clinic attendees at a tertiary hospital in Dar es salaam, Tanzania. Tanzan J Health Res. 2014;16(1):9–15.
8. Menendez C, Sanchez-Tapias JM, Kahigwa E, Mshinda H, Costa J, Vidal J, Acosta C, Lopez-Labrador X, Olmedo E, Navia M, Tanner M, Rodes J, Alonso PL. Prevalence and mother-to-infant transmission of hepatitis viruses B, C, and E in southern Tanzania. J Med Virol. 1999;58(3):215–20.
9. Manyahi J, Msigwa Y, Mhimbira F, Majigo M. High sero-prevalence of hepatitis B virus and human immunodeficiency virus infections among pregnant women attending antenatal clinic at Temeke municipal health facilities, Dar es salaam, Tanzania: a cross sectional study. BMC Pregnancy Childbirth. 2017;17(1):109.
10. Pellizzer G, Ble C, Zamperetti N, Stroffolini T, Upunda G, Rapicetta M, Chione P, Villano U, Fabris P, de Lalla F. Serological survey of hepatitis B infection in Tanzania. Public Health. 1994;108(6):427–31.
11. Nagu TJ, Bakari M, Matee M. Hepatitis a, B and C viral co-infections among HIV-infected adults presenting for care and treatment at Muhimbili National Hospital in Dar es salaam, Tanzania. BMC Public Health. 2008 Dec 19;8:416.
12. Ministry of health (MoH) Uganda, ORC Marco: Uganda HIV/AIDs Sero-behavioural survey 2994–2005, Calverton Maryland USA: MoH and ORC Marco 2006.
13. Ly KN, Kim AA, Umuro M, Drobenuic J, Williamson JM, Montgomery JM, Fields BS, Teshale EH. Prevalence of hepatitis B virus infection in Kenya, 2007. Am J Trop Med Hyg. 2016;95(2):348–53.
14. Hyams KC, Morrill JC, Woody JN, Okoth FA, Tukei PM, Mugambi M, Johnson B, Gray GC. Epidemiology of hepatitis B in eastern Kenya. J Med Virol. 1989;28:106–9.
15. Kabanga JM, Julius K, Shiramba TL, Njenga MK, Kaiguri PM, Osidiana V. Prevalence of hepatitis B virus (HBV) surface antigen and HBV-associated hepatocellular carcinoma in Kenyans of various ages. Afr J Health Sci. 2011; 18:53–61.
16. Ziraba AK, Bwogi J, Namale A, Wainaina CW, Mayanja-Kizza H. Sero-prevalence and risk factors for hepatitis B virus infection among health care workers in a tertiary hospital in Uganda. BMC Infect Dis. 2010;10:191.
17. Mueller A, Stoetter L, Kalluvya S, Stich A, Majinge C, Weissbrich B, Kasang C. Prevalence of hepatitis B virus infection among health care workers in a tertiary hospital in Tanzania. BMC Infect Dis. 2015;15:386.
18. Elavia AJ, Banker DD. Hepatitis B infection in hospital personnel. Natl Med India. 1992;5:265–8.
19. World Health Organization. Global Health sector strategy on viral hepatitis 2016–2021. WHO/HIV/2016.06 available at http://apps.who.int/iris/bitstream/10665/246177/1/WHO-HIV-2016.06-eng.pdf. Accessed 15 Dec 2017.
20. Kumar KA, Baghal PK, Shukla CB, Jain MK. Prevalence of hepatitis surface antigen (HBsAg) among health care workers. Indian J Comm Med. 2000;25:93–6.
21. Sukrit PNT, Sethi A, Angrawal K, Kumal GT. Low levels of awareness, vaccine coverage and the need for booster among health care workers in tertially care hospitals in India. J Gastro enterol Hepatol. 2008;23:1710–5.
22. Marković-Denić L, Branković M, Maksimović N, Jovanović B, Petrović I, Simić M, Lesić A. Occupational exposures to blood and body fluids among health care workers at university hospitals. Srp Arh Celok Lek. 2013;141(11–12):789–93.
23. Tafuri S, Martinelli D, Caputi G, Arbore A, Lopalco PL, Germinario C, Prato R. An audit of vaccination coverage among vaccination service workers in Puglia. Italy Am J Infect Control. 2009;37(5):414–6.
24. Karaivazoglou K, Triantos C, Lagadinou M, Bikas C, Michailidou M, Kalafateli M, Thomopoulos K, Assimakopoulos K, Nikolopoulou V, Jelastopulu E, Labropoulou-Karatza C. Acceptance of hepatitis B vaccination among health care workers in western Greece. Arch Environ Occup Health. 2014;69(2):107–11.
25. Faure E, Cortot C, Gosset D, Cordonnier A, Deruelle P, Guery B. Vaccinal status of healthcare students in Lille. Med Mal Infect. 2013;43(3):114–7.
26. Maltezou HC, Katerelos P, Poufta S, Pavli A, Maragos A, Theodoridou M. Attitudes toward mandatory occupational vaccinations and vaccination coverage against vaccine-preventable diseases of health care workers in primary health care centers. Am J Infect Control. 2013;41(1):66–70.
27. Maltezou HC, Gargalianos P, Nikolaidis P, Katerelos P, Tedoma N, Maltezos E, Lazanas M. Attitudes towards mandatory vaccination and vaccination coverage against vaccine-preventable diseases among health-care workers in tertiary-care hospitals. J Inf Secur. 2012;64(3):319–24.
28. Schenkel K, Radun D, Bremer V, Bocter N, Hamouda O.Viral hepatitis in Germany: poor vaccination coverage and little knowledge about transmission in target groups. BMC Public Health. 2008 23;8:132.
29. Vranckx R, Jacques P, De Schrijver A, Moens G. Hepatitis B vaccination coverage in Belgian health care workers. Infection. 2004;32(5):278–81.
30. Kathy K. Byrd, a Peng-jun Lu, and Trudy V. Murphy. Hepatitis B vaccination coverage among health-care personnel in the United States. Public Health Rep. 2013;128(6):498–509.
31. Suckling RM, Taegtmeyer M, Nguku PM, Al-Abri SS, Kibaru J, Chakaya JM, Tukei PM, Gilks CF. Of healthcare workers in Kenya to hepatitis B: new strategies for facilitating vaccination uptake. J Hosp Infect. 2006;64(3):271–7.
32. Braka F, Nanyunja M, Makumbi I, Mbabazi W, Kasasa S, Lewis RF. Hepatitis B infection among health workers in Uganda: evidence of the need for health worker protection. Vaccine. 2006;24(47–48):6930–7.
33. Goel V, Kumar D, Lingaiah R, Singh S. Occurrence of Needlestick and Injuries among Health-care Workers of a Tertiary Care Teaching Hospital in North India. J Lab Physicians. 2017;9(1):20–5.
34. Vardas E, Ross MH, Sharp G, McAnerney J, Sim J. Viral hepatitis in south African healthcare workers at increased risk of occupational exposure to blood-borne viruses. J Hosp Infect. 2002;50(1):6–12.
35. Assad S, Francis A. Over a decade of experience with a yeast recombinant hepatitis B vaccine. Vaccine. 1999;18(1–2):57–67.
36. Joukar F, Mansour-Ghanaei F, Naghipour M-R, Asgharnezhad M. Immune responses to single-dose versus double-dose hepatitis B vaccines in healthcare workers not responding to the primary vaccine series: a randomized clinical trial. Hepat Mon. 2016;16(2):e32799.
37. Rachiotis G, Goritsas C, Alikakou V, Ferti A, Roumeliotou A. Vaccination against hepatitis B virus in workers of a general hospital in Athens. Med Lav. 2005 Jan-Feb;96(1):80–6.
38. Stroffolini T, Guadagnino V, Rapicetta M, Menniti Ippolito F, Caroleo B, De Sarro G, Focà A, Liberto MC, Giancotti A, Barreca GS, Marascio N, Lombardo F. Staltari O; Sersale's study collaborating group. The impact of a vaccination campaign against hepatitis B on the further decrease of hepatitis B virus infection in a southern Italian town over 14 years. Eur J Intern Med. 2012;23(8):e190–2.
39. Dini G, Toletone A, Barberis I, Debarbieri N, Massa E, Paganino C, Bersi F, Montecucco A, Alicino C, Durando P. Persistence of protective anti-HBs antibody levels and anamnestic response to HBV booster vaccination: a cross-sectional study among healthcare students 20 years following the universal immunization campaign in Italy. Hum Vaccin Immunother. 2017; 13(2):440–4.
40. Kondili LA, Ulqinaku D, Hajdini M, Basho M, Chionne P, Madonna E, Taliani G, Candido A, Dentico P, Bino S, Rapicetta M. Hepatitis B virus infection in health care workers in Albania: a country still highly endemic for HBV infection. Infection. 2007;35(2):94–7.
41. Maltezou HC, Wicker S, Borg M, Heininger U, Puro V, Theodoridou M, Poland GA. Vaccination policies for health-care workers in acute health-care facilities in Europe. Vaccine. 2011;29(51):9557–62.
42. Vos D, Götz HM, Richardus JH. Needlestick injury and accidental exposure to blood: the need for improving the hepatitis B vaccination grade among health care workers outside the hospital. Am J Infect Control. 2006;34(9):610–2.
43. Falagas ME, Karydis I, Kostogiannou I. Percutaneous exposure incidents of the health care personnel in a newly founded tertiary hospital: a prospective study. PLoS One. 2007 Feb 7;2(2):e194.
44. Marinho RT, Moura MC, Pedro M, Ramalho FJ, Velosa JF. Hepatitis B vaccination in hospital personnel and medical students. J Clin Gastroenterol. 1999;28(4):317–22.
45. Joshi SC, Joshi G, Singh Y, Khalil M, Joshi A, Jha SK. Hepatitis B vaccination status among healthcare workers in a tertiary care hospital in Haldwani City of Nainital, Uttarakhand, India. Ann Trop Med Public Health. 2014;7(2):96.

6

Risk factors, person, place and time characteristics associated with Hepatitis E Virus outbreak in Napak District, Uganda

Geofrey Amanya[1], Samuel Kizito[1,3*], Immaculate Nabukenya[2], Joan Kalyango[1,3], Collins Atuheire[1], Hellen Nansumba[1], Stephen Akena Abwoye[1], Denis Nixon Opio[1], Edrisa Kibuuka[1] and Charles Karamagi[1,3]

Abstract

Background: Hepatitis E is self-limiting, but can cause death in most at risk groups like pregnant women and those with preexisting acute liver disease. In developing countries it presents as epidemic, in 2014 Hepatitis E Virus (HEV) outbreak was reported in Napak district Uganda. The role of factors in this setting that might have propagated this HEV epidemic, including host, agent, and environmental characteristics, were still not clear. This study was therefore conducted to investigate the risk factors, person, place and time characteristics, associated with the hepatitis E virus (HEV) epidemic in Napak district.

Methods: Review of line lists data for epidemiological description and matched case control study on neighborhood and age in the ratio of 1:2 were used to assess risk factors for HEV outbreak in Napak. Cluster and random sampling were used to obtain a sample size of 332, (111 cases, 221 controls). Possible interaction and confounding was assessed using conditional logistic regression.

Results: Over 1359 cases and 30 deaths were reported during 2013/2014 HEV outbreak. The mean age of patients was 29 ± years, 57.9% of cases were females. Overall case Fatality Ratio was 2.2% in general population but 65.2% in pregnant women. More than 94% of the cases were reported in the sub counties of Napak, 5.7% of cases were reported in the outside neighboring districts. The epidemic peaked in January 2014 and gradually subsided by December 2014. Risk factors found to be associated with HEV included drinking untreated water (OR 6.69, 95% CI 3.15–14.16), eating roadside food (OR 6.11, 95% CI 2.85–13.09), reported not cleaning utensils (OR 3.24, 95% CI 1.55–1.76), and being a hunter (OR 1.14, 95% CI 1.03–12.66).

Conclusion: The results of this study suggest that the virus is transmitted by the feco-oral route through contaminated water. They also suggest that active surveillance and appropriate measures targeting community and routine individual health actions are important to prevent transmission and decrease the deaths.

Keywords: Hepatitis E, Epidemic, Uganda

Background

Previously in Kitgum, Uganda reported one of the longest recorded outbreaks of Hepatitis E virus (HEV) in the history of the country [1]. HEV outbreaks occur mainly in developing countries where genotypes 1 and 2 are predominant. Although these epidemics are transmitted through feco-oral route, through fecally contaminated drinking water or food, person-to-person transmission has been reported elsewhere [1–3]. In developed countries HEV is anthropozoonotic and cases are mainly sporadic and linked to genotype 3 and 4 [4–6]. Studies of genotype 1 HEV infection have suggested that only 20–30% of infections are symptomatic [7]. Even then, HEV disease is self-limiting and usually does not result in long-term sequaele [5, 8]. The consequences of HEV infections in pregnancy are severe, and have been associated with high case fatality rates (up to 20%). In the general population a

* Correspondence: somekizito@yahoo.com
[1]Clinical Epidemiology Unit, School of Medicine, P.O Box 7072, Kampala, Uganda
[3]Makerere University College of Health Sciences, P.O Box 7072, Kampala, Uganda
Full list of author information is available at the end of the article

Case Fatality Rate (CFR) of 1% and 2% have been proven possible [8–11]. Vaccines have been developed and tested in clinical trials, however these have not been made available for public use [11, 12]. This study aimed at identifying the risk factors, person, place and time characteristics of the 2013/2014 HEV epidemic in Napak district of Uganda.

Methods

Study site and subjects

The study was carried out in Napak district, northern Uganda. It has seven sub counties, 31 parishes, and 227 villages. It is predominantly rural-nomadic with an estimated total population of 146,630 persons. Temperatures are varying from 15 to 32.5 °C depending the season. There is no month when rainfall exceeds potential evaporation. The soil are black or dark grey clays with very low organic material, they have a medium moisture storage capacity. In this Karamoja region Napak, deforestation and wild fires have left the vegetation inexistent with no green cover. Three sub counties of Lokopo, Lorengechora and Matany, accounted for the bulk cases, other isolated cases had been identified from the neighboring districts of Moroto, Nakapiripirit, Katakwi and Kotido. From an unpublished Health report in 2014 Napak district had a low latrine coverage of only 18.6% and safe water coverage of 62%. Nevertheless 44% of the safe water sources are non-functional.

Surveillance data

We obtained line listings data from the office of the district "biostatistician" for all the cases since the beginning of the outbreak from 2013 to 2014. This data was routinely collected for all the patients identified during the outbreak.

Case control study

We begun conducting a case control study in November 2014 in which we matched the cases with age and geographical location matched controls. A case patient was defined as any individual who was diagnosed with Hepatitis E basing on clinical presentation of jaundice as ascertained by a team of physicians with at least one of the accompanying symptoms (fatigue, anorexia, abdominal pain, arthralgia, fever or headache) and serological evidence of HEV infection [IgM antibody, MP Biomedical Suisse S.A. Switzerland]. The study physician excluded patients If they had jaundice of unknown etiology, or could not be contacted and reported travelled out of Napak during the review period. Case listing data missing variables of interest. Case listing data missing variables of interest, like laboratory results, were also excluded. Potential controls were individuals that had not presented with clinical picture suggestive of hepatitis E since the epidemic began. They were selected from the general population residing in the three sub counties and with each control matched to a case by neighborhood and age (±5 year's difference) on ratio of 1:2. We used random and cluster sampling to obtain a sample size of 332, (111 cases, 221 controls), 80% power to detect a minimum OR of 2.5, alpha error of 5%, design effect of 2 and a 10% none response rate.

Data collection and analysis

We developed, translated and pretested a questionnaire into the local language (Karimojong) for easy comprehension of participant's views and pretested it. We collected information on social demographic information: age, sex, pregnancy status, social economic, location of primary residence, household size (divided into tertiles) and occupation. Other culture-specific practices such as drinking locally made fermented alcoholic brew, attending ceremonies where communal hand washing was common, washing utensils, hand washing practices especially after eating and usage of toilet, the presence as well as use of soap, exposure to various animals including ownership and staying with animals in the same household.

We obtained additional environment information including the primary source of water, availability and treatment of drinking water, the type and number of drinking water storage vessels, latrine availability and use, season (dry or wet) and common bathing practices (common basin with others). Safety and confidentiality of data were ensured through use of unique identification. Collected data was kept under lock and key research assistants were trained. In a household where there were more than two, a tossup was done to select who to be interviewed.

Statistical analysis

We coded and registered the data into a computer database created using Epi-info version 7.5. We checked for errors, cleaned the data periodically and froze the data. A copy of the data was transfered to STATA version 12 for analysis. Proportions (percentages), a spot map and epidemic curve were used to describe respectively the person, place and time characteristics of the HEV outbreak in Napak district 2013/2014.

To identify the risk factors associated with the HEV outbreak, we carried out conditional logistic regression reporting odds ratios. We performed bivariate analysis and all the variables, with $p < 0.20$ were subjected to multivariate analysis; possible interactions and confounding were assessed.

Results

Description of the person, place, and time characteristics of HEV outbreak

We identified a total of 1359 cases of HEV infection from Napak district listings during this epidemic (Fig. 1).

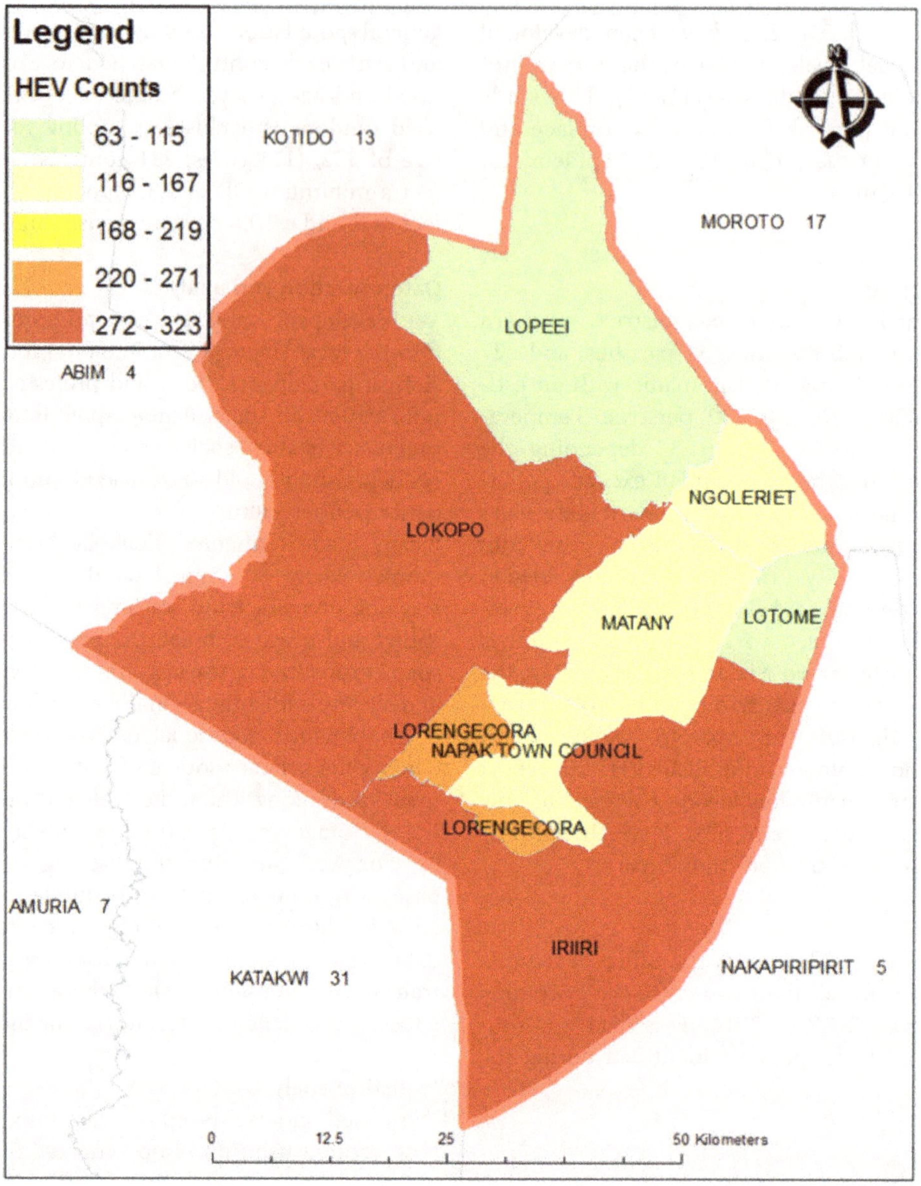

Fig. 1 Distribution of confirmed HEV cases in Napak district per Sub County, 2013/2014 -*Spot Map was GIS plotted*

The mean age of patients was 29 ± years and 57.9% (788) of the HEV cases were females. The overall CFR was 2.2%, it was highest in the 18–30 years age group (3.9%) and females (3.3%). The CFR was highest in pregnant women at 65.2%. Details are highlighted in Table 1.

Cases of HEV were first reported in January 2013 while the notification and surveillance for the epidemic began in April 2013. The HEV epidemic peaked in January 2014 and gradually subsided. By December 2014, there were no more cases reported. The median incubation period was 40 days IQR (24–53) as shown in Fig. 2.

In Table 2, Lorengechora and Ngolereit had the highest proportion of the cases in other sub counties like Lopeei (0.8%), Iriri (0.8%), Matany (0.7%), Lotome (0.5%) and Lokopo (0.02%) the CFR were below 1% of the total population.

Case control study

Four cases and 7 controls were excluded because we could not contact them. We analyzed data from a total of 107 cases, and 214 controls. With the exception of sex, the cases and controls were comparable at baseline. At bivariate (simple) analysis HEV was associated with drinking untreated water (OR 5.19, 95% CI 2.82–9.54), not cleaning their utensils (OR 2.72, 95% CI 1.60–4.61),

Table 1 Description of the person characteristics of HEV outbreak 2013/2014

Characteristic		Proportion of Cases *n* (%)	Died	CFR (%)
Age in years	<=5	51 (3.8)	0	0
	6–17	180 (13.3)	2	1.1
	18–30	594 (43.7)	23	3.9
	31–59	445 (32.7)	4	1
	60>=	89 (6.5)	0	0
Sex	Female	788 (58.0)	26	3.3
	Male	571 (42.0)	4	0.7
Pregnancy Status[a]	Yes	23 (1.7)	15	65.2
Overall Total		1359	30	2.2

[a]Subset of females who were pregnant

unsanitary (open) defecation practices (OR 2.46, 95% CI 1.47–4.12), reported frequent travels OR 2.04, 95% CI (1.14–3.63), "never" washed hands with soap after visiting the latrine (OR 1.64, 95% CI 1.01–2.65), never using soap to wash their hands before eating (OR 1.46, 95% CI 1.47–4.12), those with a well (OR 10.7, 95% CI (1.15–98.5). As shown in Table 3.

In Napak, livestock ownership is common. In this study livestock ownership was 57% among cases and 61.7% among controls. Although contact or ownership with animals were reported, there was no significant association between HEV and ownership of animals or contact with them (Table 3). We also explored for possible interactions since there was no prior knowledge of possible interaction between predictor variables. Thus, all predictor variables were Included in the model, However, there was No significant interactions were seen in relation to HEV between Sex, unsanitary defection practices, Presence of soap in Household, Cleaning utensils and hands after eating, untreated water at $P < 0.05$.

Variables like education were confounding washing of utensils and primary source of water and season were confounding occupation. At multivariate conditional logistic regression factors that were independently associated with HEV included drinking untreated water (OR 6.69, 95% CI 3.15–14.16), eating roadside food (OR 6.11, 95% CI 2.85–13.09), not cleaning utensils (OR 3.24, 95% CI 1.55–3.76) and being a hunter (OR 1.14, 95% CI 1.03–12.66). Details are shown in Table 4.

Discussion

Descriptive epidemiology

The burden of HEV outbreak is reflected by proportional morbidity from HEV at facilities and in communities. A median number of 34 cases were reported daily, female patients were observed to be more likely to be affected by the HEV outbreak. A study in Northern Namibia indicates that among patients with HEV male patients predominated over female cases 2.5:1 [13]. This distribution in females might be attributed to more severe clinical presentation in women, especially those who are pregnant [3, 8, 14]. High proportions of cases (43.7%) were adults aged between 18 and 30 years, this

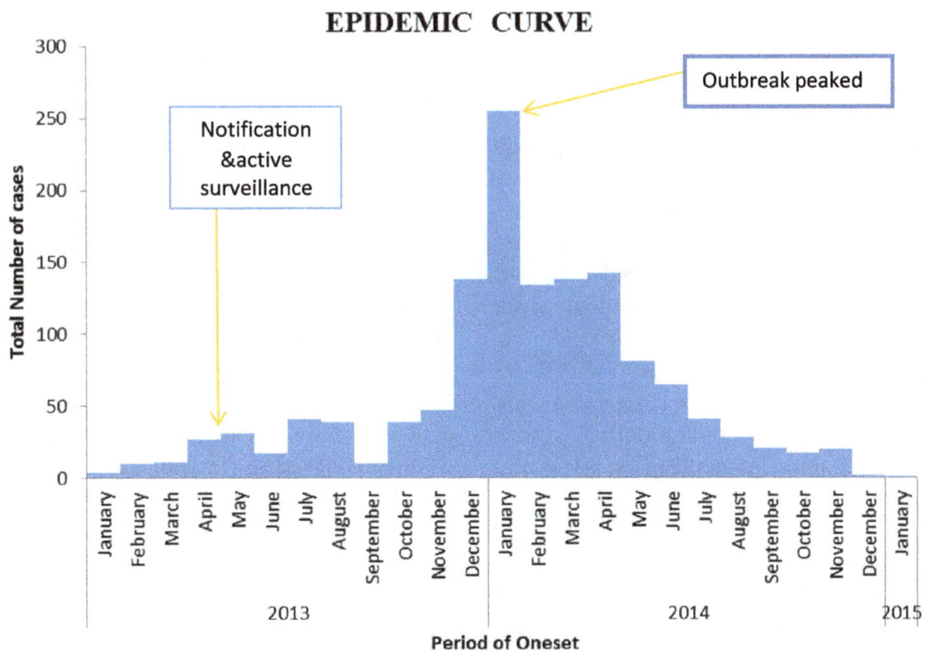

Fig. 2 Distribution of confirmed HEV cases by month of onset, Napak district (2013/2014)

Table 2 Proportion of HEV cases per sub county in Napak during 2013/2014 outbreak

Sub counties	Population estimates[a]	Cases	Proportion of cases %
Lorengchora	11,099	233	2.01
Ngolereit	10,502	126	1.20
Lopeei	13,393	104	0.77
Iriri	41,932	323	0.77
Matany	22,810	159	0.70
Lotome	11,589	63	0.54
Lokopo	21,311	288	0.02

[a]Census 2014 UNHPS

may be due to the culture differences where adults mainly search for livelihoods [15]. Contrary to these findings, in a study carried out in North India [16] showed 3.8% of the cases were aged below 5 years, indicating that also under-fives are at risk of HEV.

The high case fatality rate in the study (2.2%) is higher than that reported earlier in Uganda in 2008 (1.5%) [17], but lower than that reported in Darfur in 2004 (1.7%) [18]. With proper case management a lower CFR (<1%) could have been achieved [1]. This is likely to be due to frequent migration between dry seasons, in search for settlement areas. In this study, extremely high CFR of 65.2% was reported among pregnant women. This is higher than the 48% reported in sporadic cases in Ethiopia [6] and the 12.5% reported in Kenya in 2012 [19]. Differences in environmental factors and lack of community awareness on harmful traditional medicine like the use of local herbs to treat some complications during pregnancy could have contributed high CFR. Lorengechora being a town council, cases were most likely to be transmitted by eating roadside food [1, 2, 9]. With unsanitary food handling methods and exposure to many people, risk for HEV would be high. Ngolereit is in the north, neighboring Moroto, a very highly nomadic setting, movement could have enhanced transmission of HEV virus evidenced by number of cases reported out.

The epidemic curve was multimodal and suggestive of a propagated point source common vehicle epidemic, with the largest peak registered in the 48th epidemiologic week. Temporal peaks occurred during the 43-48th epidemiological week, coinciding with the rainy season and flooding in January. Flooding could have carried away any potential fecal substances causing contamination. Studies done in Ethiopia 2012 [6], and Uganda [2, 3] showed high proportions of cases occur in a dry season.

Risk factors for HEV outbreak

At multivariate analysis, HEV was significantly associated with eating roadside food, drinking untreated water, failure to wash utensils and being a hunter (Table 4). All these factors suggest that in this study, HEV was transmitted by the feco-oral mechanism through a waterborne route, which is typical of genotype 1 and genotype 2 as previously reported by different studies [2, 7].

The odds of having hepatitis E increased by six times among those eating roadside food. Roadside foods are easily contaminated because of unsanitary food handling methods and exposure to many people and winds. Study carried in Europe [5], confirmed food borne contamination in food handler working in a restaurant with high at risk foods.

Drinking untreated water increased the risk of HEV by almost seven times amongst the cases. This suggests that there was prior contamination of water sources and possible water-borne transmission in Napak district. This is not surprising since the situation regarding water and sanitation in this setting is very poor, this finding is confirmed elsewhere [20–22]. However, no associations with poor water and sanitation situation are reported in sporadic cases Turkmenistan [6]. Not cleaning utensils increased the risk of HEV by more than three times among the cases, unclean utensils could have acted as a reservoir for HEV. This situation was attributed to distant water sources and the scarcity of water in the areas. Cases were more likely to travel outside their homes although this finding was not significantly associated with HEV perhaps due to small numbers in strata. Previous studies have linked HEV to travel [19, 20].

Frequent travelers revealed a history of visiting an endemic country with high-risk enteric exposures prior to infection. In this study, the HEV epidemic is attributed to the nomadic livelihoods of the people in search for water, and life in camps during the dry seasons [2, 8, 19].

Unlike previous reports [1], having more than five members (larger family size) in the household was not significantly associated with HEV. These findings concur with the previous HEV outbreak in Uganda, which did not find any significant association with household size [3]. The findings in recent outbreaks in Uganda and studies done in rural Bangladesh [7, 23] and in India [14] demonstrated a strong role of person-to- person transmission in sustaining the epidemic [16]. In this study it was not evident but may have occurred. Use of unsanitary latrines i.e. like open defecation was associated with HEV at bivariate but not at multivariate analysis, perhaps due to small numbers in the strata. However previous studies from Nepal-India and Uganda confirmed a strong association between use of unsanitary latrines and HEV most probably due to fecal matter being easily washed to water sources [17, 24].

HEV was associated amongst those who reported not washing hands with soap after defecation, whose primary source of water was a well, Promiscuous defecation and improper disposal of children's feaces could have contributed to the situation. Attending social events was

Table 3 Bivariate analysis of independent factors associated with Hepatitis E Virus in Napak, 2013/2014

Variable	Cases *N* = 107(%)	Controls *N* = 214(%)	Odds Ratio (95%CI)	*P*-value
Male Sex	37 (34.6)	104 (48.6)	0.54 (0.3–0.87)	0.017*
Female not pregnant	19 (27.1)	33 (30.0)	1.55 (0.65–3.43)	0.337
Dry season	68 (63.5)	150 (70.1)	1.49 (0.83–2.52)	0.188
Live in rural setting	94 (87.8)	194 (90.6)	1.00 (0.28–3.50)	1.000
Education level				
None	78 (72.9)	172 (80.4)	1.0	
Primary	19 (17.7)	30 (14.0)	1.46 (0.75–2.85)	0.263
Secondary	7 (6.5)	9 (4.2)	2.32 (0.65–8.29)	0.193
Tertiary	3 (2.8)	3 (1.4)	2.53 (0.49–3.14)	0.267
Unsanitary (Open defecation) habits	77 (71.9)	111 (51.9)	2.46 (1.47–4.12)	0.001*
Drunk alcohol 2 weeks before outbreak.	80 (74.7)	151 (70.5)	1.24 (0.73–2.21)	0.420
No soap in the household.	56 (52.3)	89 (42.6)	1.59 (0.98–2.59)	0.060
Never wash hands with soap after defecation.	50 (46.7)	70 (35.0)	1.64 (1.01–2.65)	0.043*
Clean hands with soap before eating	69 (64.5)	141 (65.9)	0.93 (0.55–1.57)	0.789
Did not clean utensils after eating food.	70 (65.4)	94 (44.9)	2.72 (1.60–4.61)	$P < 0.001$*
Drinking untreated water.	58 (54.2)	181 (84.5)	5.19 (2.82–9.54)	$P < 0.001$*
Had contact with animals prior to epidemic.	61 (57.0)	132 (61.7)	0.81 (0.49–1.32)	0.402
Attended funerals 2 weeks before outbreak.	13 (16.6)	14 (9.2)	0.56 (0.55–3.02)	0.556
use the same basin for washing hands	42 (39.3)	75 (35.1)	1.24 (0.73–2.10)	0.420
Ate food from the roadside	43 (40.2)	39 (18.2)	2.88 (1.70–4.84)	$P < 0.001$*
Primary source of water				
Tap water	19 (17.8)	49 (22.9)	1.0	
Bore Hole	82 (76.6)	162 (75.7)	1.34 (0.69–2.58)	0.381
Well	5 (4.7)	2 (1.0)	10.7 (1.15–98.5)	0.037*
Dam	1 (1.0)	1(.5)	2.16 (0.13–34.9)	0.586
Household has no latrine	82 (76.6)	173 (80.4)	0.76 (0.42–1.37)	0.355
Have common bathing practices	59 (58.1)	124 (57.9)	1.16 (0.68–1.99)	0.587
Had recently travelled	27 (25.20)	30 (14.0)	2.04 (1.14–3.63)	0.016*
Did you own or have contacts with animals prior to the epidemic				
No	46 (43.0)	82 (38.3)		
Yes	61 (57.0)	132 (61.7)	0.81 (0.49–1.32)	0.402
If yes which animals				
Pigs	3 (4.9)	9 (6.7)	1	
Cows	24 (39.3)	38 (28.4)	1.59 (0.32–7.88)	0.570
Goats	15 (24.6)	39 (29.1)	1.36 (0.24–7.67)	0.720
Poultry	19 (31.1)	48 (35.8)	0.82 (0.18–3.70)	0.790

*Significant $P < 0.05$.Univariate conditional logistics comparing cases and controls

significantly associated with HEV at bivariate but not at multivariate analysis.

Social events like birth ceremonies, funeral ceremonies, visiting shrines and marriages can cause transmission of disease particularly through contaminated food and water [2, 11]. About 40 cases of jaundice were reported among people who attended a traditional function in Lorikitae village, in Matany Sub County. In this study, livestock ownership was high and contact with animals was common. Participants reported owning pigs (6.5%), cattle (31.8%), goats (27.9%) and chicken (34.3%).

Table 4 Multivariate analysis of independent factors associated with Hepatitis E Virus, Napak (2013/2014)

Variable	Odds Ratio	95% CI	*P*-Value
In the week before the epidemic did you eat roadside food(Yes)	6.11	2.85–13.09	*P* < 0.001*
Did you drink any untreated water(Yes)	6.69	3.15–14.16	*P* < 0.001*
Do you always clean your utensils(No)	3.24	1.55–3.760	0.002*
Education Level			
Primary	1.57	0.67–3.64	0.293
Secondary	5.57	0.94–33.0	0.059
Tertiary	1.54	0.24–9.98	0.650
Primary source of water			
Borehole	0.93	0.40–2.14	0.865
Well	2.86	0.25–32.2	0.394
Dam	1.76	0.09–31.9	0.702
Availability of soap in household(No)	1.78	0.88–3.59	0.106
Season(Wet)	1.42	0.67–3.02	0.368
Occupation-Hunter	1.14	1.03–12.66	0.013*

NB: The model was determined by means of conditional logistic regression, all variables adjusted for age, OR, confidence interval and *P*-Values

Use of Cow dung' is common, this practice consists of drying the cow dung into pieces which are then heated then used as a preservative for Beans and ataapa (Millet), what remains used for cooking. The same cow dung while still wet is used for construction of houses (Manyatas), these are considered potentially hazardous.

However, there was no significant association between HEV and livestock ownership or contact with animals at multivariate analysis. This contrasts the study done in Ghana, which reported 37% sero-prevalence in pig handlers, suggesting that the predominant HEV genotype were zoonotic [7, 25].

The less educated were more likely to confound not washing utensils. They reported poor hygiene practices, unsanitary disposal of fecal matter and also they never had permanent sources of water. Contamination was possible in these groups during the wet seasons. Hunters who had reported frequent movents were at a higher risk of HEV compared to their to their counterparts who had no occupation.

Limitations

This data had at least three limitations. First, the data was reported several months after the outbreak so they are subject to possible recall bias which might affect individual's response. Nevertheless a reference period prior the outbreak was to minimize the bias. Second, in this study we did not take water samples for detection of HEV RNA. However we were able to demonstrate and arrive at the associations in this study using the risk factors. Possible Misclassification Bias since there were no serological test done for controls, but research assistants had a clinical background, thorough screening was done to minimize potential for this bias. Third these investigations might have been susceptible to responder bias because of recently introduced interventions. This could have led to underestimation of our associations.

Conclusions

Findings from this study suggest the existence of a high proportion of cases of HEV infection in the communities of Napak district in Uganda. The detection of HEV was highly suggestive of circulation of cases in this rural population and to the neighboring districts. This epidemic curve demonstrated propagated multi model suggestive of an indirect transmission with higher proportion of cases reported in female and in adults. A high CFR was reported in pregnant women.

Results from the case-control study demonstrate that eating roadside food, drinking untreated water, not cleaning utensils and hunting was associated with increased risk of HEV infection. This suggests transmission by feco-oral route through contaminated water. Surveillance of HEV through mandatory reporting of communicable diseases should continue to enable detection and timely investigation of emerging and reemerging infections. This study supports the need of interventions like vaccines for the most at risk vulnerable groups and other interventions targeting groups such as community health education talks, and routine individual health on treating drinking water are for prevention of HEV transmission.

Abbreviations

CEU: Clinical Epidemiology Unit; CFR: Case fertility rate; CI: Confidence interval; DHO: District health officer; HEV: Hepatitis E Virus; IQR: Inter-quartile range; MoH: Ministry of Health; OR: Odds ratio; RNA: Ribonucleic acid; SOMREC: School of Medicine Research Ethics Committee; UNCST: Uganda National Council for Science and Technology; VHT: Village health Team

Acknowledgements

The authors would like to acknowledge the Makerere University Clinical Epidemiology Unit for scientific guidance, Napak district health directorate, and the research assistants for their tireless effort during the field study, and the study participants who made the study a success.

Funding

Our study was not funded.

Authors' contributions

CK (PHD) participated in the conception, design, and Implementation of the study, statistical analysis, interpretation and drafting of manuscript. KS and KE, CA, SAA, DNO HN participated in study conception, design, implementation and interpretation of the study. HRW participate in study conception, design, and interpretation of the study. JK (PHD) participated in the conception, design, statistical analysis, and interpretation of the study, NI (PHD) participated in the conception, design, interpretation and drafting of manuscript. All authors read and approved the final manuscript and interpretation of the study, NI (PHD) participated in the conception, design, interpretation and drafting of manuscript. All authors read and approved the final manuscript.

Competing interests

The authors declare that they have no competing interests.

Consent for publication

Not applicable.

Ethics approval and consent to participate

Approval to carry out the study was obtained from Makerere Clinical Epidemiology Unit (CEU) School of medicine and research committee (SOMREC), the Uganda National Council of Science and Technology (UNSCT), Ministry of Health (MOH) and Napak district health directorate. The research participants were enrolled into the study only after informed consent had been obtained. Consent for the children was obtained from the parents or guardians. Additional assent was obtained from children over 8 years of age. Consent from community leadership was through local councils. Village health teams (VHTs) identified with the communities and acted as guides to research assistants. These benefited from initial trainings.

Author details

[1]Clinical Epidemiology Unit, School of Medicine, P.O Box 7072, Kampala, Uganda. [2]Epidemiology and surveillance Division, Ministry Of Health, P.O Box 7076, Kampala, Uganda. [3]Makerere University College of Health Sciences, P.O Box 7072, Kampala, Uganda.

References

1. Gerbi GB, Williams R, Bakamutumaho B, Liu S, Downing R, Teshale EH, et al. Hepatitis E as a cause of acute jaundice syndrome in northern Uganda, 2010–2012. Am J Trop Med Hyg. 2015;92(2):411–4.
2. Cummings MJ, Wamala JF, Komakech I, Lukwago L, Malimbo M, Bakamutumaho B, et al. Hepatitis E in Karamoja, Uganda, 2009-2012: epidemiology and challenges to control in a setting of semi-nomadic pastoralism. Trans R Soc Trop Med Hyg. 2014;108(10):648–55. doi:10.1093/trstmh/tru123.
3. Teshale EH, Grytdal SP, Howard C, Barry V, Kamili S, Holmberg SD, et al. Evidence of person-to-person transmission of hepatitis E virus during a large outbreak in Northern Uganda. Clin Infect Dis. 2010;50(7):1006–10. doi:10.1086/651077.
4. Prasida HR, Ahmad I, Ahmad Z, Jameel S. Molecular virology of hepatitis E virus. Semin Liver Dis. 2013;33(1):3–14. doi:10.1055/s-0033-1338110.
5. Lewis HC, Wichmann O, Duizer E. Transmission routes and risk factors for autochthonous hepatitis E virus infection in Europe: a systematic review. Epidemiol Infect. 2010;138(02):145–66.
6. Albetkova A, Drobeniuc J, Yashina T, Musabaev E, Robertson B, Favorov M, et al. Characterization of hepatitis E virus from outbreak and sporadic cases in Turkmenistan. J Med Virol. 2007;79(11):1696–702.
7. Béji-Hamza A, Hassine-Zaafrane M, Khélifi-Gharbi H, Della Libera S, Iaconelli M, Muscillo M, et al. Hepatitis E virus genotypes 1 and 3 in wastewater samples in Tunisia. Arch Virol. 2015;160(1):183–9. doi:10.1007/s00705-014-2251-8.
8. Kim JH, Nelson KE, Panzner U, Kasture Y, Labrique AB, Wierzba TF. A systematic review of the epidemiology of hepatitis E virus in Africa. BMC Infect Dis. 2017;14:308. doi:10.1186/1471-2334-14-308.
9. Dalton HR, Hazeldine S, Banks M, Ijaz S, Bendall R. Locally acquired hepatitis E in chronic liver disease. Lancet. 2007;369(9569):1260.
10. Vitral CL, da Silva-Nunes M, Pinto MA, de Oliveira JM, Gaspar AM, Ferreira MU, et al. Hepatitis A and E seroprevalence and associated risk factors: a community-based cross-sectional survey in rural Amazonia. BMC Infect Dis. 2014;14(1):458.
11. Kmush BL, Nelson KE, Labrique AB. Risk factors for hepatitis E virus infection and disease. Expert Rev Anti-Infect Ther. 2015;13(1):41–53.
12. Purcell RH, Emerson SU. Hepatitis E: an emerging awareness of an old disease. J Hepatol. 2008;48(3):494–503.
13. Isaäcson M, Frean J, He J, Seriwatana J, Innis BL. An outbreak of hepatitis E in Northern Namibia, 1983. Am J Trop Med Hyg. 2000;62(5):619–25.
14. Begum N, Devi SG, Husain SA, Kumar A, Kar P. Seroprevalence of subclinical HEV infection in pregnant women from north India: a hospital based study. Indian J Med Res. 2009;130(6):709–13.
15. Goumba AI, Konamna X, Komas NP. Clinical and epidemiological aspects of a hepatitis E outbreak in Bangui, Central African Republic. BMC Infect Dis. 2011;11(1):93.
16. Mathur P, Arora NK, Panda SK, Kapoor SK, Jailkhani BL, Irshad M. Sero-epidemiology of hepatitis E virus (HEV) in urban and rural children of North India. Indian Pediatr. 2001;38(5):461–75.
17. Howard CM, Handzel T, Hill VR, Grytdal SP, Blanton C, Teshale E, et al. Novel risk factors associated with hepatitis E virus infection in a large outbreak in northern Uganda: results from a case-control study and environmental analysis. Am J Trop Med Hyg. 2010;83(5):1170–3.
18. Guthmann JP, Klovstad H, Boccia D, Hamid N, Pinoges L, Ciglenecki I, et al. A large outbreak of hepatitis E among a displaced population in Darfur, Sudan, 2004: the role of water treatment methods. Clin Infect Dis. 2006; 42(12):1685–91.
19. Kim JH, Nelson KE, Panzner U, Kasture Y, Wierzba TF, et al. A systematic review of the epidemiology of hepatitis E virus in Africa. BMC Infect Dis. 2014;14(1):308.
20. Khuroo MS, Kamili S. Clinical course and duration of viremia in vertically transmitted hepatitis E virus (HEV) infection in babies born to HEV-infected mothers. J Viral Hepat. 2009;16(7):519–23.
21. Kmush B, Wierzba T, Krain L, Nelson K, Labrique AB. Epidemiology of hepatitis E in low-and middle-income countries of Asia and Africa. Semin Liver Dis. 2013;33(01):015–29. Thieme Medical Publishers
22. Meng XJ. Hepatitis E virus: animal reservoirs and zoonotic risk. Vet Microbiol. 2010;140(3):256–65.
23. Labrique AB, Zaman K, Hossain Z, Saha P, Yunus M, Nelson KE, et al. An exploratory case control study of risk factors for hepatitis E in rural Bangladesh. PLoS One. 2013;8(5):e61351.
24. Shrestha A, Lama TK, Karki S, Sigdel DR, Rai U, Mishiro S, et al. Hepatitis E epidemic, biratnagar, Nepal, 2014. Emerg Infect Dis. 2015;21(4):711.
25. Adjei AA, Aviyase JT, Tettey Y, Adu-Gyamfi C, Mingle JA. Hepatitis E virus infection among pig handlers in Accra, Ghana. East Afr Med J. 2009;86(8):359.

7

Correlation between polymorphisms in toll-like receptor genes and the activity of hepatitis B virus among treatment-naïve patients: a case-control study in a Han Chinese population

Yong Lin[1,2†], Zheng-Xiang Gao[1,2†], Xu Shen[1,3†], Mei-Jun Chen[1], Yan-Ting Li[1], Shu-Lian Li[4], Hui-Ling Lin[4], Qi-Feng Zhao[1,3], Fan Liu[1,2] and Jian-Jun Niu[1,5*]

Abstract

Background: Because of the high prevalence and absence of cure for infection, chronic hepatitis B virus (HBV) infection has been acknowledged as a pressing public health issue. Toll-like receptors (TLRs) activate the human innate immune system and the polymorphisms in TLRs may alter their function. The present study aimed to investigate the association between TLR polymorphisms and disease progression of chronic HBV infection.

Methods: During the study period, 211 treatment-naïve patients with chronic HBV infection were recruited, and blood samples were collected from each individual. Matrix-assisted laser desorption/ionization time of flight mass spectrometry was employed to genotype the selected TLR polymorphisms after human genome extraction. In addition, HbsAg, TNF-α, and IL-6 levels were quantified using enzyme linked immunosorbent assay (ELISA). Statistical analyses were conducted to investigate the association between TLR polymorphisms and hepatitis activity, liver function parameters, HbsAg level, and cytokine level.

Results: We did not observe any mutations in rs4986790, rs4986791, and rs5743708 among all study subjects. A logistic regression revealed that mutations in rs3804099 and rs4696480 were associated with milder hepatitis activity. Consistent with the logistic regression, improved liver function parameters and reduced level of both HbsAg and cytokines were also correlated with the mutant carriers of rs3804099 and rs4696480.

Conclusions: TLR mutations were significantly associated with milder hepatitis activity among patients with chronic HBV infection. Therefore, we conclude that the activation of TLR pathways may further intensify the inflammation of hepatocytes, and leads to progression of disease.

Keywords: Toll-like receptors, Hepatitis activity, Immune response, Hepatitis B virus

* Correspondence: niujianjun62@163.com
[†]Equal contributors
[1]Center of Clinical Laboratory, Zhongshan Hospital, Medical College of Xiamen University, 201-209 Hubin South Road, Siming District, Xiamen City 361004, Fujian Province, People's Republic of China
[5]Fujian Provincial Key Laboratory of Chronic Liver Disease and Hepatocellular Carcinoma, Xiamen, Fujian Province, China
Full list of author information is available at the end of the article

Background

Hepatitis B virus (HBV) is a type of DNA virus that belongs to the Hepadnaviridae family, and the genome of HBV consists of small, partially double-stranded DNA containing only 3200 bp in total length. The HBV genome has four overlapping regions and encodes four genes, namely HBsAg (S), HBcAg (C), viral polymerase (P), and the X gene which is closely associated with the development of hepatocellular carcinoma [1]. Unlike most DNA viruses, the replication of HBV involves the reverse transcription of an RNA intermediate, which is more similar to retroviruses. Approximately 1×10^{11} viral particles are generated in an infected patient per day. Due to the poor fidelity of the polymerase, a large number of mutations occur during a highly active infection [2]. When compared with other DNA viruses, HBV possesses a 10-fold higher mutation rate [3]. The evidence suggests that HBV mutations are associated with increased replication activity, vaccine failure, carcinogenesis, occult infection, and drug resistance caused by the selective pressure of antiviral agents. Currently, nucleotide analogues below the cytotoxic threshold are widely applied in clinical practice to treat chronic HBV as well as HIV infection, because HBV and HIV polymerases share a similar function and structure [4]. The major advantage of nucleotide analogues is that they can reduce the viral titer directly and relatively fast; however, the application of nucleotide analogues has not been able to eradicate chronic HBV infection, and prolonged use is associated with the development of drug resistance which considerably reduces efficacy [5]. HBV mutations are the major factor affecting clinical outcome among patients with chronic HBV infection.

Chronic HBV infection is a pressing public health issue because of the large number of individuals affected, in addition to the unfavorable outcomes it causes: such as liver cirrhosis, fibrosis, and hepatocellular carcinoma. Approximately 240 million people suffer from chronic HBV infection worldwide, with deaths attributed to it totaling more than 686,000 people [6]. The prevalence of chronic HBV infection varies from 0.1% to 20% globally and about half of all chronic disease cases and mortality occur in mainland China. The rate of progression to chronic HBV infection is approximately 90% for perinatally acquired infection, from 20% to 50% for infections acquired at 1 to 5 years of age, and less than 5% for adult acquired infection [7]. Young individuals without vaccine protection are thus the highest risk population for developing chronic HBV infection.

Despite the great success yielded from the immunization program, a large number of patients suffer from chronic HBV infection and as such are at increased risk of cancer. Host immunity also plays a role in the progress and outcome of HBV infection [8, 9]. Toll-like receptors (TLRs) are pattern recognition receptors that recognize pathogen- and damage-associated molecular pattern molecules and thus activate the innate immune system. Toll-like receptor-mediated inflammatory signaling pathways have been correlated with a spectrum of liver diseases, such as hepatitis, liver fibrosis, cirrhosis, alcoholic and nonalcoholic liver disease, ischemia/reperfusion injury, liver regeneration, and hepatocellular carcinoma [10, 11]. Therefore, it is imperative to study the association between genetic variants in TLRs and HBV disease progression. To understand the role of genetic variants in TLRs in HBV disease progression, we conducted a case-control study among patients with chronic HBV infection in a Han Chinese population.

Methods

Study subjects

In total, 211 eligible subjects who were recruited from the Department of Gastroenterology, Zhongshan Hospital, Xiamen University between Nov 2015 to Jul 2016. The chronic HBV infection status was confirmed by using commercial enzyme linked immunosorbent assay kits (Wantai BioPharm, Beijing China) and quantified by using real time fluorescence quantitative PCR. Only treatment-naïve patients were enrolled to rule out the confounding effects caused by previous anti-viral treatment, allowing us to investigate the association in the chronic HBV patients with the natural state. Patients were included if following conditions were met: aged from 20 to 79 years old; HBV DNA $\geq 10^7$ copies/ml no prior history of anti-viral treatment. The exclusion criteria were as follows: the co-infection of HCV/HIV, received anti-viral treatment and refusal. All procedures involved in the present study are conformed with the Declaration of Helsinki. The study was approved by the Ethics Committee of Zhongshan Hospital, Xiamen University after formal hearing, and written, informed consent was obtained from all enrolled subjects.

Data collection

The information on gender, age, weight, height, marital status, smoking status, alcohol consumption, and family history of hepatitis was collected from face to face interview with subjects on the date of entry by extensively trained investigators. With the permission from subjects, information on HBV infection (date of HBsAg detection, HBV genotype), and the results of liver function parameters were obtained by reviewing medical records and recorded in the unified form. The precise definition of smoking and alcohol consumption was as follows: individuals who has smoked greater than 100 cigarettes (including hand rolled cigarettes, cigars, cigarillos etc) in their lifetime and has smoked in the last 28 days., and those who consumed one or more alcohol drinks a week for over 6 months were categorized as alcohol drinkers. Fibrosis stage, hepatitis activity, and inflammation grade were established using METAVIR system [12] by liver biopsy in all included subjects.

Sample and genotyping assay of TLRs polymorphisms

For each enrolled subject, a venous blood sample was collected on the date of entry. Blood samples were subjected to centrifugation at 4000 rpm for 10 min to separate serum and blood cells and stored at –78 °C prior to DNA extraction. Human genome DNA was done by using Magna Pure LC 2.0 system (Roche Applied Science, Mannheim, Germany). Six polymorphisms in TLRs including rs10759932, rs3804099, rs4696480, rs4986790, rs4986791 and rs5743708 were genotyped by employing Matrix-Assisted Laser Desorption/ Ionization Time of Flight Mass Spectrometry. All procedures were conducted strictly following the protocol as described by the manufacturer (Sequenom, San Diego CA, USA). A negative water control and reference DNA were employed as quality control measures during the genotyping assay. Moreover, approximately 5% of the samples were randomly selected and repeated for genotyping as duplicated controls. The genotyping call rate was 100% in accordance with the results generated from the platform.

Determination of HbsAg serum level

Human HbsAg ELISA kit (Wantai BioPharm, Beijing China) were used to determine the serum level of surface antigen. The sensitivity and specificity of the ELISA kit we employed for the detection of HbsAg were 100% and 99.85%, respectively. The following is the detailed procedure for HbsAg quantification: (1) Firstly mark three walls as negative control, two wells as positive control and one blank. (2) Pipette 20 µl of specimen diluent to each well except the blank. (3) Then pipette 100 µl of positive control, negative control and serum to their respective wells expect blank, cover with plate sealer and incubate at 37 °C for 1 h. (4) At the end of incubation, remove and discard the plate cover, and add 50 µL HRP-conjugate into each well except blank, and mix by tapping the plate gently. (5) Cover the plate with a new plate sealer, and incubate at 37 °C for 30 min; (6) At the end of the incubation, remove and discard the plate cover. Wash each well 5 times with diluted washing buffer. Each time allow the microwells to soak for 30–60 s. After the final washing cycle, turn down the plate onto blotting paper or clean towel and tap it to remove any remainders. (7) Add 50 µl of Chromogen A and 50 µl Chromogen B solutions into each well including the blank. Incubate the plate at 37 °C for 30 min avoiding light. The enzymatic reaction between the Chromogen solutions and the HRP-Conjugate produces blue color in positive control and HBsAg positive sample wells. (8) Using a multichannel pipette or manually, add 50 µl stop solution into each well and mix gently. Intensive yellow color develops in positive control. (9) Calibrate the plate reader with the blank well and read the absorbance at 450 nm. Calculate the Cut-off value and evaluate the results within 10 min after stopping the reaction.

Serum level of TNF-α (tumor necrosis factor-α) *and IL-6* (Interleukin-6) *assay*

Human TNF-α and IL-6 quantikine ELISA kits (R&D systems, Minneapolis, MN, USA) were employed to evaluate the serum level of corresponding protein. The sensitivity of the ELISA kits we employed for the detection of TNF-α and IL-6 were 5.5 pg/ml and 0.7 pg/ml, respectively. Following is the detailed procedure for TNF-α and IL-6 evaluation: (1) Firstly pipette 50 µl of assay diluent to each well. (2) Then pipette 200 µl of standard, control or serum sample (100 µl for IL-6) to each well, cover with plate sealer and incubate at room temperature for 2 h. (3) Aspirate each well and wash, repeating the process 3 times for a total of 4 washes. (4) Add 200 µL of Conjugate to each well. Cover with a new plate sealer, and incubate at room temperature for 2 h on the shaker. (5) Aspirate and wash for 4 times. (6) Add 200 µL substrate solution to each well. Incubate at room temperature for 30 min on the benchtop, and keep from the exposure of light. (7) Add 50 µL of stop solution to each well. Read at 450 nm within 30 min. Set wavelength correction to 540 nm or 570 nm. (8) Using the software provided by manufacturer to draw a standard curve and read the protein concentrations for each sample.

Statistical analysis

Data analysis was performed by using SPSS software version 19 (IBM, Chicago, IL, USA) unless specified. Continuous variables were presented in the form of mean and standard deviation (SD) or median. As for the categorical variables, the data was presented as frequencies. Comparison was made between carriers of different genotypes of TLR polymorphisms, and student's t-test or Mann-Whitney U test were employed to compare the continuous variables in accordance with the Gaussian distribution. Chi-squared test was used to conduct the comparison on the categorical variables. Hardy-Weinberg equilibrium (HWE) for all studied polymorphisms was calculated using an online calculator (http://scienceprimer.com/hardy-weinberg-equilibrium-calculator). Odds ratios (ORs) and 95% confidence interval (95%CI) were estimated using unconditional logistic regression analysis to evaluate the association between TLR polymorphisms and chronic HBV infection progression. The difference was considered statistically significant when the *P* value was less than 0.05.

Results

Characterization of study subjects

Study subjects included 211 treatment-naïve patients with chronic HBV infection. Among those, 151 were assigned to the mild chronic hepatitis group and the remaining 60 were assigned to the moderate to severe chronic hepatitis group in accordance with the METAVIR system. We enrolled only treatment-naïve patients to eliminate potential confounding caused by antiviral treatment. Simple statistical analyses were used to compare the demographic characteristics between two groups and the results were illustrated in Table 1. The proportion of males in the moderate to severe hepatitis group was significantly higher than the proportion of males in the mild chronic hepatitis group (61.6% vs. 83.3%, $P = 0.002$). The mean BMI in the mild chronic hepatitis group was significantly lower than in the moderate to severe chronic hepatitis group. Surprisingly, the proportion with a family history of hepatitis B was significantly higher in the moderate to severe hepatitis group as compared with the mild chronic hepatitis group (37.1% and 21.7%, respectively, $P = 0.031$). However, we observed no significant difference in age, marital status, smoking status, alcohol consumption, and HBV genotype distribution between individuals in the mild chronic hepatitis group and individuals in the moderate to severe group.

Table 1 Comparison on the characteristics of 211 treatment naïve patients by hepatitis activity

Variables	Mild chronic hepatitis Number (%)	Moderate and severe chronic hepatitis Number (%)	*P* value
Gender			
Male	93(61.6)	50(83.3)	
Female	58(38.4)	10(16.7)	0.002[a]
Age[b]	30.70(7.09)	31.10(7.86)	0.717
BMI[b]	21.40(2.94)	22.36(3.37)	0.040[a]
Marital Status			
Single	40(26.5)	19(31.7)	
Married	108(71.5)	41(68.3)	
Divorced	3(2.0)	0(0.0)	0.513
Smoking Status			
Smokers	17(11.3)	13(21.7)	
Never-smokers	134(88.7)	47(78.3)	0.051
Alcohol consumption			
No	20(13.2)	14(23.3)	
Yes	131(86.8)	46(76.7)	0.072
Family history of hepatitis B			
No	95(62.9)	47(78.3)	
Yes	56(37.1)	13(21.7)	0.031[a]
HBV genotype			
Genotype B	123(81.5)	48(80.0)	
Genotype C	28(18.5)	12(20.0)	0.808

[a] $P < 0.05$
[b] Data was presented in the form of mean (standard deviation)

TLR polymorphisms and hepatitis activity

Table 2 displays the frequency of all genotyped TLR polymorphisms in mild chronic hepatitis group and the moderate to severe chronic hepatitis group. Surprisingly, we observed no mutation in rs4986790, rs4986791, and rs5743708 in the study population; therefore, only data on rs10759932, rs3804099, and rs4696480 were presented in Table 2 and in the rest of the results section. No evidence was found for a significant difference in genotype distribution of rs1075993 between the two groups, as well as in the logistic regression ($P > 0.05$). Regarding the rs3804099 variant, we observed a protective effect against hepatitis progression in both CT heterozygous and CC homozygous (OR 0.44, 95% CI: 0.22–0.89) and (OR 0.14, 95% CI: 0.05–0.43), respectively. Similarly, the favorable genotype TT homozygous at rs4696480, which significantly reduces the possibility of disease progression, also had a protective effect (OR 0.35, 95% CI: 0.15–0.80). However, no association was found for CT heterozygous by logistic regression, and the distribution between the two groups was not significantly different ($P > 0.05$).

Comparison of liver function parameters by TLR polymorphisms

We employed the recessive model to combine homozygous wild type and heterozygotes as one group, and the

Table 2 Association between TLR polymorphisms and hepatitis activity

Genotype	Mild chronic hepatitis Number (%)	Moderate and severe chronic hepatitis Number (%)	Odds Ratio (95%CI)
rs1075993			
TT	83(55.0)	25(41.7)	1(Ref.)
CT	64(42.4)	32(53.3)	1.66(0.90–3.08)
CC	4(2.6)	3(5.0)	2.49(0.52–11.88)
rs3804099			
TT	60(39.7)	41(68.3)	1(Ref.)
CT	50(33.1)	15(25.0)	0.44(0.22–0.89)[a]
CC	41(27.2)	4(6.7)	0.14(0.05–0.43)[a]
rs4696480			
CC	83(55.0)	25(41.7)	1(Ref.)
CT	64(42.4)	32(53.3)	0.98(0.48–1.98)
TT	4(2.6)	3(5.0)	0.35(0.15–0.80)[a]

[a] $P < 0.05$

Table 3 Comparison on liver function parameters by TLR polymorphisms (rs10759932 and rs3804099) in recessive model

Variables	rs10759932 wild type	rs10759932 mutant	*P*	rs3804099 wild type	rs3804099 mutant	*P*
Total bilirubin(umol/L)	18.04(6.15)	21.87(23.24)	0.665	26.56(40.20)	20.43(15.08)	0.320
Direct bilirubin(umol/L)	3.24(2.27)	5.65(14.20)	0.655	8.45(24.88)	4.79(8.98)	0.337
Indirect bilirubin(umol/L)	14.80(5.29)	16.98(11.51)	0.618	19.98(19.24)	16.08(7.90)	0.337
ALT(U/L)	187.00(216.38)	196.13(212.91)	0.911	340.91(362.01)	156.50(123.43)	0.002[a]
AST(U/L)	220.57(228.28)	162.275(170.61)	0.380	231.42(267.27)	145.99(131.27)	0.043[a]
Total protein(g/L)	78.00(5.26)	73.79(6.45)	0.090	72.44(11.15)	74.34(4.36)	0.270
Globulin(g/L)	45.43(5.00)	41.86(4.35)	0.035[a]	41.98(7.26)	42.30(3.27)	0.996
Albumin(g/L)	32.57(3.87)	32.11(4.13)	0.772	31.27(3.50)	32.36(4.24)	0.080

[a]*P* < 0.05

rest of the statistical analysis was based on the comparison between homozygous mutation carriers and remaining subjects. The Student's t-test was employed to estimate the difference in liver function parameters between the wild type and mutant groups. As compared with rs10759932 mutants, wild type carriers had significantly higher globulin levels. As for the rs3804099, we observed significant elevation in both Alanine aminotransferase (ALT) and Aspartate aminotransferase (AST) among the wild type carriers when compared with their counterparts: the mean (and standard deviation) of ALT and AST level in wild type carriers were 340.91 (362.01) and 231.42 (267.27), respectively, while the corresponding figures were reduced to 156.50 (123.43) and 145.99 (131.27) in mutant carriers (See Table 3, Figs. 1 and 2). As shown in Table 4, we found a significant elevation in ALT level when comparing the subjects with different rs4696480 genotypes; however, no significant difference was observed in AST level. In addition, the rs4969480 mutant also maintained a higher level of albumin ($P<0.05$).

Comparison of HbsAg level by TLR polymorphisms

The difference in the HbsAg concentration between carriers with different genotypes was conducted by using Student's t-test after data normalization. As shown in Table 5 and Fig. 3, mutations in rs3804099 and rs4696480 reduced serum level of HbsAg, and the results were consistent with those generated by logistic regression. With regard to rs1075993 genotypes, no significant difference was found between groups, which was similar to previous findings.

Comparison of TNF-α and IL-6 serum level by TLR2 polymorphisms

We compared TNF-α and IL-6 levels by different TLR2 genotypes. Consistent with our previous findings in HbsAg level, we did not observe a significant difference in TNF-α or IL-6 level by rs1075993 genotypes. In addition, null association between TNF-α level and rs3804099 genotypes was also found. However, rs3804099 mutation carriers had a significantly lower level of IL-6 (5.66 ± 2.68) than the carriers of rs3804099

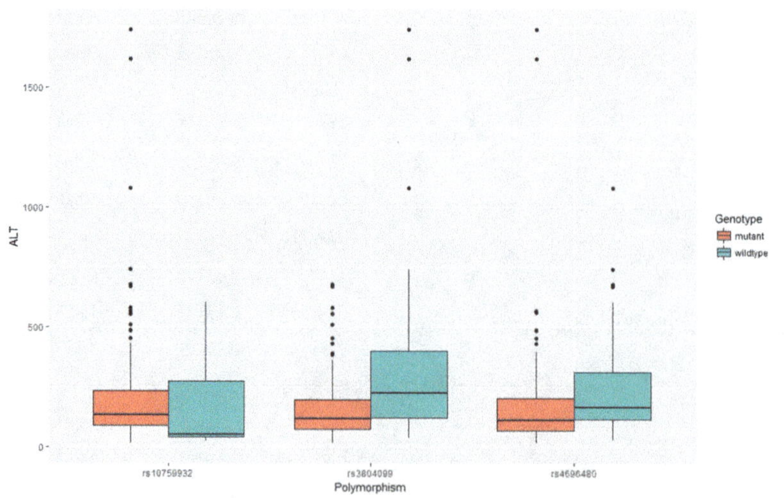

Fig. 1 Comparison of serum levels of ALT between the carriers of wild type of TLR polymorphisms and the mutants among 211 treatment naïve patients

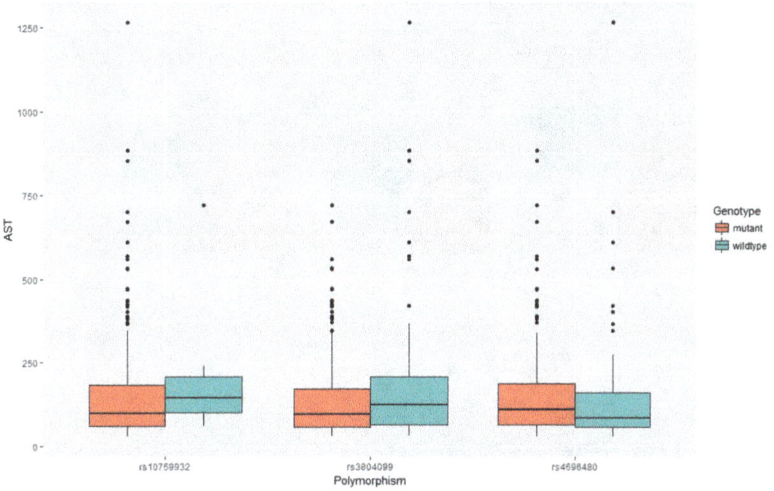

Fig. 2 Comparison of serum levels of AST between the carriers of wild type of TLR polymorphisms and the mutants among 211 treatment naïve patients

wild type (6.38 ± 2.13) ($P = 0.031$). We observed a significant reduction in both TNF-α (2.66 ± 1.09) and IL-6 (5.36 ± 1.86) level for rs4696480 genotypes, between the mutant carrier and their counterparts (TNF-α: 3.39 ± 1.60; IL-6: 6.71 ± 2.73; $P < 0.001$). Detailed data are shown in Table 6.

Discussion

We investigated the association between TLR polymorphisms and hepatitis activity, liver function parameters, and HbsAg level among patients with chronic HBV infection. As expected, we did not observe any mutation in rs4986790, rs4986791, and rs5743708 in the study population. These results are consistent with previous findings conducted by Hang et al. among Chinese cotton and silk textile workers over 20 years of observation [13]. These results are also consistent with the genotype distribution estimated in the Japanese population [14], suggesting the reliability and validity of the genotyping method we employed. Despite the absence of a mutation on several polymorphisms we investigated, the principle finding of this study is that both rs3804099 and rs4696480 in TLR2 mutant carriers present improved liver function parameters and reduced level of HbsAg, suggesting the mutations on TLR genes may have the potential to reduce the inflammatory damage that occurs in chronic HBV infection. The logistic regression results further demonstrate that the mutation in rs3804099 and rs4696480 were inversely associated with hepatitis activity as evaluated by METAVIR.

There has been substantial research undertaken on the role of TLRs related immune response with presence of pathogens, such as HBV. TLR2 has been correlated with the inhibition of HBV replication in human hepatoma cells [15]. However, our results indicate that both synonymous mutation and polymorphism in the promoter of TLR2 were associated with milder hepatitis activity. The concept of TLR2 activation as a protective factor has been recently challenged: Isogawa et al. [16] demonstrated that

Table 4 Comparison on liver function parameters by TLR polymorphism rs4696480 in recessive model

Variables	rs4696480 wild type	rs4696480 mutant	*P*
Total bilirubin(umol/L)	21.29 ± 20.31	21.96 ± 24.13	0.840
Direct bilirubin(umol/L)	5.47 ± 12.62	5.62 ± 14.64	0.941
Indirect bilirubin(umol/L)	17.33 ± 12.60	16.70 ± 10.73	0.706
ALT(U/L)	244.61 ± 198.66	171.61 ± 215.66	0.018[a]
AST(U/L)	152.33 ± 190.18	170.11 ± 163.32	0.482
Total protein(g/L)	73.39 ± 4.88	74.21 ± 7.10	0.386
Globulin(g/L)	42.53 ± 3.27	41.71 ± 4.86	0.204
Albumin(g/L)	30.86 ± 4.09	32.76 ± 3.99	0.001[a]

[a]*P < 0.05*

Table 5 Association between normalized HbsAg level and TLR polymorphisms

Genotypes	Normalized HbsAg level (ng/ml)
rs1075993 wild type	4.69(0.57)
rs1075993 mutant	4.11(0.77)
P	0.051
rs3804099 wild type	4.37(0.78)
rs3804099 mutant	4.07(0.76)
P	0.014[a]
rs4696480 wild type	4.35(0.80)
rs4696480 mutant	4.02(0.73)
P	0.003[a]

[a]*P < 0.05*

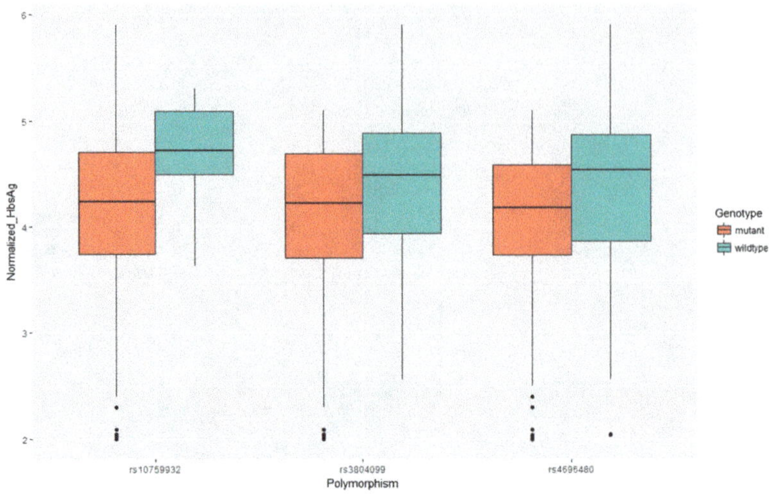

Fig. 3 Comparison of serum levels of HbsAg between the carriers of wild type of TLR polymorphisms and the mutants among 211 treatment naïve patients

TLR2 activation was not able to restrain HBV infection in mice in vivo. Moreover, TLR2 activation leads to the production of pro-inflammatory cytokines such as IL-6 and TNF-α in hepatic non-parenchymal cells and hepatocytes [17], and it has been generally acknowledged that chronic inflammation is closely associated with cellular damage and even carcinogenesis in the presence of HBV infection. Our findings are consistent with previous studies. We found that the mutations in rs3804099 and rs4696480 were associated with a suppressed level of TNF-α and IL-6 among patients with chronic HBV infection as compared with wild type carriers. Further, no significant difference was observed in comparison of TNF-α and IL-6 level by rs1075993 genotypes, which was similar to the results of the liver function parameter comparison. In sum, our results indicate that the mutation in rs3804099 and rs4696480 leads to relieved inflammation, and the pro-inflammatory cytokines were also reduced in the TLR2 mutant carriers. Others have found evidence of increased TLR2 level associated with higher serum ALT concentration and advanced hepatitis activity in an Iranian population [18]. Consistent with the literature, improved liver function parameters were observed among those with the TLR2 mutation. Although the mutations we investigated were either synonymous mutations or in the promoter region, a possible explanation for our results is that the mutations are associated with down-regulated transcription of TLR2, and with reduced TLR2 level. Under such circumstances, the pro-inflammatory cytokines were partially inhibited. Consequently, the inflammation and damage were relieved by the TLR2 mutation.

Table 6 Comparison on TNF-α and IL-6 level by TLR polymorphisms

Genotypes	TNF- α(pg/ml)	IL-6(pg/ml)
rs1075993 wild type	2.94 ± 1.48	6.18 ± 2.47
rs1075993 mutant	3.13 ± 1.34	5.87 ± 2.39
P	0.330	0.357
rs3804099 wild type	3.13 ± 1.47	6.38 ± 2.13
rs3804099 mutant	2.91 ± 1.35	5.66 ± 2.68
P	0.262	0.031 [a]
rs4696480 wild type	3.39 ± 1.60	6.71 ± 2.73
rs4696480 mutant	2.66 ± 1.09	5.36 ± 1.86
P	<0.001 [a]	<0.001 [a]

[a] $P < 0.05$

There is a consensus that HbsAg is the most abundant protein and classic hallmark of HBV infections. The concentration of HbsAg has been correlated with disease progression, as well as with copies of HBV DNA in serum [19], and thus eradicating HbsAg has been the ultimate purpose of antiviral treatment against HBV infection. We found that TLR2 mutations were inversely associated with HbsAg level, a finding supported by Visvanathan et al. [20]. The enhanced HBV replication was associated with up-regulation of the TLR2 pathway leading to increased TNF-α production. Thus, it seems likely that such connections existing between TLR2 and hepatitis activity were mediated by the production of pro-inflammatory cytokines.

Conclusions

We observed a positive association between TLR2 polymorphisms and hepatitis activity. With the evidence acquired from this study, it is possible to identify the patients among those with chronic HBV infection that are likely to progress to an advanced stage, in order to provide targeted interventions. The underlying mechanism between cytokines and TLR2 polymorphisms has yet to be identified. Therefore, further investigation is needed to address this question.

Abbreviations

ALT: Aspartate transaminase; AST: Alanine transaminase; DNA: Deoxyribonucleic acid; ELISA: Enzyme-linked immunosorbent assay; HbsAg: Hepatitis B surface antigen; HBV: Hepatitis B virus; HCV: Hepatitis C virus; HIV: Human immunodeficiency virus; HWE: Hardy-Weinberg equilibrium; RNA: Ribonucleic acid; TLR: Toll-like receptors

Acknowledgements

We are truly grateful to the study participants for their invaluable contribution to this study. The authors would also like to express gratitude to Zhi-Nan Guo and Hong-Fei Mi for their great effort in field investigation. We also would like to express our gratitude to CapitalBio Corporation, Beijing for their assistance on SNP genotyping assay.

Funding

This work was supported by the National Natural Science Foundation of China (No.81471970), the Projects of Xiamen Science and Technology Program (No.3502Z20144022, 3502Z20154015, WSK2010-01), the Natural Science Foundation of Fujian Province (No.2015 J01529), The funders had no role in study design, data collection and analysis, decision to publish, or preparation of the manuscript.

Authors' contributions

JN and FL designed the study and provide the support. YL, ZXG and XS were involved with the execution of the study, include field investigation, data analysis and manuscript preparation. MJC and YTL were involved with the laboratory experiments. SLL, HLL and QFZ were mainly contributed to the sample collection and subject recruitment. All authors have approved the manuscript before submission.

Consent for publication

Not applicable.

Competing interests

The authors declare that they have no competing interests.

Author details

[1]Center of Clinical Laboratory, Zhongshan Hospital, Medical College of Xiamen University, 201-209 Hubin South Road, Siming District, Xiamen City 361004, Fujian Province, People's Republic of China. [2]Institute of Infectious Disease, Medical College of Xiamen University, Xiamen, Fujian Province, China. [3]School of Public Health, Fujian Medical University, Fuzhou, Fujian Province, China. [4]Xiamen Huli District Maternity and Child Care Hospital, Xiamen, Fujian Province, China. [5]Fujian Provincial Key Laboratory of Chronic Liver Disease and Hepatocellular Carcinoma, Xiamen, Fujian Province, China.

References

1. Wang Q, Xu Y, Zhou W, Zhong L, Wen Z, Yu H, et al. The viral oncoprotein HBx of hepatitis B virus promotes the growth of hepatocellular carcinoma through cooperating with the cellular oncoprotein RMP. Int J Biol Sci. 2014;10(10):1181–92.
2. Coleman PF. Detecting hepatitis B surface antigen mutants. Emerg Infect Dis. 2006;12(2):198–203.
3. Datta S, Chatterjee S, Veer V, Chakravarty R. Molecular biology of the hepatitis B virus for clinicians. J Clin Exp Hepatol. 2012;2(4):353–65.
4. Bartholomeusz A, Tehan BG, Chalmers DK. Comparisons of the HBV and HIV polymerase, and antiviral resistance mutations. Antivir Ther. 2004;9(2):149–60.
5. Baxa DM, Thekdi AD, Golembieski A, Krishnan PV, Sharif O, Kizy A, et al. Evaluation of anti-HBV drug resistant mutations among patients with acute symptomatic hepatitis B in the United States. J Hepatol. 2013;58(2):212–6.
6. GBD 2013 Mortality and Causes of Death Collaborators. Global, regional, and national age-sex specific all-cause and cause-specific mortality for 240 causes of death, 1990-2013: a systematic analysis for the global burden of disease study 2013. Lancet. 2015;385(9963):117–71.
7. Busch K, Thimme R. Natural history of chronic hepatitis B virus infection. Med Microbiol Immunol. 2015;204(1):5–10.
8. Lauret E, González-Diéguez ML, Rodríguez M, Rodríguez M, González M, Melón S, et al. Long-term outcome in Caucasian patients with chronic hepatitis B virus infection after HBsAg seroclearance. Liver Int. 2015;35(1):140–7.
9. Milosevic I, Delic D, Lazarevic I, Pavlovic IP, Korac M, Bojovic K, et al. The significance of hepatitis B virus (HBV) genotypes for the disease and treatment outcome among patients with chronic hepatitis B in Serbia. J Clin Virol 2013; 58(1):54-8.
10. Roh YS, Seki E. Toll-like receptors in alcoholic liver disease, non-alcoholic steatohepatitis and carcinogenesis. J Gastroenterol Hepatol. 2013;28(Suppl 1):38–42.
11. Chen Y, Sun R. Toll-like receptors in acute liver injury and regeneration. Int Immunopharmacol. 2011;11(10):1433–41.
12. The French METAVIR Cooperative Study Group. Intraobserver and interobserver variations in liver biopsy interpretation in patients with chronic hepatitis C. Hepatology. 1994;20(1):15–20.
13. Hang J, Zhou W, Zhang H, Sun B, Dai H, Su L, et al. TLR4 Asp299Gly and Thr399Ile polymorphisms are very rare in the Chinese population. J Endotoxin Res. 2004;10(4):238–40.
14. Tahara T, Arisawa T, Shibata T, Hirata I, Nakano H. Absence of common polymorphisms of toll like receptor 4 (TLR4): Asp299Gly, Thr399Ile in patients with Gastroduodenal diseases in Japan. J Clin Biochem Nutr. 2007;40(1):62–5.
15. Zhang X, Ma Z, Liu H, Liu J, Meng Z, Broering R, et al. Role of toll-like receptor 2 in the immune response against hepadnaviral infection. J Hepatol. 2012;57(3):522–8.
16. Isogawa M, Robek MD, Furuichi Y, Chisari FV. Toll-like receptor signaling inhibits hepatitis B virus replication in vivo. J Virol. 2005;79(11):7269–72.
17. Wu J, Meng Z, Jiang M, Zhang E, Trippler M, Broering R, et al. Toll-like receptor-induced innate immune responses in non-parenchymal liver cells are cell type-specific. Immunology. 2010;129(3):363–74.
18. Moradzadeh M, Tayebi S, Poustchi H, Sayehmiri K, Shahnazari P, Naderi E, et al. The possible role of TLR2 in chronic hepatitis B patients with Precore mutation. Adv Virol. 2013;2013:780319.
19. Kim YJ, Cho HC, Choi MS, Lee JH, Koh KC, Yoo BC, et al. The change of the quantitative HBsAg level during the natural course of chronic hepatitis B. Liver Int. 2011;31(6):817–23.
20. Visvanathan K, Skinner NA, Thompson AJ, Riordan SM, Sozzi V, Edwards R, et al. Regulation of toll-like receptor-2 expression in chronic hepatitis B by the precore protein. Hepatology. 2007;45(1):102–10.

8

The current incidence, prevalence, and residual risk of hepatitis B viral infections among voluntary blood donors in China

Ling Li[1†], Tingting Han[2†], Liang Zang[3], Libin Niu[4], Weifang Cheng[5], Hongkeng Lin[6], Ka Yi Li[7], Ruan Cao[8], Binghai Zhao[9], Yuqiang Liu[10], Guojin Ou[1], Xiao Liu[11], Yingjie Qi[12], Yanhua Li[13] and Zhong Liu[1,14*]

Abstract

Background: There are few data available on the prevalence, incidence, and residual risk of transfusion-transmitted HBV (TT-HBV) infections among Chinese blood donors. This study investigated the demographic characteristics of blood donors, as well as the prevalence, incidence, and residual risk (RR) of TT-HBV infections in six large blood centers in different regions of China.

Methods: The demographic characteristics and HBV screening test results of blood donors from six blood centers in different regions in China were collected and analyzed. The hepatitis B surface antigen (HBsAg) yield approach was used to estimate the incidence of HBV. Then, the RR of TT-HBV infections was evaluated using the incidence-window period model.

Results: The majority of donors were between 18 and 35 years old (including 35), with the exception of the Changzhi Blood Center where a majority of donors were between 35 and 55 years old (including 55). The prevalences of HBV were 0.13%, 0.078%, 0.16%, 0.07%, 0.20%, 0.25% in Hefei, Dalian, Changzhi, Kaifeng, Mianyang and Fujian, respectively. The estimated corresponding incidences were 213.44, 161.59, 989.80, 278.05, 125.31 and 352.19 per 10^5 person-years. Using an infectious window period of 59 days, the RR for HBV was estimated to be 34.14, 25.85, 158.35, 44.48, 20.04 and 56.35 per 10^5 person-years in Hefei, Dalian, Changzhi, Kaifeng, Mianyang and Fujian, respectively.

Conclusion: Despite the introduction of more sensitive assays in blood screening, our data revealed that the current residual risk of TT-HBV infection was still high (overall 56.53 per 10^5 py). A continuous monitoring of the residual risk of transfusion-transmitted infections is crucial for safe blood management.

Keywords: HBV, Residual risk, Transfusion, Donors

Background

Blood donor screening practices for the hepatitis B virus (HBV) infections vary from country to country both in terms of the manufacturers of the reagents and the testing methods. Over the past 30 years, the risk of TT-HBV has markedly decreased due to the development of more sensitive hepatitis B surface antigen (HBsAg) tests, the introduction of screening for antibodies against the hepatitis B core antigen (anti-HBc) in some countries, the use of nucleic acid tests (NAT), and improved volunteer donor recruitment processes [1–3]. In recent years, the government of China has taken several measures to improve the safety of the blood supply, which included promulgating a new blood donation law in 1998 [4] and revising standard protocols for donor screening and donation screening processes in 2012 [5]. However, in China, the risk of TT-HBV still remains higher than that of other routinely screened viruses, such as HCV and HIV. When using only HBsAg tests for HBV infection screening, the risk of TT-HBV is high because donors may appear HBsAg-negative but are actually

* Correspondence: liuz@ibt.pumc.edu.cn
†Equal contributors
[1]Institute of Blood Transfusion, Chinese Academy of Medical Sciences and Peking Union Medical College, Chengdu, Sichuan, China
[14]26 Huacai Rd, Longtan Industry Zone, Chenghua District, Chengdu, Sichuan, People's Republic of China
Full list of author information is available at the end of the article

HBV infected, such as those currently in the window period (WP) or at the late stage of infection. This is especially true for the areas with both a high prevalence of HBV and a lack of NAT screening [6]. Also, there is an additional risk associated with chronic OBI. OBI is usually defined (in the blood donor screening context) as an HBV infection without detectable HBsAg, usually presenting itself as anti-HBc positive and, typically, with low levels of HBV DNA. Liang et al. reported that the prevalence of HBsAg in the general population in China fell to 7.2% from 9.8% after the implementation of vaccination against hepatitis B [7], which has played an important role in decreasing the rate of HBV infection.

The residual risk (RR) is different with different blood screening strategies. Using NAT for donor screening can shorten the window period and identify occult HBV infections (OBI) which cannot be detected by HBsAg tests [6]. In terms of the risk for TT-HBV, it is a problem particularly in the countries and/or areas with both a high prevalence of HBV and where NAT for HBV is not used routinely for donor screening [8]. Despite the implementation of donor screening by NAT, there are still a number of countries where there is a residual risk for TT-HBV [9–11].

China still is a developing country with most areas undeveloped economically. At present, most blood centers cannot afford NAT, thus most donations are routinely screened with two ELISA tests for HBsAg in China. This issue has been brought to the attention of the relevant authorities of the Chinese Government, which have decided to pilot NAT testing for HBV, HCV, and HIV in all provincial blood centers in 2015 during blood donor screening [12]. This study aims to evaluate the residual risk (RR) of HBV infections in China before the implementation of NAT. This study will provide helpful data to assess the effectiveness of the implementation of NAT in China. Available data about the prevalence, incidence, and RR of HBV infections among Chinese blood donors is limited. In 2013, Wuping Li and his colleagues reported their findings on the prevalence, incidence, and residual risk of HBV infections in the Anhui Blood Center from 2009 to 2011 [13]. However, that study was based on the data from one single blood center, which is the limitation of that study.

The present study involves six blood centers located in different regions of China (Fig. 1).Hopefully this study was therefore more representative. The aims of the present study were to evaluate the current prevalence, incidences and RR of HBV infections of blood donors among the six blood centers, and to provide guidance for developing and monitoring evidence-based blood donor management strategies to improve the safety of the blood supplies regarding the RR of TT-HBV infections.

Methods

Ethics statement

This study was approved by the Ethics Committee of the Institute of Blood Transfusion, of the Chinese Academy of Medical Sciences & Peking Union Medical College. Written informed consent was obtained from each study participant before the interview, sample collection and testing.

Participants and study procedure

This study was a collaborative effort between the Institute of Blood Transfusion (IBT) of the Chinese

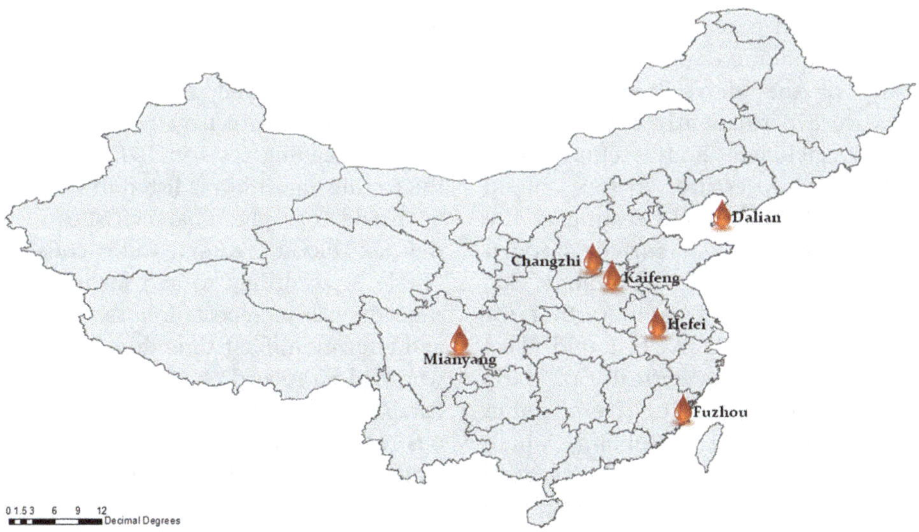

Fig. 1 Geographic Distribution of the Six Blood Centers and the Institute of Blood Transfusion

Academy of Medical Sciences and six blood centers located in different regions of China. The six Chinese regional blood centers were the Anhui Blood Center (Hefei, Anhui, located in the east), Fujian Blood Center (Fuzhou, Fujian, located in the south), Dalian Blood Center (Dalian, Liaoning, located in the north), Changzhi Blood Center (Changzhi, Shanxi, located centrally), Kaifeng Blood Center (Kaifeng, Henan, located centrally) and Mianyang Blood Center (Mianyang, Sichuan, located in the west). Figure 1 shows the geographic distribution of the six blood centers. The study population consisted of all blood donors who donated at one of the six participating blood centers or at one of their mobile blood collection vehicles between July 1, 2014 and June 30, 2015. All blood donations were screened with the serological tests for HIV, HBV, HCV and syphilis. All samples of HBsAg reactive screening were sent to the IBT national reference laboratory for blood donor testing, and then were subjected to the HBsAg neutralization test and anti-HBc tests. Residual risks could be calculated by the HBV yield approach as Li et al. described [13].

History questionnaire and rapid pre-donation screening

Following the "Technical and Operational Guidelines and Procedures for Blood Centers" issued by the Chinese Ministry of Health on December 31, 2011 [12], all six blood centers had the same approach for blood donor screening, requiring all blood donors to pass a routine pre-donation screening process that consisted of a medical history questionnaire, a brief physical examination, and pre-donation rapid screening. The medical history questionnaire included questions about their histories of sexually transmitted diseases, hepatitis, illegal parenteral drug use, sex with multiple partners, and men who had sex with men (MSM). If any of the above items screened positive, the donors were permanently deferred. The physical examination included body temperature, body weight, and blood pressure. Before blood collection, all donors underwent rapid testing at the collection sites for the hepatitis B surface antigen (HBsAg, Rapid Test Kit, Aikang Bio-technology Co., Ltd., Hangzhou, China) as well as rapid testing for Alanine Aminotransferase (ALT) (ALT Rapid Test Kit, Rongsheng Biological Pharmaceutical Co., Ltd., Shanghai, China) and hemoglobin (Hb) (Hemoglobin Assay Kit, Amyjet Scientific Inc., Wuhan, China). The donors with increased ALT levels or a reactive HBsAg result would be temporarily deferred, the samples and information were saved if donors tested HBsAg positive on the rapid test.

Routine screening tests for the HBV infection

All successful donations were subjected to tests on two different HBsAg assays by an enzyme-linked immuno sorbent assay (ELISA). If both testing on the two different HBsAg assays were reactive, the screening test was defined as reactive. If the results from either one of two tests was reactive, the sample was retested in duplicate on the same assay and/or another appropriate kit. The screening test was defined as reactive if either one or two positive reactive results were obtained during retesting of the HBsAg ELISA tests. If both tests showed non-reactive results, the screening test was defined as non-reactive, and the corresponding donation was qualified for transfusion.

All test kits were approved and licensed by the Chinese State Food and Drug Administration (or Food and Drug Administration, FDA). The reagents used for donor screening tests are listed in Table 1, and the assays were performed following the manufacturer's instructions.

Confirmation testing

All HBsAg screening reactive samples, including pre-donation rapid screening and after-donation reactive testing by ELISA, were sent to the IBT national reference laboratory for donor testing where they were tested for HBsAg, via the ELISA test (MONOLISA TM HBsAg ULTRA, BIO-RAD, California, USA), and anti-HBc antibodies (HBcAb ELISA Kit, Beijing WANTAI Biological Pharmacy Enterprise Co. Ltd., Beijing, China). When the signal to cutoff ratio (S/CO) for the HBsAg test was greater than or equal to 1.0, the ELISA for HBsAg tests were considered as reactive, after which they were confirmed with a neutralization assay (Reagent Kit for the Confirmation of the HBV Surface Antigen, ZHUHAI LIVZON DIAGNOSTICS INC., Zhuhai, China). If there was a positive confirmed result by neutralisation, the sample was confirmed as HBsAg-positive; if a negative neutralisation result was obtained, the samples were considered HBsAg-negative. The reagents used for donor screening tests in IBT are listed in Table 2, and the testing algorithm is listed in Fig. 2.

The demographic characteristics of all donors among the six blood centers were collected and analyzed (Table 3) according to and including donor status (first time donors vs repeat donors), gender, age, occupation and education. First-time donors were defined as donors who had no record on file according to the blood center databases. Repeat donors were donors who had a previous record in the databases of the blood centers.

HBsAg-positive donors and/or donations were defined by neutralization assay. The prevalence of HBV infections was calculated by the number of HBsAg positive donations divided by the number of total donations.

Table 1 Screening Test Kits for HBsAg Used at Each Blood Center

Blood Center	First Assay		Second Assay	
	Test Kit	Sensitivity (%) / Specificity (%) / Limit (ng/ml)	Test Kit	Sensitivity (%) /Specificity (%) / Limit (ng/ml)
Anhui	WANTAI (Beijing)	99.5 / 98.5 / 0.03	BIO-RAD (United States)	100 / 97.55 / ND
Fujian	BIO-RAD (United States)	100 / 97.55 / ND	WANTAI (Beijing)	99.5 / 98.5 / 0.03
Dalian	InTec (Xiamen, China)	100 / 98.6 / ND	BIO-RAD (United States)	100 / 97.55 / ND
Changzhi	BIO-RAD (United States)	100 / 97.55 / ND	InTec (Xiamen, China)	100 / 98.6 / ND
Kaifeng	BIO-RAD (United States)	100 / 97.55 / ND	WANTAI (Beijing)	99.5 / 98.5 / 0.03
Mianyang	WANTAI (Beijing)	99.5 / 98.5 / 0.03	BIO-RAD (United States)	100 / 97.55 / ND

ND no data
WANTAI Beijing WANTAI Biological Pharmacy Enterprise Co., Ltd.
BIO-RAD BIO-RAD Clinical Diagnostics
InTec Xiamen InTec Biological Pharmacy Enterprise Co., Ltd.

The incidence rate of HBV was determined by using the HBsAg yield approach as previously described [10]. In the process of the HBV infection, HBsAg becomes detectable earlier than anti-HBc. HBsAg may be transient, while anti-HBc can persist for a long time. Therefore, donations confirmed as HBsAg-positive but non-reactive for anti-HBc can be regarded as newly infected cases that are considered to be HBsAg yield cases. The number of HBsAg yield cases divided by the total number of donations is equal to the HBsAg yield rate. The quotient divided by the length of time a patient has been HBsAg-positive prior to anti-HBc seroconversion (termed the HBsAg yield window, calculated as 44 days) gives an incidence estimate for HBV infections among blood donors [14].

The RR attributable to WP donations was calculated using the following equation:

$$\begin{aligned}\text{HBsAg new infection rate} \\ = \text{Number of HBsAg positive but anti–HBc–negative} \\ / \text{ The total number of donations;}\end{aligned}$$

the ratio of HBsAg new infection rate = HBsAg new infection rate of first – time donors over HBsAg new infection rate of repeat donors;

Table 2 Screening Test Kits Used for IBT

Kit Name	Company	Sensitivity / Specificity (%)
Diagnostic Kit for HBV Surface Antigen (ELISA)	BIO-RAD (United States)	100 / 97.55
HBsAg Neutralization, Antibody to Hepatitis B Surface Antigen (Human)	Livzon (Zhuhai)	no data
Diagnostic Kit for Antibody to Hepatitis Core Antigen (ELISA)	WANTAI (Beijing)	99.4 / 99.1

$$\begin{aligned}\text{Incidence rate for HBV infection} = \text{HBsAg new infection rate} \\ /\text{HBsAg yield window (44 days);}\end{aligned}$$

$$\begin{aligned}\text{RR} = \text{incidence rate for HBV infection} \\ \times \text{ window period (0.16 years or 59 days);}\end{aligned}$$

Data were statistically analyzed using computer software (SPSS 17.0, SPSS, Chicago, IL). An approximate 95% confidence interval (95% CI) was obtained using the Poisson distribution model. The Chi-square test was performed to assess the association between the categorical variants. A *P*-value of <0.05 was used as the cut-off level for significance.

Results

Demographic characteristics of blood donors

From July 1, 2014 to June 30, 2015, a total of 558,089 blood donations were collected at six blood centers located in different areas of China *(see* Figure 1). The demographic characteristics of all of the donors at the six blood center were collected, and the distributions of all demographic characteristics were examined *(see* Table 3). Among the Anhui, Dalian and Fujian Blood Centers, almost 60% of all donations came from donors aged between 18 and 35 years old, while almost 40% at Changzhi, Kaifeng and Mianyang blood centers were of this age group. Across all of the blood centers, the proportions of male and female donors were 63% and 37%, respectively. Donors with a high school education or less contributed to 70% of all donations. Overall, more than half of the donors were employees and students. There were significant differences in the constitutions of donors in terms of their demographic characteristics across the six blood centers in this study.

Serologic prevalence of HBV infections confirmed by the neutralization assay

In this study there were 558,089 donor samples, of which there were 1664 donor samples found to be HBsAg

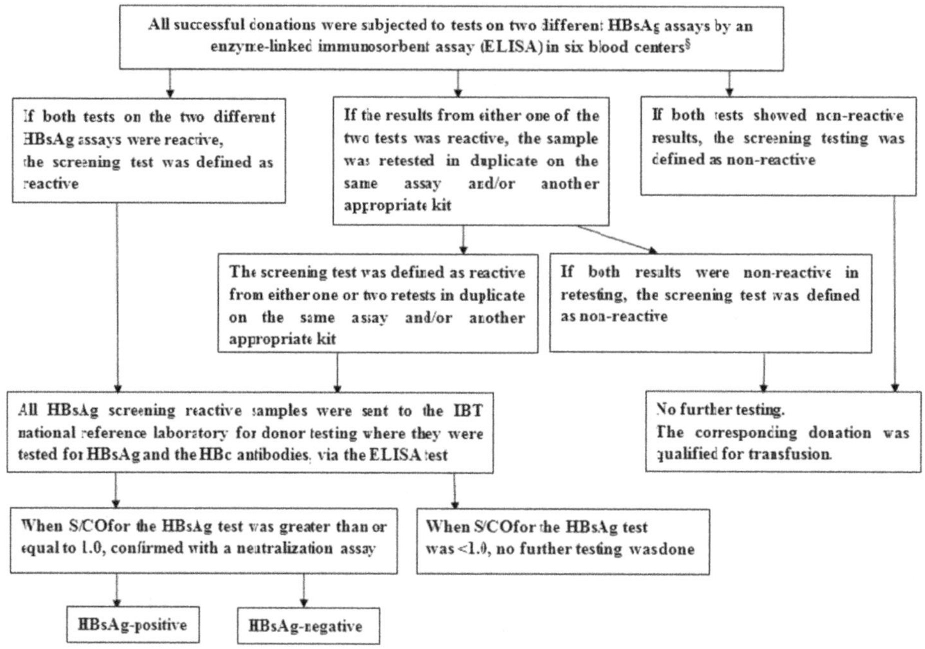

Fig. 2 Testing Algorithm. Note: §: We do not take into account the risk from OBI. HBsAg: Hepatitis B surface Antigen. HBc antibody: Hepatitis B core antibody. ELISA: Enzyme-Linked Immuno Sorbent Assay. IBT: Institute of Blood Transfusion. S/CO: the signal to cutoff ratio

reactive. All of the 1664 samples were tested for anti-HBc and HBsAg and confirmed by neutralisation, and those that were HBsAg positive and anti-HBc positive totaled 484, while those that were HBsAg positive and anti-HBc negative totaled 94; those that were HBsAg negative and anti-HBc positive totaled 326, and those that were HBsAg negative and anti-HBc negative totaled 760. 746 of the 1664 were repeat donors, the mean of interdonation interval for repeat donors was about 11.9 months, and the inter-donation interval data for all 746 repeat donors is shown in Table 4.

Overall, the serologic prevalence of confirmed HBV infections from first-time and repeat donations is shown in Tables 5 and 6. In all, 578 samples were HBsAg positive, confirmed by neutralization assay. The overall prevalence was 0.15%. The seroprevalence of HBsAg was estimated to be 0.13%, 0.078%, 0.16%, 0.07%, 0.20%, and 0.25% at the Hefei, Dalian, Changzhi, Kaifeng, Mianyang and Fujian Blood Centers, respectively. The prevalence of HBsAg varied significantly among the six blood centers, and the prevalence in Fujian was much higher (0.25%) than all of the other blood centers. By contrast, the prevalence in Kaifeng was the lowest (0.07%) among all of the blood centers. Of all 578 reactive samples, 520 (98.5%, 520/528) were from first-time donors.

Estimated incidence of HBV infection using the HBsAg yield approach

In order to estimate HBV incidence accurately, an HBsAg yield window of 44 days was used as described in a previous study [11]. The ratio of HBsAg new infection rate of donations from first-time donors to repeat donors was 6.97, 6.57, 6.94, 4.41, 9.04 and 15.43, at the Hefei, Dalian, Changzhi, Kaifeng, Mianyang and Fujian Blood Centers, respectively. Overall, the estimated incidence rate was 213.44, 161.59, 989.80, 278.05, 125.31 and 352.19 (per 100,000 person-years) in Hefei, Dalian, Changzhi, Changzhi, Kaifeng, Mianyang and Fujian, respectively (*see* Table 7).

RR estimates obtained using the HBsAg yield approach

The residual risk of HBV infection was estimated by applying the refined infectious window-period estimate of 0.16 years (or 59 days) [15] to the derived incidence estimates. The residual risk of HBV infection among blood donations from the participating blood centers is shown in Table 8. The estimated residual risks were 34.14, 25.85, 158.35, 44.48, 20.04 and 56.35 (per 100,000 person-years) in Hefei, Dalian, Changzhi, Kaifeng, Mianyang and Fujian, respectively. The residual risk of Dalian was the highest, approximately 6 times that of Fujian, which had the lowest residual risk.

Discussion

In China, most donations were routinely subjected to screening for HBsAg by ELISA twice. The remaining few blood centers screen HBV infection by ELISA(×1) plus NAT. However, due to the transient nature of the HBsAg detectable period during the HBV infection process, and also due to the lack of routine screening

Table 3 Demographic Characteristics of all Donors Across Six Blood Centers from June, 2014 to July, 2015

Blood Centers	Anhui	Dalian	Changzhi	Kaifeng	Mianyang	Fujian
Donors Status						
First-Time	60,812(62.26%)	38,503(49.75%)	10,643(32.43%)	40,227(67.11%)	18,889(41.52%)	43,384(51.92%)
Repeat	36,856(37.74%)	38,892(50.25%)	22,174(67.57%)	19,711(32.89%)	26,605(58.48%)	40,170(48.08%)
Gender						
Male	65,105(66.66%)	48,496(62.66%)	20,790(63.35%)	38,942(64.97%)	27,742(60.98%)	50,124(59.99%)
Female	32,563(33.34%)	28,899(37.34%)	12,027(36.65%)	20,996(35.03%)	17,752(39.02%)	33,430(40.01%)
Age Group						
18~25	42,212(43.22%)	32,597(42.12%)	2701(8.23%)	11,688(19.50%)	9313(20.47%)	28,450(34.05%)
25~35	27,328(27.98%)	21,421(27.68%)	7269(22.15%)	15,740(26.26%)	10,150(22.31%)	21,933(26.25%)
35~45	18,762(19.21%)	15,439(19.95%)	13,199(40.22%)	19,234(32.09%)	16,005(35.18%)	20,989(25.12%)
45~55	8907(9.12%)	7536(9.74%)	8765(26.71%)	11,976(19.98%)	9276(20.39%)	10,854(12.99%)
55~60	459(0.47%)	402(0.52%)	883(2.69%)	1301(2.17%)	751(1.65%)	1329(1.58%)
Occupation						
Farmers	5801(5.94%)	3243(4.19%)	12,270(37.39%)	16,405(27.37%)	5687(12.50%)	2565(3.07%)
Workers	10,206(10.45%)	12,027(15.54%)	5907(18.00%)	11,286(18.83%)	4841(10.64%)	2423(2.90%)
Students	23,020(23.57%)	18,103(23.39%)	1414(4.31%)	5580(9.31%)	4599(10.11%)	14,647(17.53%)
Soldiers	1845(1.89%)	859(1.11%)	98(0.30%)	623(1.04%)	641(1.41%)	1504(1.80%)
Teachers	2724(2.79%)	410(0.53%)	755(2.30%)	468(0.78%)	1210(2.66%)	/
Civil Servants	3437(3.52%)	186(0.24%)	1195(3.64%)	336(0.56%)	1843(4.05%)	4278(5.12%)
Doctors	4189(4.29%)	573(0.74%)	597(1.82%)	2242(3.74%)	3071(6.75%)	3175(3.81%)
Staff	24,026(24.60%)	2748(3.55%)	2110(6.44%)	22,914(38.23%)	3662(8.05%)	19,518(23.36%)
Other	22,414(22.95%)	39,247(50.71%)	8470(25.81%)	84(0.14%)	19,940(43.83%)	35,444(42.42%)
Education						
Below High School	18,645(19.09%)	22,174(28.65%)	15,765(48.04%)	21,799(36.37%)	14,185(31.18%)	31,458(37.65%)
High School and	42,662(43.68%)	21,733(28.08%)	14,407(43.90%)	30,784(51.36%)	22,893(50.32%)	23,111(27.66%)
Associate Degree						
Bachelor's Degree	22,044(22.57%)	20,726(26.78%)	2543(7.75%)	5556(9.27%)	7670(16.86%)	28,525(34.14%)
Master's Degree	3340(3.42%)	805(1.04%)	30(0.09%)	1091(1.82%)	669(1.47%)	460(0.55%)
Others	10,977(11.24%)	11,958(15.45%)	72(0.22%)	707(1.19%)	77(0.17%)	/
Sum up	97,668	77,395	32,817	59,938	45,494	83,554
Total	396,866					

testing for anti-HBc antibodies, the residual risk of HBV infection has remained high in China [8, 13, 16]. In order to develop an evidence-based, efficient and safe blood donor screening strategy and/or policies to decrease the RR of HBV infections, it is essential to have epidemiological information regarding the prevalence, incidence and RR of HBV infections and the associated demographic characteristics of both high-risk and low-risk populations of voluntary blood donors. The demographic characteristics of volunteer blood donors in different blood centers in China were quite different. For example, the percent of the first time donors among the six blood centers ranged from 32.43% to 67.11% of all donations. The proportion of young donors 18 to 25 years old was 43.22% of all donations at the Anhui Blood Center, but only 8.23% at the Changzhi Blood

Table 4 The interdonation interval data for all 746 repeat donors

The interdonation interval (month)	6-9(including 9)	9-12	12-15	15-18	18-21	21-24	>24 Total
Donors	339	194	62	34	41	57	19,746
Mean(month)	11.9						

Table 5 HBsAg Prevalence by Blood Center / Bank Among all Donors (First-Time and Repeat)

Blood Center	Donations (Total)	First-Time			Repeat			Prevalence(%) (Among all Donors)
		Donations	Number of HBsAg Confirmed Positive	Prevalence (%) (95% Confidence Intervals)	Donations	Number of HBsAg Confirmed Positive	Prevalence (%) (95% Confidence Intervals)	
Hefei	97,668	60,812	115	0.19 (0.15-2.23)	36,856	10	0.027 (0.01-0.04)	0.13 (0.11-0.15)
Dalian	77,395	38,503	52	0.14 (0.09-0.17)	38,892	8	0.02 (0.01-0.04)	0.08 (0.06-0.09)
Changzhi	32,817	10,643	40	0.38 (0.26-0.49)	22,174	12	0.05 (0.02-0.08)	0.16 (0.12-0.20)
Kaifeng	59,938	40,227	36	0.09 (0.06-0.12)	19,711	4	0.02 (0.004-0.04)	0.07 (0.05-0.09)
Mianyang	45,494	18,889	77	0.41 (0.32-0.50)	26,605	12	0.05 (0.02-0.07)	0.20 (0.16-0.24)
Fujian	83,554	43,384	200	0.46 (0.40-0.52)	40,170	12	0.03 (0.013-0.05)	0.25 (0.22-0.29)
Total	396,866	212,458	520	0.24 (0.22-0.27)	184,408	58	0.03 (0.02-0.04)	0.15 (0.13-0.16)

Center. Meanwhile, the proportion of middle aged donors 35 to 55 years old was 28.33% of all donations at the Anhui Blood Center, but was 66.93% at the Changzhi Blood Center. There were also some differences in the occupations and education levels at the different blood centers. For instance, 37.39% of donors were farmers, 18.00% were workers and 4.31% were students at the Changzhi Blood Center, while these proportions were 3.07%, 2.9% and 17.53%, respectively, at the Fujian Blood Center. 91.94% of donors had either received an Associate's degree, a high school diploma or below at the Changzhi Blood Center, while this figure was 56.68% at the Dalian Blood Center. However, some similarities were noted among different blood centers regarding the gender of the donors; namely male donors comprised the majority of donors (with a mean of 61%) at all of the blood centers. In addition, more than half of all donors at all of the blood centers were under 35 years old in this study except for those at the Changzhi Blood Center (see Table 3).

The differences found in the demographic characteristics at different blood centers may have contributed to the differences of estimated residual risks at the blood centers. A higher RR was found at Changzhi (158.35 per 100,000 donations per year), while the lowest was found at Mianyang (20.04 per 100,000 donations per year) (see Table 7). According to the characteristics of the blood donors, most of the blood donors were first-time donors, and only Changzhi had the most repeat blood donors, reaching 67.57%. Theoretically, and according to published data, repeat donors have a lower RR for infectious diseases [12, 14]. However, the results of this study showed that the HBV incidence and residual risks at Changzhi were the highest. With regards to the age of the blood donors, most of them were under the age of 35, but most (70%) donors at Changzhi were over 35 years old. China began nationwide hepatitis B vaccinations in 1992, so the residual risk of donors under 35 years old is lower than that of donors above 35 years old. Perhaps this is thus a major cause of Changzhi having the highest residual risk. This data also proved that the HBV vaccine in China has been successful, and it shows that hepatitis B vaccination can effectively reduce residual risks. Second, the proportion of farmers at the Changzhi Blood Center was 37.39%, much higher than the proportions at the other five blood centers. (These proportions ranged from 3.07% at the Fujian Blood Center to 27.37% at the Kaifeng Blood Center. See Table 3). Due to economic barriers and other multivariate factors, farmers had the lowest vaccination rate, which again could have led to their higher susceptibility to HBV infections. Third, the

Table 6 HBV Prevalence for Blood Donors Above and Below 35 Years Old

Blood Center	Donations	Below 35			Over 35			P-value	Total Prevalence
		Donations	Number of HBsAg confirmed positive	Prevalence	Donations	Number of HBsAg Confirmed Positive	Prevalence		
Hefei	97,668	69,540	38	0.06%	28,128	87	0.31%	<0.001	0.13%
Dalian	77,395	54,018	16	0.03%	23,377	44	0.19%	<0.001	0.08%
Changzhi	32,817	12,671	11	0.09%	20,146	41	0.20%	0.01	0.17%
Kaifeng	59,938	27,428	12	0.04%	32,510	28	0.09%	0.045	0.07%
Mianyang	45,494	19,463	21	0.11%	26,031	68	0.26%	<0.001	0.20%
Fujian	83,554	50,383	55	0.11%	33,171	157	0.47%	<0.001	0.25%
Total	396,866	233,503	153	0.07%	163,363	625	0.38%	<0.001	0.20%

Table 7 HBsAg Incidence by Blood Center/ Bank Among First-Time and Repeat Donors

Blood Center	First-Time		Repeat			Ratio of[a] HBsAg new infection rate	Yield Window (year)	Incidence (per 10^5 py)
	Number of HBsAg Confirmed Positive, Anti-HBc Negative	Incidence (per 10^5 py)	Number of HBsAg Confirmed Positive, Anti-HBc Negative	Yield Rate (per 10^5 py)	Incidence (per 10^5 py)			
Hefei	13	315.39	2	5.43	45.25	6.97	0.12	213.3
Dalian	36	281.52	2	5.14	42.85	6.57	0.12	161.59
Changzhi	5	2347.34	9	40.59	338.23	6.94	0.12	989.80
Kaifeng	10	372.89	2	10.15	84.56	4.41	0.12	278.05
Mianyang	2	261.14	5	3.47	28.89	9.04	0.12	125.31
Fujian	6	640.19	2	4.98	41.19	15.43	0.12	352.19
Total	72	773.49	22	11.93	99.42	7.78	0.12	197.38

[a]The HBsAg new infection rate in repeat donors is the HBsAg+/HBc antibody- prevalence, and the incidence for HBV infections in first-time donors is equal to the incidence for HBV infections in repeat donors multiplied by the ratio of HBsAg new infection rate (the ratio of HBsAg new infection rate = HBsAg new infection rate of first-time donors over HBsAg new infection rate of repeat donors). The overall incidence for HBV infections in all donors is the percentage of incidence in first-time donors plus the percentage of incidence in repeat donors. For Hefei, $315.18 \times 10^{-5} \times 0.6226$ (Number of first-times / number of first-times + number of repeats = 60,812 / 97,668) + $45.22 \times 10^{-5} \times 0.3774 = 196.23 \times 10^{-5} + 17.07 \times 10^{-5} = 213.3 \times 10^{-5}$)
The residual risk calculation model used in this study is one of the more suitable computational models in the absence of nucleic acid detection. Based on the results of the last two blood tests, it is possible to extrapolate whether the recent donors have a new infection. However, for the first-time donors, the new infection ratio cannot be determined or calculated directly. Therefore, this model is adopted to indirectly establish the incidence and residual risk of the first-time donors

proportion of donors without a high school education was relatively high at the Changzhi Blood Center. These donors may have had a relatively low level of health knowledge, which also could have accounted for their elevated rates of HBV infection. The findings in this study are very interesting, because the evidence above indicates that the evaluation of residual risks should take into consideration not only the proportions of first time and repeat donors, but also their ages, occupations and education backgrounds.

TT-HBV can still occur after transfusion, even though the carrier blood has tested negative for HBsAg. Apart from occult HBV infections, there remains a limitation in the model that was used to estimate the residual risk of HBV, because neither the window period nor the incidence of donor HBV infections is precisely known. Thus, theoretically, the actual infection risk may be underestimated, which might not accurately reflect infectivity. However, the estimated result of Li's model can still be used to evaluate the safety of blood supplies.

Some countries and/or regions have low prevalence of HBV infections, such as Canada and Hong Kong. These two locations exhibit low residual risks of 1:1,700,000 [17] and 1:22,000 [9], respectively, whereas China has a moderate-to-high residual risk for HBV infections (about 1:13,670 in Shanghai) [18]. Although the prevalence of HBsAg in the Chinese population has dropped to 7.2% in 2006 from 9.8% since the implementation of the nation-wide HBV vaccination program in 1992, the prevalence of HBV infections in China is still high [7, 8, 13, 18]. Continued efforts are still needed in donor education, improving donor recruitment and screening strategies. The incidence window period model used in this study can also be used to evaluate the potential impact of HBV NAT implementation by calculating the expected percentage residual risk reduction and yield of a particular assay system [19]. Per the request of the Chinese Ministry of Health, NAT testing for HBV, HCV, and HIV will have been piloted in all provincial blood centers by 2015 [9]. This may decrease the residual risk of TT-HBV markedly.

Table 8 HBsAg Residual Risk by Blood Center/ Banks Among First-Time and Repeat Donors

Blood Center	First-time		Repeat		Window Periods in Year	Overall (per 10^5 py)
	Incidence (per 10^5 py)	Residual risk (per 10^5 py)	Incidence (per 10^5 py)	Residual risk (per 10^5 py)		
Hefei	315.39	50.46 (6.13-182.04)	45.25	7.24 (0.88-26.12)	0.16	34.14
Dalian	281.52	45.04 (5.46-162.62)	42.85	6.85 (0.83-24.75)	0.16	25.85
Changzhi	2347.34	375.57 (64.40-721.85)	338.23	54.12 (9.28-104.01)	0.16	158.35
Kaifeng	372.89	59.66 (7.22-215.38)	84.56	13.53 (1.64-48.84)	0.16	44.48
Mianyang	261.14	41.78 (3.98-65.31)	28.89	4.62 (0.44-7.22)	0.16	20.04
Fujian	640.19	102.43 (12.39-369.78)	41.19	6.59 (0.80-23.96)	0.16	56.35
Average	703.08	112.49 (15.04-187.96)	96.83	15.49 (1.93-24.16)	0.16	56.53

Limitations

This study may underestimate the incidence of HBV infections due to its definition of an infection incident and because its risk estimates do not take into account the risk from OBI. The numbers of HBsAg positive and anti-HBc negative tests in each region are low, leading to a general lack of precision in RR calculations (see the wide 95% CIs). In terms of limitations, the incidence calculations are sensitive to assumptions around the window period. In addition, the study may have a number of other limitations around window period estimates. Although, this study included six different locations of blood centers from a diversity of geographical areas, it still may not be representative of all of China.

Conclusion

Despite the introduction of more sensitive assays in blood donor screening, our data revealed that the current residual risk of transfusion-transmitted HBV infection is still high (overall 56.53 per 10^5 py). To improve the safety of blood supplies, we need to continue to educate blood donors and improve donor recruitment and screening strategies. NAT for blood donor screening is needed in China, which may markedly decrease the RR for HBV infections and improve the safety of blood supplies. It is worth considering testing for anti-HBc during blood donor screening in China.

Abbreviations

ALT: Alanine aminotransferase; ELISA: Enzyme-linked immuno sorbent assay; HBc antibody: Hepatitis B core antibody; HBsAg: Hepatitis B surface antigen; NAT: Nucleic acid tests; OBI: Occult HBV infection; RR: Residual risk; S/CO: The signal to cutoff ratio; TTHBV: Transfusion-Transmitted HBV; WP: Window period

Acknowledgements

The authors would like to thank all of the people working at the Anhui Blood Center, Fujian Blood Center, Dalian Blood Center, Changzhi Blood Center, Kaifeng Blood Center and Mianyang Blood Center for collecting samples and information on donors. The authors also want to thank Dr. Yonghua Yin for providing help on this manuscript.

Funding

This study was funded by the PUMC Youth Fund (3332015121) and the CAMS Initiative for Innovative Medicine (2016-I2M-3-024).

Consent to publish

Not Applicable.

Authors' contributions

LL and TH conceived and designed the experiments and gave their critical views on the writing of the manuscript. LZ, LN, CW, LH, CR, BZ, YL1 (Yuqiang Liu) and YQ collected samples and acquired the data. KL analyzed the data and revised the manuscript. GO and XL performed the experiments and analyzed the data. ZL and YL2 (Yanhua Li) also gave their critical views on the writing of the manuscript. All of the authors read and approved of the final manuscript.

Competing interests

The authors declare that they have no competing interests.

Author details

[1]Institute of Blood Transfusion, Chinese Academy of Medical Sciences and Peking Union Medical College, Chengdu, Sichuan, China. [2]No. 1 People's Hospital of Anqing, Anqing, Anhui, China. [3]Dalian Blood Center, Dalian, Liaoning, China. [4]Changzhi Blood Center, Changzhi, Shanxi, China. [5]Anhui Blood Center, Hefei, Anhui, China. [6]Fujian Blood Center, Fuzhou, Fujian, China. [7]Cooper Medical School of Rowan University, Camden, USA. [8]Mianyang Blood Center, Mianyang, Sichuan, China. [9]Nanchong Blood Center, Nanchong, Sichuan, China. [10]Kaifeng Blood Center, Kaifeng, Henan, China. [11]No. 1 People's Hospital of Deyang, Deyang, Sichuan, China. [12]Anhui Provincial Infection Hospital, Hefei, Anhui, China. [13]Department of Pathology, New York University School of Medicine, NYU Langone Health, New York, USA. [14]26 Huacai Rd, Longtan Industry Zone, Chenghua District, Chengdu, Sichuan, People's Republic of China.

References

1. Candotti D, Allain JP. Transfusion-transmitted hepatitis B virus infection. J Hepatol. 2009;51(4):798–809.
2. Niederhauser C. Reducing the risk of hepatitis B virus transfusion-transmitted infection. J Blood Med. 2011;2:91–102.
3. Alter HJ, Houghton M. Hepatitis C virus and eliminating post-transfusion hepatitis. Nat Med. 2000;6(10):1082–6.
4. Blood Donation Law [Internet]. Beijing: NHFPC; 1997. Available from: http://www.gov.cn/banshi/2005-08/01/content_18963.htm. Accessed 20 Mar 2016.
5. Technical and operational guidelines and procedures for blood centers [Internet]. Beijing: MOH; 2012. Available from: www.gov.cn/gzdt/2012-02/28/content_2078097.htm. Accessed 1 Jan 2016
6. Allain JP. Occult hepatitis B virus infection: implications in transfusion. Vox Sang. 2004;86(2):83–91.
7. Liang XBS, Yang W, Wang L, et al. Evaluation of the impact of hepatitis B vaccination among children born during 1992-2005 in China. J Infect Dis. 2009;200:39–47.
8. Li C, Xiao X, Yin H, He M, Li J, Dai Y, et al. Prevalence and prevalence trends of transfusion transmissible infections among blood donors at four Chinese regional blood centers between 2000 and 2010. J Transl Med. 2012;10:176. https://doi.org/10.1186/1479-5876-10-176.
9. Tsoi W-C, Lelie N, Lin C-K. Enhanced detection of hepatitis B virus in Hong Kong blood donors after introduction of a more sensitive transcription-mediated amplification assay. Transfusion. 2013;53:2477–88.
10. Weusten J, van Drimmelen H, Vermeulen M, Lelie N. A mathematical model for estimating residual transmission risk of occult hepatitis B virus infection with different blood safety scenarios. Transfusion. 2017;57:841–9.
11. Seed CR, Kiely P. A method for estimating the residual risk of transfusion-transmitted HBV infection associated with occult hepatitis B virus infection in a donor population without universal anti-HBc screening. Vox Sang. 2013; 105:290–8.
12. National blood banks will use nucleic acid test to reduce the risk of infection in 2015 [Internet]. Beijing: NHFPC; 2015. Available from: http://www.gov.cn/xinwen/2015-01/12/content_2803435.htm. Accessed 21 Jan 2016
13. Li W, Gao Z, Yang C, Li J, Li L, Lv R, et al. The estimation of prevalence, incidence, and residual risk of transfusion-transmitted human hepatitis B infection from blood donated at the Anhui blood center, China, from 2009 to 2011. PLoS One. 2013;8(9):e73472.
14. Taira R, Satake M, Momose S, Hino S, Suzuki Y, Murokawa H, et al. Residual risk of transfusion-transmitted hepatitis B virus (HBV) infection caused by blood components derived from donors with occult HBV infection in Japan. Transfusion. 2013;53(7):1393–404.
15. Schreiber GB, Busch MP, Kleinman SH, Korelitz JJ. The risk of transfusion-transmitted viral infections. The retrovirus epidemiology donor study. N Engl J Med. 1996;334(26):1685–90.

16. Centers for Disease Control and Prevention (CDC). Progress in hepatitis B prevention through universal infant vaccination. Morb Mortal Wkly Rep. 2007;56(18):441–5.
17. O'Brien SF, Yi Q-L, Fan W, Scalia V, Fearon MA, Allain J-P. Current incidence and residual risk of HIV. HBV HCV Canadian Blood Services Vox Sanguini. 2012;103:83–6.
18. Liu Y, Xu W, Jia Y, Wu X, Cai J, Liu X, Zhihua S. The residual risk of hepatitis B infection among repeat blood donors in shanghai Fengxian region. Chin J Blood Transfus. 2012;25(1):50–2.
19. Kleinman SH, Busch MP. Assessing the impact of HBV NAT on window period reduction and residual risk. J Clin Virol. 2006;35:34–40.

9

Guillain-Barre syndrome caused by hepatitis E infection

Xiaoqin Zheng, Liang Yu, Qiaomai Xu, Silan Gu and Lingling Tang*

Abstract

Background: Hepatitis E infection is a global disorder that causes substantial morbidity. Numerous neurologic illnesses, including Guillain–Barre syndrome (GBS), have occurred in patients with hepatitis E virus (HEV) infection.

Case presentation: We report a 58 year-old non-immunocompromised man who presented with progressive muscle weakness in all extremities during an episode of acute HEV infection, which was confirmed by measuring the anti-HEV IgM antibodies in the serum. Both cerebrospinal fluid examination and electrophysiological study were in agreement with the diagnosis of HEV-associated GBS. Following the treatment with intravenous immunoglobulin, the patient's neurological condition improved rapidly.

Conclusions: HEV infection should be strongly considered in patients with neurological symptoms, especially those with elevated levels of liver enzymes.

Keywords: Hepatitis E infection, Guillain–Barre syndrome, Viral hepatitis, Extra-hepatic manifestations

Background

Hepatitis E virus (HEV) infection, one of the most common causes of acute viral hepatitis, is an important public-health concern and leads to substantial morbidity [1]. HEV causes acute and chronic hepatitis, but most of these infections are asymptomatic [2]. In symptomatic patients, HEV can cause fulminant acute hepatitis, fibrosis, or cirrhosis [3, 4] Numerous extra-hepatic manifestations, including many neurological illnesses, are associated with acute or chronic hepatitis E [5]. In this article, we report a rare case of a patient clinically diagnosed with Guillain-Barre syndrome (GBS) due to acute HEV infection. We also reviewed English language scientific literature for the clinical characteristics of HEV associated with GBS.

Case presentation

A 58 year-old non-immunocompromised man presented general fatigue, anorexia, cough, mild jaundice, and excretion of tea-colored urine for 7 days. He was referred to a local hospital, wherein his liver function tests showed elevated levels of aspartate aminotransferase (AST) at 273 U/L, alanine aminotransferase (ALT) at 664 U/L, total bilirubin at 51.8 μmol/L, and conjugated bilirubin at 20.5 μmol/L. Serological study was positive for IgM antibodies for HEV. A working diagnosis of acute hepatitis E was performed, and liver protection treatment was applied to the patient. However, on the 4th day of admission, the patient complained about progressive muscle weakness on his lower limbs, numbness, and abnormal pinprick sensation in his plantar that render him unable to walk. The patient was subsequently transferred to our hospital for further treatment because of the rapidly progressive symmetrical weakness of his lower and upper limbs.

The patient had a history of recovered schistosomiasis. He had never been exposed to a polluted environment or affected animals. He also had no history of blood transfusions, risky sexual behavior, or drug addiction.

Upon admission, general examination on the patient revealed unremarkable findings. His temperature was 36.4 °C, and his blood pressure was 130/99 mmHg. Physical examination showed asthenia, jaundice, blepharoptosis, and paresthesia. His cranial nerve

* Correspondence: 1196040@zju.edu.cn
Zhejiang University First Affiliated Hospital State Key Laboratory for Diagnosis and Treatment of Infectious Diseases, Hangzhou, Zhejiang, China

examination showed unilateral facial nerve palsy, Romberg's sign and the straight leg raising test was positive. Motor weakness was present in all limbs, with power of 4/5 in the upper limbs and 2/5 in the lower limbs. His triceps, biceps, and brachioradialis reflexes were normal, whereas his patellar and Achilles tendon reflexes were absent bilaterally. Two days after admission, he developed dysphagia, choking, areflexia and labored breathing. Neurological examination showed and unilateral cranial palsy with left blepharoptosis, flat nasolabial fold and incomplete eyelid closure of right side. Muscle weakness in his four limbs progressed rapidly. The power of the upper extremity was 2/5 for the proximal muscles and 4/5 for the distal muscles. The power grade of both proximal and distal legs was 1/5. GBS was suspected, and lumbar puncture was conducted on the 2nd day. Cerebrospinal fluid (CSF) examination showed 0/μL monocyte, 4.6 mmol/L glucose level, and 275.3 mg/dL protein level, which suggested albuminocytologic dissociation. Nerve conduction studies showed evidence of demyelinating neuropathy with dysfunction of motor and sensory nerve fibers.

Laboratory investigations showed 20 μmol/L total bilirubin, 10 μmol/L conjugated bilirubin, 126 U/L alanine aminotransferase, and 160 U/L gamma-glutamyl transpepidase. Serologic studies for IgM and IgG anti-HEV were both positive. No serological evidence was found for hepatitis A virus, hepatitis B virus, hepatitis C virus, hepatitis D virus, and syphilis or human immunodeficiency virus. Epstein–Barr virus and cytomegalovirus serology indicated positive IgG. Serum antibodies to anti-ganglioside antibodies GM1 and GM2 were negative, while the level of serum immunoglobulin G was increased.

Cerebral computed tomography and magnetic resonance imaging scans indicated normal results. (The clinical course is summarized in Fig. 1).

The clinical history, physical examination, and biochemical findings of the patient were consistent with the diagnosis of acute HEV-associated GBS. He was treated with intravenous immunoglobulin at a dose of 0.4 mg/kg per day for 5 days. Meanwhile, methylprednisolone were also used to suppress inflammatory response. Glycyrrhizin, glutathione, and ademetionine were simultaneously administered for liver therapy. During the next 2 weeks, his clinical condition and muscle power improved gradually, and the patient had no complaints of respiratory distress or malaise. Repeat CSF examination 2 weeks after admission revealed 10/μL monocyte and 85.7 mg/dL protein level. At discharge, the patient had 5/5 power bilaterally in his arms and 4/5 power bilaterally in his legs. A month later, his liver function substantially improved, and his serum levels of AST and ALT were nearly normal. Six months after discharge, serological study (Wantai HEV-IgM ELISA) showed that IgM anti-HEV antibodies became negative, which suggested full recovery from the acute phase of hepatitis E. The patient responded well to treatment with his muscle power returning to normal, but still felt weakness in his right arm.

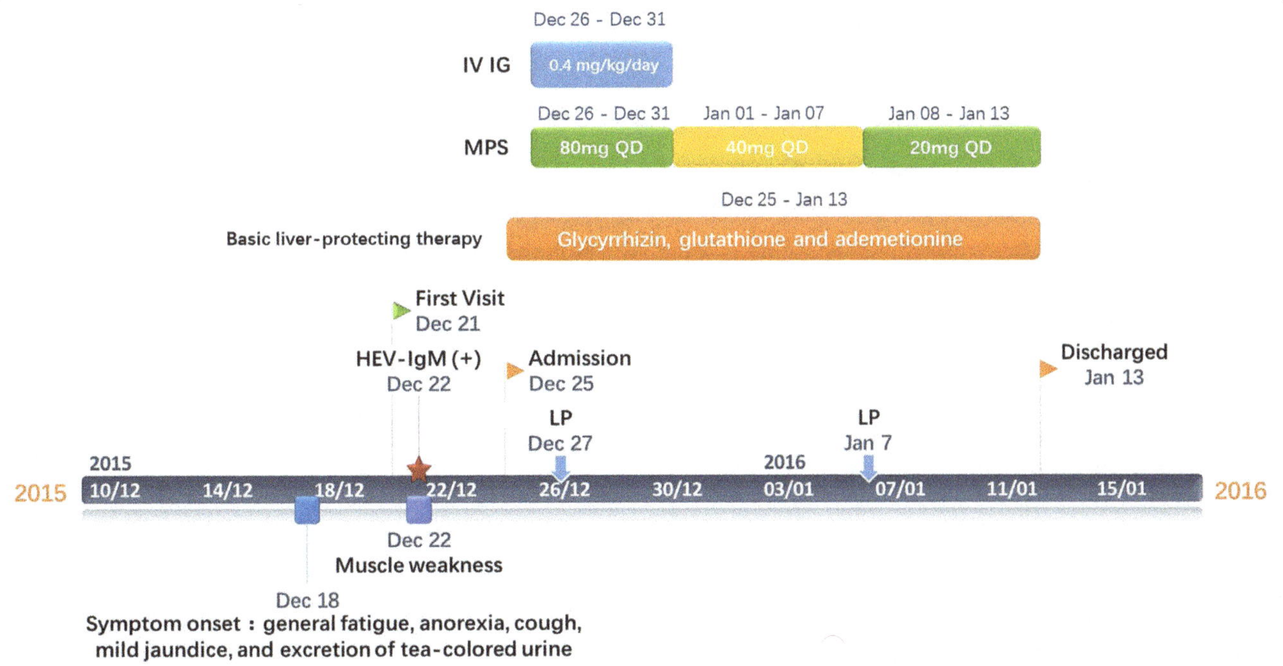

Fig. 1 Medical History. IVIg: intravenous immunoglobulin; MPS: Methylprednisolone; LP: lumbar puncture

Table 1 Clinical characteristics of HEV-associated GBS

Reference	Country	No. of cases	Age	Sex	Delay hepatitis neurological manifestation	Nerve conduction study	Anti-glycoprotein antibody	IgM	HEV RNA
Sood 2000 [13]	India	1	50	M	5 days	AIDP	NT	+	NT
Kumar 2002 [16]	India	1	35	M	17 days	AMSAN	NT	+	NT
Kamani 2005 [12]	India	1	58	F	9 days	NT	NT	+	NT
Khanam 2008 [19]	Bangladesh	1	20	M	10 days	AIDP&AMSAN	NT	+	NT
Loly 2009 [14]	Belgium	1	66	M	Few days	AIDP	GM2+	+	NT
Cronin 2011 [15]	Ireland	1	40	M	Concomitant	AIDP	GM2+	+	NT
Kamar 2011 [7]	France	1	60	F	Concomitant	AIDP	NT	+	Serum+ CSF-
Maurissen 2012 [17]	Belgium	1	51	F	Concomitant	AIDP	GM1&GM2+	+	Serum+
Del Bello 2012 [20]	France	1	65	M	Concomitant	AIDP	NT	+	Serum+
Tse 2012 [21]	Hong Kong	1	60	F	3 days	AIDP	NT	+	NT
Santos 2013 [22]	Portugal	1	58	M	17 days	AIDP	NT	+	Serum+
Sharma 2013 [23]	India	1	27	M	40 days	AIDP	NT	+	NT
Geurtsvan-Kessel 2013 [24]	Bangladesh	11	mean: 24	NM	NM	NM	NT	+	Serum+($n = 1$)
van den Berg 2014 [25]	Netherlands	10	mean: 54	6 M, 4F	Mean: 5 days	AIDP($n = 5$) AMAN($n = 1$) AMSAN($n = 1$) Equivocal($n = 2$) Inexcitable($n = 1$)	NT	+	Serum+($n = 3$) CSF-($n = 10$)
Chen 2014 [26]	China	1	64	M	5 days	AIDP	GM2+	+	NT
Scharn 2014 [27]	Germany	1	50	M	7 days	AIDP & AMAN	–	+	Serum+ CSF-
Woolson 2014 [28]	NM	1	42	M	NM	NM	NT	+	Serum+
Comont 2014 [29]	France	1	73	M	Concomitant	NM	GM1+	+	Serum+ CSF+

Table 1 Clinical characteristics of HEV-associated GBS *(Continued)*

Bandyopadhyay 2015 [30]	Japan	1	43	F	14 days	AIDP & AMAN	GM1+	+	Serum+CSF-
Higuchi 2015 [31]	Japan	1	49	M	10 days	AIDP	–	+	Serum+
Perrin 2015 [32]	France	2	Mean: 57	1F, 1 M	Few days	AIDP	NT	+	Serum+($n = 1$)
Fukae 2016 [33]	Japan	3	Mean: 53	3 M	NM	AIDP($n = 1$) MSF($n = 1$)	GM1 + ($n = 1$) GQ1b + ($n = 1$)	+	Serum+($n = 1$)
Ji 2016 [34]	South Korea	1	58	M	75 days	NM	NT	+	NT
Lei 2017 [35]	China	1	30	M	Concomitant	AIDP	NT	+	NT
Stevens 2017 [36]	Belgium	6	Mean:61	4 M, 2F	NM	AIDP($n = 1$) AMSAN($n = 1$) Equivocal($n = 1$) Demyelinating($n = 2$) Sensory neuropathy($n = 1$)	–	+	Serum+($n = 2$)
Our case	China	1	58	M	11 days	AIDP	–	+	NT

Table 1 Clinical characteristics of HEV-associated GBS *(Continued)*

HEV genotype	ALT (IU/L)	Bilirubin(μmol/L)	CSF Protein level, mg/dL	CSF Cell count (×10^6/L)	Treatment	Recovery/Delay	Comorbidity
NT	114	242.82	186	0	Supportive	Full/1 month	None
NT	752	91.8	NT	NT	MV/IVIg	Full/2 weeks	None
NT	1448	40.7	80	2	IVIg/PP	Full/12 days	None
NT	2509	61.56	190	0	MV	Full/12 days	None
NT	1813	NM	172.2	NM	IVIg	Full/4 months	None
NT	57	NM	>500	0	MV/IVIg/PP	Full/6 months	None
3f	384	35	200	14	IVIg	Partial/18 months	None
NT	2704	NM	61	15	IVIg	Full/1 week	None
3f	2000	NM	64	0	MV/IVIg/Ribavirin	partial/2 month	Severe myositis
NT	2858	60	NM	NM	PP	Full/1 month	None
3a	2320	114.74	181	4	MV/IVIg	partial/2 month	None
NT	NM	NM	243	<5	IVIg	Full/NM	None
1($n = 1$)	NM	NM	NM	NM	NM	NM	None
3	Mean: 160.9	Mean: 13.3	NM	Mean:4.2	NM	NM	NM
NT	1461	156.9	88	10	MV/IVIg	Full/12 months	Encephalitis
3c	334	NM	81	<1	IVIg	Partial/5 months	None
3	623	16	127	145	NM	Full/3 months	None
3f	822	101	137	NM	IVIg	Full/2 months	None
3	1950	85.5	350	12	MV/IVIg	Partial/NM	None
3	1246	15.4	102	7	IVIg	Full/3 months	None
3f	Mean:216	Mean:20.6	Mean:173	NM	IVIg	Partial ($n = 2$)/Mean: 9 weeks	None
NT	Mean: 230.3	NM	Mean: 91	Mean:5	IVIg	Full ($n = 2$) partial($n = 1$)/NM	None
NT	525	23.59	44.6	0	IVIg	Full/12 months	None
NT	4502	83.96	344.19	0	IVIg	Full/3 months	None
NT	Mean:762	Mean:39.27	Mean:69.4	Mean:4.8	IVIg($n = 4$) PP($n = 1$) supportive($n = 1$)	Partial ($n = 5$)/3–6 months Death($n = 1$)/1 month	NM
NT	664	51.8	275.3	0	IVIg	Full/6 months	None

F female, *M* male, *HEV* hepatitis E virus, *ALT* alanine aminotransferase, + positive, – negative, *CSF* cerebrospinal fluid, *AIDP* acute inflammatory demyelinating polyneuropathy, *AMAN* acute motor axonal neuropathy, *AMSAN* acute motor-sensory axonal neuropathy, *MSF* Miller Fisher syndrome, *NM* not mentioned, *NT* not tested, *MV* mechanical ventilation, *IVIg* intravenous immunoglobulin, *PP* plasmapheresis

Discussion and conclusions

HEV, previously known as waterborne or enterically transmitted viral hepatitis, is hyper-endemic in many developing countries and endemic in developed countries [6]. Aside from hepatitis symptoms, HEV-associated neurological injuries also cause significant morbidity. Neurologic complications develop in 7 (5.5%) out of 126 patients with acute and chronic HEV infections in the United Kingdom and France [7]. The clinical spectrum of neurological injury is broad. GBS and neuralgic amyotrophy are the most frequently reported conditions [8]. Other neurological disorders include transverse myelitis, encephalitis, cranial nerve palsy, and meningoradiculitis [9, 10].

GBS is an acute immune-mediated polyradiculoneuropathy that results in rapidly progressing symmetric motor paralysis, limb palsy, hypoflexia, areflexia, and other neurological disorders. GBS is also a heterogeneous disorder with several forms, including acute inflammatory demyelinating polyneuropathy (AIDP), acute motor axonal neuropathy (AMAN), acute motor–sensory axonal neuropathy (AMSAN), and Miller Fisher syndrome (MFS). GBS is usually preceded by an infection, which evokes an immune response that cross-reacts with peripheral nerve components via molecular mimicry [11]. Anti-ganglioside GM1or GM2 positive has been measured in three out of six cases of HEV-associated GBS. This condition may lead to autoimmune inflammatory polyneuropathy [12–17].

A literature review was performed using the PubMed database to identify other published cases and clarify the clinical characteristics of HEV-associated GBS. We used combinations of keywords, including hepatitis E and Guillain–Barre syndrome, and hepatitis E and MFS. Fifty-two cases described HEV-associated GBS. With the addition of our patient, 53 cases were counted, and the clinical characteristics of these cases are summarized in Table 1. The mean age of the reported patients was 47 years (20–73 years), and most of them are middle-aged men (30 men out of 53 cases: 57.7%). These patients developed HEV-associated GBS within an acute onset and have experienced hepatitis symptoms, including jaundice, malaise, nausea, and vomiting. GBS symptoms include motor weakness, cranial nerve palsy, and sensory disorder, which usually manifest after the occurrence of hepatitis symptoms. The mean delay between acute hepatitis E and GBS symptoms was 12 days (with a range of 3–73). Genotyping was performed among 11patients. Most of these patients revealed type 3, which suggested that HEV3 had high tropism of GBS. Most of our reviewed cases were found in Western Europe and Southern and Eastern Asia, where genotype 3 is prevalent. HEV RNA was found in the serum of 17 patients. Furthermore, HEV RNA was positive in the serum and the CSF of one patient.

Among the 47 cases with available details of nerve conduction studies, 23(48.9%) had experienced AIDP. Other variants of GBS, including AMAN, AMSAN, and sensory neuropathy, were also detected. Anti-ganglioside GM1, anti-ganglioside GM2, and GQ1b were detected in eight patients. Thus, the pathogenesis of GBS-associated HEV may be related to GM1, GM2, and GQ1b antibodies. Among the 31 cases with available details of treatments, 25 used intravenous immunoglobulin (IVIg), 4 used plasmapheresis (PP), and 1 used ribavirin. Some patients recovered spontaneously without IVIg or PP administration. Mechanical ventilation was performed in seven patients due to the involvement of respiratory muscles. Almost all the reviewed patients achieved complete neurological recovery within several weeks to several months, which suggested good prognosis for HEV-associated GBS. However, one patient died after cardiac arrest 1 month after the onset of neurological symptoms.

In conclusion, GBS is an emerging extrahepatic manifestation of HEV infection. HEV infection should be strongly considered in patients with neurological symptoms, especially those with elevated levels of liver enzymes. In our case, HEV infection was confirmed by IgM anti-HEV in the serum. This infection could also be supported by HEV RNA. CSF examination showed an increased level of proteins alongside with pleocytosis, which is supported with the suspicion of GBS. Nevertheless, the elevation of CSF proteins is frequent in encephalitis or encephalopathy as well. Thus, the diagnosis of GBS should be cautious. In removes under other resembling disease's premise. Testing for HEV genotype and anti-ganglioside antibodies will likely help in further studying the pathogenesis of HEV-associated GBS.

HEV infection is a self-limiting disorder, and most patients require no treatment. IVIg and PP are both effective treatments for GBS. However, IVIg has replaced PP as the first line of treatment in most hospitals due to the convenience and availability of the former [18]. There is no significant difference between intravenous methylprednisolone with IVIg or IVIg alone.

Additional files

Additional file 1: Table S1. Liver function after admission in our hospital. The patient's liver function tests showed showed 20 μmol/L total bilirubin, 10 μmol/L conjugated bilirubin, 126 U/L alanine aminotransferase, and 160 U/L gamma-glutamyl transpepidase.

Additional file 2: Table S2. Serologic studies for hepatitis virus. Serologic studies for IgM and IgG anti-HEV were both positive. No serological evidence was found for hepatitis A virus, hepatitis B virus, hepatitis C virus, hepatitis D virus.

Additional file 3: Table S3. Serological study for HBV, HCV, Syphilis and HIV. Serologic studies for hepatitis B virus, hepatitis C virus, syphilis or human immunodeficiency virus was negative.

Additional file 4: Table S4. Serological study for Epstein–Barr virus and cytomegalovirus. Epstein–Barr virus and cytomegalovirus serology indicated positive IgG.

Additional file 5: Table S5. The first cerebrospinal fluid (CSF) examination. Cerebrospinal fluid (CSF) examination showed 0/μL monocyte, 4.6 mmol/L glucose level, and 275.3 mg/dL protein level.

Additional file 6: Table S6. The second cerebrospinal fluid (CSF) examination. Cerebrospinal fluid (CSF) examination revealed 10/μL monocyte and 85.7 mg/dL protein level.

Additional file 7: Table S7. Liver function (one month later after discharge). A month later, the liver function of the patient substantially improved, and his serum levels of AST and ALT were nearly normal.

Additional file 8: Table S8. Serological study for HEV(six months later). Six months after discharge, serological study showed IgM anti-HEV antibodies became negative.

Abbreviations

AIDP: Acute inflammatory demyelinating polyneuropathy; ALT: Alanine aminotransferase; AMAN: Acute motor axonal neuropathy; AMSAN: Acute motor-sensory axonal neuropathy; AST: Aspartate aminotransferase; CSF: Cerebrospinal fluid; GBS: Guillain–Barre syndrome; HEV: Hepatitis E virus; IVIg: Intravenous immunoglobulin; MFS: Miller Fisher syndrome; PP: Plasmapheresis

Acknowledgements
Not applicable.

Funding
Not applicable.

Authors' contributions

XZ carried out the data collection, literature review and drafting of the manuscript. LY and QX contributed to the drafting of the manuscript and aided in the literature review. SG participated in the data collection and the drafting of the manuscript. LT help to draft the manuscript and revised the final version of the manuscript. All authors read and approved the final manuscript.

Consent for publication
Written informed consent was obtained from the patient for publication of this case report and any accompanying images. A copy of the written consent is available for review by the Editor-in-Chief of this journal.

Competing interests
The authors declare that they have no competing interests.

References
1. Dalton HR, Bendall R, Ijaz S, Banks M. Hepatitis E: an emerging infection in developed countries. Lancet Infect Dis. 2008;8(11):698–709.
2. Zhu FC, Zhang J, Zhang XF, Zhou C, Wang ZZ, Huang SJ, Wang H, Yang CL, Jiang HM, Cai JP, et al. Efficacy and safety of a recombinant hepatitis E vaccine in healthy adults: a large-scale, randomised, double-blind placebo-controlled, phase 3 trial. Lancet. 2010;376(9744):895–902.
3. Bazerbachi F, Haffar S. Acute fulminant vs. acute-on-chronic liver failure in hepatitis E: diagnostic implications. Infect Dis (Lond). 2015;47(2):112.
4. Kamar N, Izopet J, Dalton HR. Chronic hepatitis e virus infection and treatment. J Clin Exp Hepatol. 2013;3(2):134–40.
5. Dalton HR, Kamar N, van Eijk JJ, Mclean BN, Cintas P, Bendall RP, Jacobs BC. Hepatitis E virus and neurological injury. Nat Rev Neurol. 2016;12(2):77–85.
6. Lee GY, Poovorawan K, Intharasongkroh D, Sa-Nguanmoo P, Vongpunsawad S, Chirathaworn C, Poovorawan Y. Hepatitis E virus infection: epidemiology and treatment implications. World J Virol. 2015;4(4):343–55.
7. Kamar N, Bendall RP, Peron JM, Cintas P, Prudhomme L, Mansuy JM, Rostaing L, Keane F, Ijaz S, Izopet J, et al. Hepatitis E virus and neurologic disorders. Emerg Infect Dis. 2011;17(2):173–9.
8. Cheung MC, Maguire J, Carey I, Wendon J, Agarwal K. Review of the neurological manifestations of hepatitis E infection. Ann Hepatol. 2012;11(5): 618–22.
9. Mandal K, Chopra N. Acute transverse myelitis following hepatitis E virus infection. Indian Pediatr. 2006;43(4):365–6.
10. Bazerbachi F, Haffar S, Garg SK, Lake JR. Extra-hepatic manifestations associated with hepatitis E virus infection: a comprehensive review of the literature. Gastroenterol Rep (Oxf). 2016;4(1):1–15.
11. Yuki N, Hartung HP. Guillain-Barre syndrome. N Engl J Med. 2012;366(24): 2294–304.
12. Kamani P, Baijal R, Amarapurkar D, Gupte P, Patel N, Kumar P, Agal S. Guillain-Barre syndrome associated with acute hepatitis E. Indian J Gastroenterol. 2005;24(5):216.
13. Sood A, Midha V, Sood N. Guillain-Barre syndrome with acute hepatitis E. Am J Gastroenterol. 2000;95(12):3667–8.
14. Loly JP, Rikir E, Seivert M, Legros E, Defrance P, Belaiche J, Moonen G, Delwaide J. Guillain-Barre syndrome following hepatitis E. World J Gastroenterol. 2009;15(13):1645–7.
15. Cronin S, McNicholas R, Kavanagh E, Reid V, O'Rourke K. Anti-glycolipid GM2-positive Guillain-Barre syndrome due to hepatitis E infection. Ir J Med Sci. 2011;180(1):255–7.
16. Kumar R, Bhoi S, Kumar M, Sharma B, Singh B, Gupta B. Guillain-Barré syndrome and acute hepatitis E: a rare association. JIACM. 2002;4(3):389–91.
17. Maurissen I, Jeurissen A, Strauven T, Sprengers D, De Schepper B. First case of anti-ganglioside GM1-positive Guillain-Barre syndrome due to hepatitis E virus infection. Infection. 2012;40(3):323–6.
18. van Doorn PA, Ruts L, Jacobs BC. Clinical features, pathogenesis, and treatment of Guillain-Barre syndrome. Lancet Neurol. 2008;7(10):939–50.
19. Khanam RA, Faruq MO, Basunia RA, Ahsan AA. Guillain-Barré syndrome associated with acute HEV hepatitis. Med Coll J. 2008;1(2):32–4.
20. Del Bello A, Arne-Bes MC, Lavayssiere L, Kamar N. Hepatitis E virus-induced severe myositis. J Hepatol. 2012;57(5):1152–3.
21. Tse AC, Cheung RT, Ho SL, Chan KH. Guillain-Barre syndrome associated with acute hepatitis E infection. J Clin Neurosci. 2012;19(4):607–8.
22. Santos L, Mesquita JR, Rocha PN, Lima-Alves C, Serrao R, Figueiredo P, Reis J, Simoes J, Nascimento M, Sarmento A. Acute hepatitis E complicated by Guillain-Barre syndrome in Portugal, December 2012–a case report. Euro Surveill. 2013;18(34):6–9.
23. Sharma B, Nagpal K, Bakki SR, Prakash S. Hepatitis E with Gullain-Barre syndrome: still a rare association. J Neuro-Oncol. 2013;19(2):186–7.
24. Geurtsvankessel CH, Islam Z, Mohammad QD, Jacobs BC, Endtz HP, Osterhaus AD. Hepatitis E and Guillain-Barre syndrome. Clin Infect Dis. 2013; 57(9):1369–70.
25. van den Berg B, van der Eijk AA, Pas SD, Hunter JG, Madden RG, Tio-Gillen AP, Dalton HR, Jacobs BC. Guillain-Barre syndrome associated with preceding hepatitis E virus infection. Neurology. 2014;82(6):491–7.
26. Chen XD, Zhou YT, Zhou JJ, Wang YW, Tong DM. Guillain-Barre syndrome and encephalitis/encephalopathy of a rare case of northern China acute severe hepatitis E infection. Neurol Sci. 2014;35(9):1461–3.
27. Scharn N, Ganzenmueller T, Wenzel JJ, Dengler R, Heim A, Wegner F. Guillain-Barre syndrome associated with autochthonous infection by hepatitis E virus subgenotype 3c. Infection. 2014;42(1):171–3.
28. Woolson KL, Forbes A, Vine L, Beynon L, McElhinney L, Panayi V, Hunter JG, Madden RG, Glasgow T, Kotecha A, et al. Extra-hepatic manifestations of autochthonous hepatitis E infection. Aliment Pharmacol Ther. 2014;40(11–12):1282–91.
29. Comont T, Bonnet D, Sigur N, Gerdelat A, Legrand-Abravanel F, Kamar N, Alric L. Acute hepatitis E infection associated with Guillain-Barre syndrome in an immunocompetent patient. Rev Med Interne. 2014;35(5):333–6.
30. Bandyopadhyay D, Ganesan V, Choudhury C, Kar SS, Karmakar P, Choudhary V, Banerjee P, Bhar D, Hajra A, Layek M, et al. Two uncommon causes of Guillain-Barre syndrome: hepatitis E and Japanese encephalitis. Case Rep Neurol Med. 2015;2015:759495.

31. Higuchi MA, Fukae J, Tsugawa J, Ouma S, Takahashi K, Mishiro S, Tsuboi Y. Dysgeusia in a patient with Guillain-Barre syndrome associated with acute hepatitis E: a case report and literature review. Intern Med. 2015;54(12): 1543–6.
32. Perrin HB, Cintas P, Abravanel F, Gerolami R, D'Alteroche L, Raynal JN, Alric L, Dupuis E, Prudhomme L, Vaucher E, et al. Neurologic disorders in Immunocompetent patients with autochthonous acute hepatitis E. Emerg Infect Dis. 2015;21(11):1928–34.
33. Fukae J, Tsugawa J, Ouma S, Umezu T, Kusunoki S, Tsuboi Y. Guillain-Barre and miller fisher syndromes in patients with anti-hepatitis E virus antibody: a hospital-based survey in Japan. Neurol Sci. 2016;37(11):1849–51.
34. Ji SB, Lee SS, Jung HC, Kim HJ, Kim HJ, Kim TH, Jung WT, Lee OJ, Song DH. A Korean patient with Guillain-Barre syndrome following acute hepatitis E whose cholestasis resolved with steroid therapy. Clin Mol Hepatol. 2016; 22(3):396–9.
35. Lei JH, Tian Y, Luo HY, Chen Z, Peng F. Guillain-Barre syndrome following acute co-super-infection of hepatitis E virus and cytomegalovirus in a chronic hepatitis B virus carrier. J Med Virol. 2017;89(2):368–72.
36. Stevens O, Claeys KG, Poesen K, Saegeman V, Van Damme P. Diagnostic challenges and clinical characteristics of hepatitis E virus-associated Guillain-Barre syndrome. Jama Neurol. 2017;74(1):26–33.

10

Hepatitis B reactivation characterized by HBsAg negativity and anti-HbsAg antibodies persistence in haematopoietic stem cell transplanted patient after lamivudine withdrawal

C. Cerva[1], G. Maffongelli[1*], V. Svicher[2], R. Salpini[2], L. Colagrossi[2], A. Battisti[2], B. Mariotti[3], R. Cerretti[3], L. Cudillo[3] and L. Sarmati[1]

Abstract

Background: HBV reactivation is associated with high mortality rates in hematopoietic stem cell transplantation (HSCT) and prophylactic lamivudine (LMV) treatment is suggested to prevent this phenomenon. However, the duration of LMV treatment in HSCT patients is not fully defined and the time of immune recovery is considered the best parameter for a drug to be safely interrupted. In patients undergoing allogeneic HSCT, the time of immune recovery is not easy to define and may take years after transplantation and prolonged LMV treatments, which can lead to drug-resistant viral strains.

Case presentation: An anti-HBc-positive hematological patient who was undergoing prolonged immunosuppression and who experienced HBV reactivation 3 months after the suspension of a prolonged LMV prophylaxis is described. HBV-DNA matching an atypical serological profile characterized by HbsAg negativity and anti-HBs positivity was detected in the patient. The genotypic analysis of the HBV strain identified T127P, F170FL and S204R mutations of HbsAg, which can hinder HBsAg recognition in a diagnostic assay.

Conclusions: HBV reactivation in the HSCT host can be sustained by HBsAg viral variants with characteristics of altered immunogenicity that cannot be detected by usual laboratory tests. This clinical case description suggests the importance of screening for serum HBV-DNA levels in the diagnosis of HBV reactivation and monitoring HBV-DNA after prophylaxis suspension, particularly in HSCT subjects who have undergone prolonged periods of LMV treatment.

Keywords: HBV reactivation, Hbv DNA, Prophylaxis, Hepatitis B, Hematopoietic stem cell transplantation

Background

HBV reactivation is a complication of immunosuppressive treatments and is associated with high mortality [1]. Patients undergoing allogeneic hematopoietic stem cell transplantation (allo-HSCT) are considered at major risk for HBV reactivation [1–6], with a mortality rate of up to 40% [3]. A number of national and international guidelines [7–9] have addressed the prophylaxis of HBV reactivation in an immunocompromised host. Nonetheless, several aspects of HBV prevention, such as prophylaxis duration and virological monitoring after prophylaxis suspension, remain poorly defined, particularly in HSCT cases, where HBV reactivation may occur several years after the start of immunosuppressive treatments [10]. Prolonged lamivudine (LMV) prophylaxis is associated with the occurrence of LMV resistance at a rate that increases to 60% in immunocompromised patients [11]. Viral variants, both resistant and sensitive to LMV, can develop in patients under anti-viral treatment and may lead to HBsAg amino acid changes with altered antigenicity, also known as

* Correspondence: maffongelligaetano@gmail.com
[1]Clinical Infectious Disease, Department of Systems Medicine, Tor Vergata University, Rome, Italy
Full list of author information is available at the end of the article

immune escape mutants. The modified HBsAg produced by these viruses is not detectable by current commercial assays.

Here, we report the case of a severely immunocompromised allo-HSCT patient who experienced reactivation of HBV infection a few months after the withdrawal of a very long-term LMV prophylaxis, without the reappearance of HBsAg and with the persistence of high titer anti-HBs antibodies.

Case presentation

The patient is a 59-year-old Italian male who received a diagnosis of non-Hodgkin's lymphoma (NHL) (stage IV) in May 2003. Histological diagnosis indicated a small B-cell lymphoma. From September 2003 to January 2004, he underwent 6 R-CHOP courses (rituximab, cyclophosphamide, doxorubicin, vincristine and prednisone), which were followed by complete disease remission. In March 2005, the patient experienced an NHL relapse. Therefore, fludarabine treatment (4 courses) was started, and the treatment again resulted in complete remission. In November 2005, he underwent an autologous HSCT. In May 2010, a second relapse of NHL was diagnosed, and a treatment regimen with Rituximab-Bendamustine (R-Bendamustine) was started. After 6 courses of R-Bendamustine, a partial response was obtained. The disease had progressed again by October 2011, and an R-DHAP (rituximab, cisplatin, cytosine arabinoside and dexamethasone) treatment was started. Because of renal toxicity, the R-DHAP was replaced with Alentuzumab, obtaining a partial response. In February 2012, the disease had progressed again. Ofatumumab treatment (9 courses) was initiated with no clinical response. In November 2012, the patient underwent an allo-HSCT by a matched unrelated donor (MUD) as a curative option due to refractory disease. The patient received a reduced intensity condition regimen ([TBF-RIC] consisting of thiotepa, busulfan, and fludarabine plus anti-thymocyte globulin). Graft versus host disease (GvHD) prophylaxis consisted of cyclosporine and methotrexate. The engraftment for neutrophils >500/mmc and platelets >20,000/mmc occurred 20 and 24 days after the allo-HSCT, respectively. The post-transplant course was complicated by Aspergillus pneumonia (day 19 post allo-HSCT), for which the patient underwent prolonged antifungal treatment. In July 2013, the patient had the residual pulmonary nodule surgically removed. In the context of the fungal nodule, a lung adenocarcinoma was histologically present.

After allo-HSCT, the patient achieved a stable, complete remission of hematological disease (last follow-up visit in May 2016). At the HBV screening, the patient was identified as positive for anti-HBs, anti-HBc and anti-HBe, and negative for HBV-DNA. The HBV donor serology showed no previous HBV infection (anti-HBc/anti-HBs negative). An HBV DNA test was performed that resulted in a negative outcome. He was not vaccinated for HBV.

Therefore, LMV prophylaxis was started in 2010. The patient continuously received LMV for up to 24 months after the allo-HSCT (January 2015), at which point the prophylaxis was suspended. During the LMV prophylaxis, he remained positive for anti-HBs, anti-HBc and anti-HBe, and HBV-DNA was consistently undetectable. Three months after the suspension of LMV treatment (March 2015), he experienced virological HBV reactivation (serum HBV DNA 42 IU/mL), and no other HBV serological variations were present. Despite HBV reactivation, HBsAg remained negative, and the anti-HBs titers remained consistently high (482 mIU/ml in November 2014, 505 mIU/ml in March 2015, 457 mIU/ml in April 2015, 576 mIU/ml in June 2015 and 542 mIU/ml in July 2015).

A genotypic test (based on the sequencing of HBV reverse transcriptase and HBsAg) was performed during the HBV reactivation diagnosis. The test did not reveal the presence of LMV resistance mutations but showed the presence of three mutations in HbsAg: T127P, F170FL and S204R.

Due to the persistence of quantitative HBV DNA (35 IU/mL), antiviral therapy was started with 245 mg tenofovir. After 2 weeks, the patient underwent a bone density test that documented osteopenia, while the glomerular filtration rate remained stable, although reduced. Tenofovir treatment was interrupted and 0.5 mg entecavir was started. The patient is now in complete hematological remission, and the quantitative HBV DNA is undetectable (see Fig. 1).

Conclusions

This paper describes the clinical case of an anti-HBc-positive and anti-HBs-positive patient undergoing prolonged immunosuppression who developed HBV reactivation 3 months after the suspension of prolonged (4 years) LMV prophylaxis. At HBV reactivation, the patient showed an atypical serological profile characterized by HBsAg negativity and anti-HBs positivity (with a high antibody titer of 505 mIU/ml). These results corroborate recently published studies showing that a substantial proportion (10% to 80%) of patients who tested positive for anti-HBc and anti-HBs remained HBsAg-negative despite the reuptake of viral replication [12–14]. Overall, our results suggest that this immunological profile is critical in the management of patients who are at risk of HBV reactivation and strongly support the use of serum HBV-DNA (rather than HBsAg) for the diagnosis of HBV reactivation.

HBsAg negativity may be related to the high degree of genetic variability in HBsAg observed in patients who develop immunosuppression-driven HBV reactivation,

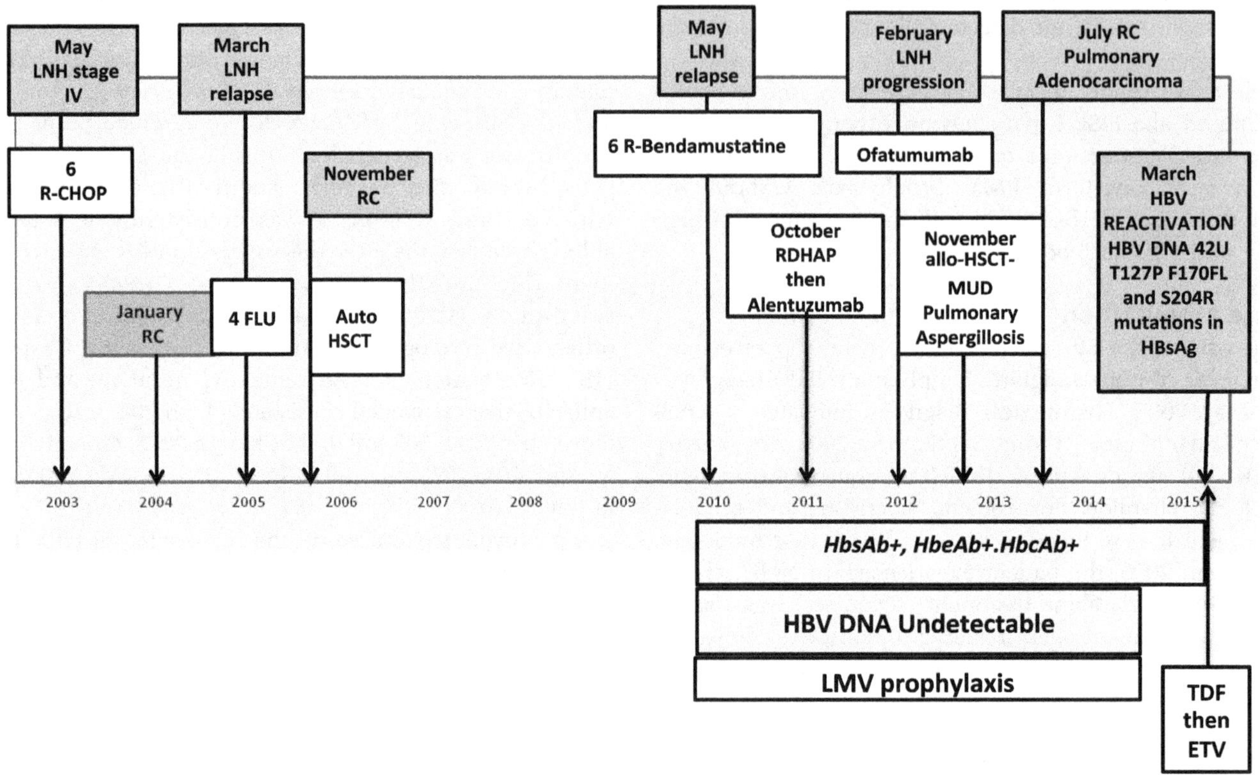

Fig. 1 Medical History. LNH: non-Hodgkin's lymphoma; R-CHOP: rituximab, cyclophosphamide, doxorubicin, vincristine and prednisone; FLU: fludarabine treatment; RC: complete remission of disease; Auto HSCT: autologous peripheral blood stem cell transplantation; R: rituximab; RDHAP: rituximab, cisplatin, cytosine arabinoside and dexamethasone; Allo-HSCT: allogenic peripheral blood stem cell transplantation; MUD: matched unrelated donor

which may hinder HBsAg recognition by the antibodies used in the diagnostic assay [12, 13]. In particular, a previous study has shown the enrichment of additional N-linked glycosylation sites in the major hydrophilic HBsAg region in patients who remained HbsAg-negative despite HBV reactivation [10]. In vitro studies have shown the ability of these glycosylation sites to hamper or abrogate the recognition and quantification of HBsAg by the currently available diagnostic test. In the current clinical case, the HBsAg mutation S204R was detected. This mutation was localized in the C-terminal transmembrane domain, which is known to play an important role in the modulation of HBsAg secretion and viral particle assembly [15]. The acquisition of a positively-charged amino acid (Arginine [R] at position 204) in this transmembrane domain might alter the HBsAg structure to result in i) HBsAg negativity in the currently available diagnostic test and ii) HBV escape from a high anti-HBs titer. This mutation may also affect the viral particle release, resulting in HBV reactivation that is characterized by a low level of serum HBV DNA, as demonstrated in our clinical case. This concept agrees with a previous study, which showed that the viral clones encoding S204R (lysine [S] substitution with arginine [R] at position 204) and G145R (glycine [G] substitution with arginine [R] at position 145) exhibited an approximately 60% viral secretion defect compared with the wild-type. According to this result, the authors proposed that the basic arginine residues may be important for HBsAg retention within the endoplasmic reticulum [16].

Finally, the genotypic testing also highlighted the presence of two HBV RT mutations (S135Y and I233V) that are potentially involved in resistance to first-generation nucleos(t)ide RT inhibitors [17, 18]. The role of these genetic mutations in facilitating HBV evasion from LMV warrants further investigation.

This clinical case also demonstrates the challenges of determining the proper duration of prophylaxis. The current guidelines recommend suspending prophylaxis from the immunosuppressive treatments after 12–18 months [19]. However, in the setting of HSCT, the risk of HBV reactivation can persist for several years after transplantation due to the long delays in immune reconstitution. In this context, Hammond et al. [20] showed that the cumulative probability of HBV reactivation increases from 9%, 1 year after transplantation, to 43%, 4 years after transplantation. Thus, the duration of prophylaxis needs to be extended further in the setting of profound immunosuppression to prevent late HBV reactivation episodes. In addition, these findings also highlight the need for markers that can predict the full immune reconstitution against HBV.

In conclusion, the described case demonstrates that HBV reactivation in the immunocompromised host is a complex phenomenon often sustained by virus strains with virological characteristics that can prevent the recognition of the virus by specific antibodies and by the usual laboratory tests. Therefore, we recommend the careful consideration of the duration of HBV prophylaxis and the subsequent virological monitoring, which should also include the measurement of viral DNA in these patients.

Abbreviations

HSCT: Hematopoietic stem cell transplantation; MUD: Matched unrelated donor; NHL: Non-Hodgkin's lymphoma; PBSCT: Peripheral blood stem cell transplantation; R: Rituximab; R-CHOP: Rituximab, cyclophosphamide, doxorubicin, vincristine and prednisone; RDHAP: Rituximab, cisplatin, cytosine arabinoside and dexamethasone; TBF-RIC: Thiotepa, busulfan, and fludarabine reduced intensity condition regimen

Acknowledgements

None.

Funding

None.

Authors' contributions

CC and MG carried out the case conception and design, and drafted the manuscript. MB and SR participated in the acquisition of data. CR and CL were involved in the clinical management of patients. SR, CL and BA participated in the analysis and interpretation of data. SL, CL, and SV critically revised the manuscript and approved the final version.

Authors' information

SL is a respected consultant in infectious diseases who works in the hematology department and is responsible for the management and prevention of infection during transplant procedures. GM and CC are her young collaborators. VS is a respected researcher who works in the field of virology on chronic viral infections. SR, CL and BA are her young collaborators. CR and CL are medical hematologists who address the management of transplantation patients, MB is their young collaborators.

Consent for publication

Written informed consent for the publication of his clinical details was obtained from the patient. A copy of the consent form is available for review by the Editor of this journal.

Competing interests

The authors declare no conflicts of interest related to this manuscript. However, LS has received funds for attending symposia, speaking, grant research support, consultancy and advisory, and board membership from *ABBOTT, BRISTOL, GILEAD, MERCK, JANSSEN CILAG, PFIZER, ROCHE, and ViiV HEALTHCARE.*

Author details

[1]Clinical Infectious Disease, Department of Systems Medicine, Tor Vergata University, Rome, Italy. [2]Department of Experimental Medicine and Surgery, Tor Vergata University, Rome, Italy. [3]Department of Hematology, Stem Cell Transplant Unit, Tor Vergata University, Rome, Italy.

References

1. Oketani M, Ido A, Nakayama N, et al. Intractable Hepato-Biliary diseases study Group of Japan. Etiology and prognosis of fulminant hepatitis and late-onset hepatic failure in Japan: summary of the annual nationwide survey between 2004 and 2009. Hepatol Res. 2013;43(2):97–105.
2. Reactivation of hepatitis B. American Association for the Study of Liver Diseases Emerging Trends Conference; Arlington, Virginia, March 21–22, 2013: American Association for the Study of Liver Diseases; 2013.
3. Liang R, Lau GKK, Kwong YL. Chemotherapy and bone marrow transplantation for cancer patients who are alsochronic hepatitis B carriers. J Clin Oncol. 1999;17:394–8.
4. Koo YX, Tay M, Teh YE, et al. Risk of hepatitis B virus (HBV) reactivation in hepatitis B surface antigen negative/hepatitis B core antibody positive patients receiving rituximab-containing combination chemotherapy without routine antiviral prophylaxis. Ann Hematol. 2011;90(10):1219–23.
5. Seto WK, Chan TS, Hwang YY, et al. Hepatitis B reactivation in patients with previous hepatitis B virus exposure undergoing rituximab-containing chemotherapy for lymphoma: a prospective study. J Clin Oncol. 2014; 32(33):3736–43.
6. Dong HJ, Ni LN, Sheng GF, Song HL, Xu JZ, Ling Y. Risk of hepatitis B virus (HBV) reactivation in non-Hodgkin lymphoma patients receiving rituximab-chemotherapy: a meta-analysis. J Clin Virol. 2013;57(3):209–14.
7. Reddy KR, Beavers KL, Hammond SP, Lim JK. Falck-Ytter YT; American Gastroenterological Association Institute. American Gastroenterological Association Institute guideline on the prevention and treatment of hepatitis B virus reactivation during immunosuppressive drug therapy. Gastroenterology. 2015;148(1):215–9.
8. Marzano A, Angelucci E, Andreone P, et al. Italian Association for the Study of the liver. Prophylaxis and treatment of hepatitis B in immunocompromised patients. Dig Liver Dis. 2007;39(5):397–408.
9. European Association For The Study Of The Liver. EASL clinical practice guidelines: management of chronic hepatitis B virus infection. J Hepatol. 2012;57(1):167–85. Erratum in: J Hepatol. 2013 Jan;58(1):201
10. Schubert A, Michel D, Mertens T. Late HBsAg seroreversion of mutated hepatitis B virus after bone marrow transplantation. BMC Infect Dis. 2013;13:223.
11. Matthews GV, Bartholomeusz A, Locarnini S, Ayres A, Sasaduesz J, Seaberg E, Cooper DA, Lewin S, Dore GJ, Thio CL. Characteristics of drug resistant HBV in an international collaborative study of HIV-HBV-infected individuals on extended lamivudine therapy. AIDS. 2006;20(6):863–70.
12. Salpini R, Colagrossi L, Bellocchi MC, et al. Hepatitis B surface antigen genetic elements critical for immune escape correlate with hepatitis B virus reactivation upon immunosuppression. Hepatology. 2015;61(3):823–33.
13. Colson P, Borentain P, Coso D, et al. Hepatitis B virus reactivation in HBsAg-negative patients is associated with emergence of viral strains with mutated HBsAg and reverse transcriptase. Virology. 2015;484:354–63.
14. Seto WK. Hepatitis B virus reactivation during immunosuppressive therapy: appropriate risk stratification. World J Hepatol. 2015;7(6):825–30.
15. Bruss V. Envelopment of the hepatitis B virus nucleocapsid. Virus Res. 2004;106(2):199–209.
16. Sterneck M, Kalinina T, Günther S, et al. Functional analysis of HBV genomes from patients with fulminant hepatitis. Hepatology. 1998;28(5):1390–7.
17. Tan J, Degertekin B, Wong SN, Husain M, Oberhelman K, Lok AS. Tenofovir monotherapy is effective in hepatitis B patients with antiviral treatment failure to adefovir in the absence of adefovir-resistant mutations. J Hepatol. 2008;48(3):391–8.
18. Schildgen O, Sirma H, Funk A, et al. Variant of hepatitis B virus with primary resistance to adefovir. N Engl J Med. 2006;354(17):1807–12.
19. Hwang JP, Lok AS. Management of patients with hepatitis B who require immunosuppressive therapy. Nat Rev Gastroenterol Hepatol. 2014;11(4):209–19.
20. Hammond SP, Borchelt AM, Ukomadu C, Ho VT, Baden LR, Marty FM. Hepatitis B virus reactivation following allogeneic hematopoietic stem cell transplantation. Biol Blood Marrow Transplant. 2009;15:1049–59.

11

Assessing the knowledge of expectant mothers on mother-to-child transmission of viral hepatitis B in Upper West region of Ghana

Frederick Dun-Dery[1*], Martin Nyaaba Adokiya[1], Williams Walana[2], Ernestina Yirkyio[3] and Juventus B. Ziem[2,3]

Abstract

Background: Viral Hepatitis B is of a major public health concern globally, especially in developing countries. Expectant mothers' knowledge of Mother-To-Child Transmission (MTCT) of the disease is significant in preventing the spread from an infected mother to her child. This study sought to assess the expectant mothers' knowledge of Mother-To-Child Transmission of viral hepatitis B in the Wa Municipality and Lawra District of Upper West Region, Ghana.

Methods: A descriptive cross-sectional study with a multi-stage sampling technique was employed to select a total of 450 study respondents (expectant mothers), and a semi-structured questionnaire was used for the data collection. Respondents were interviewed using face-to-face interview technique.

Results: Majority (54.0%) of the respondents were aged between 25 and 35 years and the results were similar in both districts. Overall, 62.4% (281/450) of the respondents had at least Junior High level education, and 76.2% (343/450) were multigravida. Educational levels among respondents in the two areas were above 50.0% and considered relatively high. Respondents' general knowledge of hepatitis B infection and disease was 46.0% (208/450). However, there was a slight difference between the two districts (40.1% in Lawra District and 51.6% in Wa Municipality). The overall knowledge level on MTCT of viral hepatitis B among the respondents was 34.7% (156/450): the Wa Municipality recorded higher knowledge (43.3%) compared to 24.8% in Lawra District.

Conclusion: The knowledge level of the expectant mothers on MTCT of viral hepatitis B is relatively low in Upper West Region, Ghana. Majority of the respondents had some form of formal education. The age, marital status, education, occupation, gravity and family setup were found to be associated with knowledge of Hepatitis B infection and MTCT. Thus, there is urgent need to intensify efforts of health staff to educate expectant mothers. In addition, home education and outreach activities should be intensified on HBV infection as well as MTCT. Consequently, planning, implementation and execution of preventive activities, especially in the antenatal clinics should critically consider the social and demographic variations of mothers.

Keywords: Knowledge, Hepatitis B, Mother-to-child transmission, Expectant mothers, Ghana

* Correspondence: kuanufred@gmail.com
[1]Department of Community Health, School of Allied Health Sciences, University for Development Studies (UDS), Tamale, Ghana
Full list of author information is available at the end of the article

Background

Ghana is considered as endemic for hepatitis B infection with an estimated national prevalence of 10% [1–3]. Hepatitis refers to the inflammation of the liver. There are several types of hepatitis and its infectious causes include viral hepatitis A, B, C, D, E, G and other non-viral and non-infectious causes. The Hepatitis B virus (HBV) is most common in developing countries and causes infection which can lead to death resulting from liver cirrhosis, cancer and liver failure [4]. Universally, an average of 2 billion people are infected with the HBV and well over 240 million of this number have developed chronic liver infection, with an estimated annual mortality of 1 million [5]. Sub-Saharan Africa, comparatively, has the most predominant prevalence rate of chronic hepatitis B infection among its mature population, of about 5 to 10% [6]. A major route of HBV transmission, especially in endemic areas is Mother-To-Child Transmission (MTCT), also known as the perinatal transmission [7]. MTCT of HBV refers to a positivity of the hepatitis B surface antigen or the HBV-DNA at 6 to 12 months of a child's life born to an infected mother [8]. Higher percentage of the global chronic carrier cases of HBV, especially in children, is due to MTCT. There is about 80–90% chance of developing chronicity and possible liver complications later in life [9]. There are few reported studies on the knowledge of HBV infection among expectant women [10], particularly in developing countries where illiteracy still remains a major challenge. In spite of the fact that, infection with the HBV remains a universal public health concern, not much is known about its epidemiology for the duration of pregnancy in sub-Saharan Africa [11]. Evidence from Kenya, Cameroon, and Nigeria, recorded limited knowledge of the occurrence of HBV infection among expectant mothers [11–14], though a simple clinical test for HBV infection is available in many countries.

In Ghana, there is a compulsory component of the array of medical tests required of every expectant woman who visits a health facility for antenatal services including clinical test for HBV infection. Thus, it is expected that all pregnant women will be screened for HBV surface antigen and also have some knowledge of HBV disease, especially the perinatal route of transmission [10]. With the existence of a potent vaccine against HBV infection, it is expected that good knowledge of the disease coupled with strict adherence to antenatal and postnatal policy measures would lead to the establishment of HBV-free generation. The Upper West Region is among the poorest regions with relatively high illiteracy rate in the country. The study therefore hypothesized low knowledge of HBV infection among expectant mothers, and relatively high carrier rate. Thus, the objective of this study was to assess the knowledge of expectant mothers' on Mother-To-Child Transmission of viral Hepatitis B in Upper West Region, Ghana.

Methods

Study area

Two (2) of the eleven (11) districts in the Upper West Region of Ghana were selected for the study: namely; Wa Municipality and Lawra District. The Wa Municipality lies in the South Western part of the Upper West Region between Longitudes 9° 32″ W and 10° 20″W and Latitudes 1° 40″N and 2°45″N while the Lawra District is located between longitudes 2° 25″W and 2° 45″W and Latitudes 10° 20″ N and 11° 00″N [15]. The Wa Municipality and Lawra District have an estimated total land area of 579.86 and 483.6 km^2 respectively. Projecting from the 2010 Population and Housing Census, an estimated population of 107,214, comprising of 52,996 males and 54,218 females, and 50,703, comprising 23,628 males and 27,075 females have been recorded for Wa Municipality and Lawra District respectively. The Wa Municipality had an estimated population density of 185 persons/km^2 and the population of Women In Fertility Age (WIFA) was 29,396 whiles the Lawra District had a population density of 105 persons/km^2 and the population of WIFA was 13,185 as at December 2014 [16, 17]. The Wa Municipality has been subdivided in six (6) Sub-Municipals with a total of 26 government health facilities including Community-based Health Planning and Services (CHPS) and 4 private facilities. However, there were 22 active government and 4 private health facilities that offered Antenatal Care (ANC) services as at December 2014 [16]. The Lawra District on the other hand has been sub-divided into five (5) Sub-Districts with a total of 16 government health facilities and 1 private health facility which provide ANC services [17]. The following is a summary of the 6 Sub-Municipals for the Wa Municipality and the 5 Sub-Districts from the Lawra District and their respective number of active ANC health facilities:

Study design

This was a descriptive cross-sectional study conducted in the antenatal clinic service facilities in Wa the Municipality and Lawra District from April to May 2014. The study population included all expectant mothers in the study area who were registered as ANC clients during the period of the study. Information on socio-demographic and obstetric characteristics of the respondents were collected as well as information on their general knowledge of the HBV infection and disease before proceeding to assess their specific knowledge of MTCT. The input variables included the socio-demographic and obstetric characteristics of the expectant mothers: age, educational background, occupation, family setup, average monthly income, marital status, rural-urban residence, gravidity and parity. The output variable included the knowledge on MTCT of HBV infection. For instance, an expectant mother's obstetric characteristic of gravidity can directly influence her knowledge of the HBV infection and disease through the ANC education and counseling services.

Sample size determination

In accordance with [18], the following logical arithmetic procedure N = $\{Z^2 * (PQ)/d^2\}$ was used to compute the desired sample size for the study. Where *N* is the desired sample size, *Z* is the confidence level of 95%, *P* is the prevalence rate (19.0% and 15.1%) of hepatitis B in the Wa Municipality and Lawra Districts respectively. *Q* is a constant computed as 1-P, and *d* is (5%) the set of margin of error. Therefore, for the Wa Municipality, giving hepatitis B prevalence of 19.0%, the sample size was calculated as:

$$N = \frac{Z^2 \times PQ}{d^2} = \frac{\{(1.96)^2 * (0.19(1-0.19))\}}{0.05^2} = \frac{0.5912}{0.0025} = 236$$

Assuming a 5%, non-response rate, 12 respondents were added to arrive at a sample size (248) in the Wa Municipal.

Similarly for the Lawra District, assuming hepatitis B prevalence of 15.1%, the sample size was calculated as:

$$N = \frac{Z^2 \times PQ}{d^2} = \frac{\{(1.96)^2 * (0.15(1-0.15))\}}{0.05^2} = \frac{0.489804}{0.0025} = 199$$

Assuming a 5%, non-response rate, 11 respondents were added to the sample size (210) in the Lawra district. These resulted in an overall sample size of 458.

Sampling procedures

A three-stage random sampling procedure was used to select the sub-districts, health facilities (HFs) and individual respondents for the study. At the first stage of sampling, all sub-districts in Wa Municipality and Lawra District were included in the study. That is, six sub-districts in Wa Municipality and five sub-districts in Lawra District. At the second stage of sampling, the HFs were selected per sub-district respectively. Selection of the HFs was done at the sub-district levels. For each sub-district, list of all HFs where ANC services are available was compiled and through the lottery method, one HF was randomly selected from the lists respectively. However, due to the fact that majority of women visit the Wa Regional and Lawra District Hospitals respectively, the two were purposively included in the study. This is because the two hospitals are situated in the capital towns of areas that are of comparatively high population densities in their respective districts. The Municipal hospital also serves as the regional hospital where as the hospital in Lawra sub-district also doubles as the district hospital. As such, they are well resourced with staff and equipment such as HBV test equipment, ultrasound scan machines, etc. as compared to the other health facilities. In all, thirteen (13) HFs were selected for the study; seven (7) HFs in the Wa Municipality and six (6) HFs in the Lawra District (see Table 1).

The third stage involved the selection of respondents at the HF level using the quota sampling method. For each of the study areas, a calculated sample size was allocated among the selected HFs in proportion to their past ANC attendance. All selected HFs were visited by the field team during ANC days. As a routine at the facility level, pregnant women who attend ANC for services usually sit in queues on the basis of first-come-first-served. They then file in one after the other to consult the ANC nurse for assessment and counseling where necessary. Each time a facility was visited, respondents were recruited by consecutive sampling, as and when the pregnant women arrived for their scheduled ANC services. Pregnant women who arrived earlier than the research team were usually prompted to participate in the study after going through their ANC schedule if they had some time to spare. This was done to ensure that every pregnant woman who attended the facility for ANC services at the time of this study was given opportunity to participate in the study. This recruitment procedure was usually done until the quota for that facility was met, if not, subsequent visits were made until the quota for that facility was exhausted. At the ANC level in each health facility, the study protocol was clearly

Table 1 ANC Health facilities in Wa Municipality and Lawra District in 2014

Municipal/District	Sub-Municipal/ Sub-district	Number of ANC HFs	Number sampled
Wa Municipality	Wa Central Sub	5	2
	Kambali Sub	4	1
	Bamahu Sub	4	1
	Charia Sub	2	1
	Charingu Sub	5	1
	Busa Sub	3	1
Lawra District	Lawra Sub	7	2
	Babile Sub	3	1
	Eremon Sub	2	1
	Domwini Sub	3	1
	Zambo Sub	2	1
Total ANC HFs		40	13

Source: Extracts from [16, 17]

explained to the expectant mothers in the English language and/or in a local dialect for those who did not understand the English language. At the individual level, their voluntary participation in the study was sought and only those who agreed to participate were recruited. Post-natal mothers and other women who were at the facilities but were not confirmed ANC registrants were excluded from this study.

Research Assistants were recruited among university students with health background from the study areas. This was to ensure that the recruits had adequate understanding of the HBV disease concept as an infectious communicable disease. They were trained on the purpose of the study, the methodology, socio-cultural norms and questionnaire administering techniques. A pretesting of the questionnaire was done before the main data collection started. The study used a semi-structured questionnaire to collect the information from the pregnant women at the ANC facilities. In addition, the antenatal cards of expectant women were also sought and assessed to confirm the information provided. To avoid misclassification bias in designing the questionnaire for the study, the questions on knowledge were purposefully extracted from peer reviewed journal articles on the general knowledge of HBV infection and also on specific knowledge on MTCT of HBV. Further review and classification assistance was sought from a clinical professor. Further information on data collection can be found in Additional file 1.

Data analysis

The data was entered into Microsoft Office Excel for Windows version 2010 and checked for data inaccuracies and errors to ensure consistency. Though the study sampled 458 respondents, only 450 were included in the analyses following the data cleaning process; the 8 respondents were found to be incomplete and were excluded from the analysis. It was then exported to Statistical Package for Social Sciences (SPSS) software version 20.0 for Windows for analysis. The data was analyzed and presented in the form of frequencies, percentages, proportions and tabulations.

Results

Socio-demographic characteristics of respondents

Table 2 shows the socio-demographic characteristics of the respondents. A total of 450 respondents were included in the analysis and majority (54.0%) were within the ages of 25–35 years. The proportion of respondents who had some level of formal education was 62.4% with nearly 20.0% higher in Wa Municipality compared to Lawra District. Approximately, 76.2% of the respondents were multigravida with similar results in Wa and Lawra Districts. In terms of respondents' occupational status, majority (56.0%) were unemployed. However, majority (56.2%) of the employed respondents were in the Wa Municipality as against 30.0% in the Lawra District. Polygamy was generally practiced by 33.6% of the respondents though monogamy was predominant (58.0%). In terms of income, nearly all (95.3%) expectant mothers earned an average monthly income of either GHC500 or less.

Table 3 presents the number of respondents that were recruited from the 13 ANC health facilities in the respective sub-municipals and sub-districts. Two ANC facilities were sampled in the Wa Sub-Municipality: the Wa regional hospital in the Wa Municipality was a constant and the Wa Central HC which was randomly sampled. Similarly in the Lawra district, two ANC facilities were sampled under the Lawra Sub-district: the Lawra district hospital was a constant and the Lawra Sub HC which was randomly sampled.

Table 4 shows the respondents' knowledge about hepatitis B infection and disease. In total, less than half of the respondents, 46.2% (208) knew about hepatitis B infection and its disease. Knowledge of the infection and disease was lower in Lawra District (40.1%) compared to Wa Municipality (51.6%). Overall, respondents' knowledge of liver damage/cirrhosis as a consequence of hepatitis B infection was 47.1%. The knowledge was higher in Lawra District (50.0%) compared to Wa Municipality (45.0%). About half of the respondents, 49.0% (219) of respondents knew that the HBV can be transmitted through blood and/or blood products. Respectively in the Lawra District and Wa Municipality, 35.2% (74) and 60.4% (145) of the respondents knew that HBV infection could occur through contact with blood or blood products. In total, 42.8% (193) of the respondents knew that unprotected sex could lead to HBV transmission. The awareness was higher in Wa Municipality compared to Lawra district (57.0% vs. 26.7%) (See Table 4).

Respondents' knowledge of mother-to-child transmission of HBV

Table 5 shows the average knowledge level of Mother-To-Child Transmission of viral hepatitis B among respondents was 34.7%. This is comparatively higher in the Wa Municipality (43.3%) than Lawra District (24.8%). In some specific cases, only 1.8% of respondents knew that breast milk poses no verified risks of transmitting HBV, and 76.2% knew that an HBV carrier expectant mother can pass on the virus to her child during or after delivery. In total, 39.3% of the respondents also knew that a child who is not vaccinated against the HBV can still be infected after birth from an infected mother. Meanwhile, 56.7% of the respondents in Wa Municipality as compared to 19.5% in Lawra District knew that a child who is not vaccinated against HBV can still be infected after birth from an infected mother. However, 16.7% of the respondents agreed that HBV vaccine was

Table 2 Socio-demographic characteristics of respondents

Variable	Total		Wa Municipality		Lawra District	
	N	%	N	%	N	%
Age group (years)						
≤24	137	30.4	64	26.7	73	34.8
25–35	243	54.0	140	58.3	103	49.0
>35	70	15.6	36	15.0	34	16.2
Total	450	100.0	240	100.0	210	100.0
Marital Status						
Married	382	84.9	209	87.1	173	82.4
Not Married	68	15.1	31	12.9	37	17.6
Total	450	100.0	240	100.0	210	100.0
Occupation						
Unemployed	252	56.0	105	43.8	147	70.0
Employed	198	44.0	135	56.2	63	30.0
Total	450	100.0	240	100.0	210	100.0
Educational level						
Educated	281	62.4	171	71.2	110	52.4
Uneducated	169	37.6	69	28.8	100	47.6
Total	450	100.0	240	100.0	210	100.0
Gravidity						
Primidgravida	105	23.3	57	23.8	48	22.9
Multigravida	343	76.2	182	76.2	161	76.6
Total	448	99.5	240	100.0	209	99.5
Average monthly income						
≤ GHC500	429	95.3	227	94.5	202	96.2
GHC501–1000	17	3.8	9	3.8	8	3.8
> GHC1000	4	0.9	4	1.7	0	0.0
Total	450	100.0	240	100.0	210	100.0
Family Set-up						
Polygamous	151	33.6	89	37.1	62	29.5
Monogamous	261	58.0	132	55.0	129	61.4
Other	37	8.2	18	7.5	19	9.0
Total	449	99.8	239	99.6	210	100.0

safe, protects against HBV infection, and poses no harm to the unborn baby. This was similar among respondents in Wa Municipality and Lawra District.

Respondents' socio-demographic characteristics and their knowledge about MTCT of HBV

Table 6 presents finding on how the socio-demographic characteristics of respondents were associated with their knowledge about MTCT of HBV infection in the study area. Each socio-demographic factor was analyzed using binary regression model to determine its relationship with their knowledge about MTCT of HBV infection. In the combination of the two districts (Wa Municipal and Lawra District), married (P = 0.007 and OR = 2.13), uneducated (P = 0.007 and OR = 1.83), unemployed (P = <0.001 and OR = 2.46) and primigravida (P = 0.008 and OR = 1.92) had statistically significant association with their general knowledge of MTCT of HBV compared to unmarried, educated, employed and multigravida respondents.

When it was analyzed by separate districts, the Wa Municipality found married (P = 0.02 and OR = 0.27), polygamous family setup (P = 0.015 and OR = 2.44) and primigravida (P = 0.003 and OR = 2.99) were statistically significant associated with their knowledge of MTCT of HBV compared to unmarried, monogamous family setups, and multigravida. While in the Lawra District, only uneducated (P = 0.017 and OR = 0.49) and unemployed (P = 0.015 and OR = 0.42) had statistical significant evidence of association with their knowledge of MTCH of HBV compared to educated and employed (see Table 6).

Discussion

Expectant mothers' knowledge of HBV infection is very critical in eliminating the transmission cycle of the virus in newborns. In contrast, majority of the respondents in this study had some formal education above primary level and yet their knowledge was generally low. Generally, the study revealed a relatively low general knowledge of the HBV infection and disease (46.2%) and MTCT of HBV (34.7%) among the expectant mothers in the study area. Specifically, less than half (39.3%) of the overall respondents knew that newborns to HBV infected mothers are at risk of contracting the HBV. Few (1.8%) of the mothers correctly said that the transmission could possibly occur via breast milk, especially if the mother is also tested positive of the Hepatitis B envelop antigen (HBeAg). Majority of the respondents did not know their HBV status or their spouse's. This finding should be a major concern for the health authority in the two districts. Expectant mothers with high HBeAg values could be transmitting the infection to their babies in ignorance. The observation of relatively low knowledge made in this study supports that of [19] who found that overall knowledge among their respondents regarding hepatitis B was poor and inaccurate. It however differed from a study conducted by Adeyemi and colleagues who found that majority of their study respondents didn't have formal education with responding low level of knowledge about HBV transmission [14].

Majority of the respondents were within the ages of 20 to 35 years, which is similar to findings reported in other studies [14, 20–22]. They found that majority of their respondents were within a youthful age of 25 to 35 years. Many studies assessing the knowledge and prevalence of HBV infection, especially among pregnant women affirm

Table 3 List of health facilities sampled and the quota of sample size

Sno	Sub-District	Health Facility	ANC Attendance	% of Total Attendance	Quota Sampled
Wa Municipality					
1	Kambale Sub	Kambale HC	697	5.64	14
2	Bamahu Sub	Bamahu HC	407	3.30	8
3	Charingu Sub	Charingu HC	282	2.28	6
4	Busa Sub	Busa HC	279	2.26	5
5	Wa Sub	Wa Reg. Hospital	8942	10.87	180
6	Wa sub	Wa Central HC	1341	72.50	27
7	Charia Sub	Dobile CHPS	392	3.18	8
Total			12,340	100.00	248
Lawra District					
8	Eremon Sub	Eremon HC	107	8.89	19
9	Lawra Sub	Lawra Dist. Hosp	715	59.43	125
10	Lawra Sub	Lawra Sub HC	28	2.33	5
11	Babile Sub	Babile Polyclinic	194	16.13	34
12	Domwini Sub	Domwini HC	42	3.49	7
13	Zambo Sub	Zambo HC	117	9.73	20
Total			1203	100.00	210

Quota sample is the product percentage of respective ANC attendance and the Sample Size

that, women <30 years of age are at a higher risks of being infected with the HBV [10–14, 23, 24]. This has been attributed to unsafe sexual practices among such people which predisposes them to sexually transmitted infections [25].

Literacy rate among respondents was generally high as majority had some form of formal education above primary school level. This result could be due to the fact that Ghana has an overall literacy rate of 56.3% and female literacy rate of about 47% [26] while the Lawra District has a female literacy rate of 59.7% [27]. The Wa Municipality is a relatively urban setting with a comparatively educated population in that, approximately 70% of persons who are older than 14 years and living in urban areas of Ghana are literate [26]. In addition, there is about 44% Secondary School enrolment participation ratio among females in Ghana [28], with relatively higher proportions in urban areas. The interplay of these factors possibly account for the relatively high literacy rate among the respondents since majority of the sample were resident in the central sub-districts of the two areas.

Majority of the respondents earned monthly income of 500 Ghana cedis (GHC 500) or less on an average - approximately 125 United States Dollars (USD 125.00) and above the national poverty line of GHC 106 per month

Table 4 Knowledge of Hepatitis B infection and disease

General knowledge of HBV infection & disease	Overall	Wa Municipality	Lawra District
	N (%)	*N* (%)	*N* (%)
HBV is more Infectious than HIV/AIDS	132 (29.3)	62 (25.8)	70 (33.3)
HBV can lead to liver damage/cirrhosis	212 (47.1)	107 (44.6)	105 (50.0)
There's blood test for HBV infection	341 (75.8)	199 (82.9)	142 (67.6)
HBV can be transmitted via blood/products	219 (48.7)	145 (60.4)	74 (35.2)
HBV infection is possible via sharing of food, drinks, witchcraft, etc.	40 (8.9)	21 (8.8)	19 (9.0)
The HBV can be transmitted through unprotected sex with an infected person	193(42.8)	137(57.0)	56(26.7)
An HBV infected infant may not show any sign and symptoms	349 (77.5)	189 (78.8)	160 (76.2)
Knowledge of your HBV status?	349 (77.5)	131 (54.6)	48 (22.9)
Percentage Knowledgeable	208 (46.2)	124 (51.6)	84 (40.1)
Total number of respondents	450[a]	240[a]	210[a]

[a]Percentages do not add up to 100% due to multiple responses

Table 5 Expectant mothers' knowledge of mother-to-child transmission of HBV

Knowledge about MTCT of HBV	Correct response only *N* (%)		
	Total N (%)	Wa Municipality	Lawra District
An HBV infected Mother can infect her baby in the uterus (intrauterine) before birth	343(76.2)	202 (84.2)	141(67.1)
Breast milk can transmit HBV	8(1.8)	3(1.2)	5(2.4)
Newborns are too young to contract HBV from infected mothers	177(39.3)	136 (56.7)	41(19.5)
The HBV vaccine is harmful to the unborn	75(16.7)	51 (21.1)	24 (11.4)
HBV infection of the child cannot occur after the child is born to an infected mother.	175(38.9)	128 (53.3)	47(22.4)
Average Knowledge about MTCT (sum of % N/5)	156(34.7)	104 (43.3)	52 (24.8)
Total number of respondents	450	240[a]	210[a]

[a]Percentages do not add up to 100 due to multiple responses

per individual [29]. This might imply that on an average, majority of the expectant mothers in the Wa Municipality may be unable to afford basic health care services such as blood screening for HBV, and the cost of the HBV vaccination for themselves as individuals. The average household density as revealed by the study was five persons in the Wa Municipality and seven in Lawra District. This does not include indirect dependents as it is usually the case in most developing countries. The financial demands on these mothers are relatively high, thereby affecting their health seeking behaviors [30]. Maternal access to comprehensive blood screening test and vaccination cover for the whole family against HBV infection could be challenging, especially in the comparatively larger homes.

The association between maternal age distribution and their knowledge of MTCT of HBV particularly in the Wa Municipality, is similar to the findings that maternal age below 35 years is a strong predictor of knowledge of MTCT of HBV [11, 13, 14, 31]. Though majority of the respondents were educated, no significant association was found between educational status and knowledge level of MTCT of HBV in the Wa Municipality, contrary to reports by [10, 24]. However in the Lawra District,

Table 6 Socio-demographic determinants of knowledge about MTCT of HBV using Binary logistics regression analysis

	Overall		WMHD		LDHD	
	P-value	OR(95%CI)	*P*-value	OR(95%CI)	*P*-value	OR(95%CI)
Age						
≥ 30 years		1.0		1.0		1.0
≤ 30 years	0·472	1·24(0·69, 2·20)	0·404	1·60(0·53, 4·82)	0·13	0·56(0·27, 1·19)
Marital status						
Not Married		1.0		1.0		1.0
Married	0·007	2·13(1·23, 3·69)	0·002	0·27(0·12, 0·62)	0·48	0·77(0·37, 1·60)
Education						
Educated		1.0		1.0		1.0
Not Educated	0·007	1·83(1·18, 2·84)	0·977	0·99(0·46, 2·12)	0·017	0·49(0·27, 0·88)
Occupation						
Employed		1.0		1.0		1.0
Not Employed	<0·001	2·46(1·54, 3·95)	0·122	0·58(0·29, 1·16)	0·015	0·42(0·21, 0·85)
Family Setup						
Monogamous		1.0		1.0		1.0
Polygamous	0·965	1·01(0·65, 1·57)	0·015	2·44(1·19, 4·99)	0·092	0·59(0·32, 1·09)
Gravidity						
Multigravida		1.0		1.0		1.0
Primigravida	0·008	1·92(1·82, 3·10)	0·003	2.99(1·43, 6·24)	0·272	1·45(0·75, 2·84)
Income						
≥ GHS500		1.0		1.0		1.0
≤ GHS500	0·998	5·37(0·00, 0·00)	0·999	3·24(0·00, 0)	0·999	8·38(0·00, 0)

there was an association between respondents' educational background and their knowledge of MTCT of HBV. This indicates that more expectant mothers in the Lawra District who were educated had correct knowledge about MTCT of HBV unlike their uneducated colleagues. This is also similar to the finding of many other studies around the globe [10, 11, 14, 20, 32].

The finding with regards to the association between respondents' marital status and their knowledge of MTCT of HBV in the Wa Municipality in particular, contradicts the finding by [19] who reported no association between marital status and knowledge about HBV infection. The current findings predict that married respondents were knowledgeable than their unmarried colleagues could be a quantitative difference since there were many married respondents who were also younger in age than the unmarried. In the case of the Lawra District however, there was no association between respondents' marital status and their knowledge about MTCT of HBV which rather agrees with the report of [19].

The study also found an association between respondents' family setup and their knowledge of MTCT of HBV infection among the respondents in the Wa Municipality unlike in the Lawra District. This is an important indicator for the current study because many studies that have explored knowledge about HBV infection among expectant mothers did not discuss this relationship. In 2014, a knowledge assessment study among Cameroonian pregnant women captured the indicator of family setup but did not find any significant association between that and knowledge of HBV among the respondents [11].

The occupational status of our respondents in the Lawra District was also associated with their knowledge of MTCT of HBV unlike in the Wa Municipality. The probable reason for this relationship could be linked to respondents' educational background. The educational background of respondents in the Lawra District was also found to be significantly associated with their knowledge of MTCT of HBV. This contradicts the findings of [13, 20, 29], and yet agrees with other findings in similar studies around the globe [30, 31].

The obstetric gravidity of the respondents in the Wa Municipality was also significantly associated with their knowledge of MTCT of HBV infection. This could result from the assumption that the expectant mothers in the Wa Municipality were regular to their ANC schedules as expected and benefited from the regular education provided at the ANC clinics. This finding conforms to the finding of [19] who reported significant relationship between the knowledge of their respondents and their obstetric gravidity. The absence of association between respondents' gravidity and their knowledge as in the Lawra District agrees with reports by [31] which did not also find any significant linkage between gravidity and knowledge among Nigerian expectant mothers. Unlike the finding of [20], the finding of no significant relationship between expectant mothers' educational background and their knowledge about MTCT of HBV infection agrees with [11]. Generally, there was no significant association between the respondents' monthly income and their knowledge of MTCT of HBV infection as also reported by [32].

Conclusion

The knowledge of MTCT of HBV among expectant mothers in the Upper West Region was low in general. Majority of the respondents had some form of formal education. The age, marital status, education, occupation, gravity and family setup were found to be significantly associated with knowledge of Hepatitis B infection and MTCT in the Upper West Region. Thus, there is urgent need to intensify the efforts of health staff to educate more expectant mothers. In addition, home education and outreach activities should be intensified on HBV infection as well as MTCT. Consequently, planning, implementation and execution of preventive activities, especially in the antenatal clinics should critically consider the social and demographic variations of mothers.

Abbreviations

ANC: Antenatal Care; CHPS: Community-based Health Planning and Services; GHC: Ghana Cedis; GHS: Ghana Health Service; HBeAg: Hepatitis B 'envelop' Antigen; HBV: Hepatitis B Virus; HBV-DNA: Hepatitis B Virus Deoxyribonucleic Acid; HC: Health Center; HF: Health Facility; HFs: Health Facilities; HIV/AIDS: Human Immunodeficiency Virus/Acquired Immune Deficiency Syndrome; LDHD: Lawra District Health Directorate; MTCT: Mother-to-Child Transmission; OR: Odds Ratio; SPSS: Statistical Package for Social Sciences; UDS: University for Development Studies; USD: Unite States Dollars; WIFA: Women in Fertility Age; WMHD: Wa Municipal Health Directorate

Acknowledgements

We would like to thank the Regional, Municipal and District Health Directorates of the Upper West Region, as well as all the study participants. Their support made the study a success.

Funding

The authors declare that they did not request or receive any funding from any organization, institution or individual to conduct part or whole of this study.

Authors' contributions

JBZ and FD-D conceived and designed the study. FD-D and EY collaborated to do the field work: recruitment and training of research assistants and data collection. FD-D, MNA, and WW analyzed the data. The first draft manuscript was developed by FD-D and EY. Further revisions of the manuscript were done by JBZ, MNA and WW. All authors have read and approved the final manuscript.

Competing interests
The authors declare that they have no competing interests.

Consent for publication
Not applicable.

Ethics approval and consent to participate
Prior to data collection, an introductory letter obtained from the Department of Community Health, School of Allied Health Sciences, University for Development Studies, Tamale was sent to the Upper West Regional Health Directorate to request for permission to carry out the study. At the Municipal and District levels, permission was also sought from the Wa Municipal and Lawra Health Directorates, Sub-municipals and the HF managements respectively before commencing the study. At the individual level, written informed consent was sought. The rationale of the study, the study design and procedure were explained to all respondents in a language they understood and only those who agreed and signed or thumb-printed the consent forms to participate were included in the study. Each time a facility was visited, a written permission was obtained from the facility management. Respondents could freely opt out of the study, even though their full participation was encouraged.

Author details
[1]Department of Community Health, School of Allied Health Sciences, University for Development Studies (UDS), Tamale, Ghana. [2]Department Clinical Microbiology, School of Medicine and Health Sciences, UDS, Tamale, Ghana. [3]Clinical Laboratory Department, Tamale Teaching Hospital, Tamale, Ghana.

References
1. World Health Organization. Hepatitis B vaccines: WHO position paper. Wkly Epidemiol rec [Internet] 2009;84(40):405–420. Available from: http://www.who.int/wer/2009/wer8440.pdf?ua=1.
2. WHO. WHO | Hepatitis B Fact Sheet 204 [Internet]. World Health Organization; 2015 [cited 2015 Jan 21]. Available from: http://www.who.int/mediacentre/factsheets/fs204/en/.
3. WHO-WPRO. WPRO | Hepatitis B [Internet]. WPRO | WHO Western Pacific Region; 2015 [cited 2015 May 15]. Available from: http://www.wpro.who.int/mediacentre/factsheets/fs_20120219_hepb/en/.
4. Dongdem JT, Kampo S, Soyiri IN, Asebga PN, Ziem JB, Sagoe K. Prevalence of hepatitis B virus infection among blood donors at the Tamale Teaching Hospital, Ghana (2009). BMC Res Notes [Internet]. 2012 Jan [Cited 2015 Jan 21];5:115. Available from: https://www.ncbi.nlm.nih.gov/pmc/articles/PMC3392729/?tool=pmcentrez.
5. Rufai T, Mutocheluh M, Kwarteng K, Dogbe E. The prevalence of hepatitis B virus E antigen among Ghanaian blood donors. Pan Afr Med J [Internet], 24 [Cited 2015 May 15];17(53):1–4. 2014 Jan; Available from: http://www.panafrican-med-journal.com/content/article/17/53/full/#.WS3oHWiGPIU.
6. Walana W, Hokey P, Ahiaba S. Sero-prevalence of hepatitis B virus infection among blood donors : a retrospective study in the Kintampo municipal hospital. Ghana Open J med Microbiol. 2014;4(March):64–9.
7. Custer B, Sullivan SD, Hazlet TK, Iloeje U, Veenstra DL, Kowdley K V. Global Epidemiology of Hepatitis B Virus. Vol. 38, Journal of Clinical Gastroenterology. 2004. p. S158–68.
8. Gentile I, Borgia G. Vertical transmission of hepatitis B virus: challenges and solutions. Int J Womens Health [Internet]. 2014 Jan [Cited 2015 May 15];6: 605–11. Available from: https://www.ncbi.nlm.nih.gov/pmc/articles/PMC4062549/?tool=pmcentrez.
9. Siakwa M, Kpikpitse D, Ankobil A, Mupepi S, John ME, Doe PF, et al. EFFECTS OF CHRONIC HEPATITIS B INFECTION ON PREGNANCY AND BIRTH OUTCOMES IN GHANA. Int Jounal Res Med Heal Sci. 2014;4(5).
10. Chan OK, Lao TT, Suen SSH, Leung TY. Deficient Knowledge on Hepatitis B Infection in Pregnant Women and Prevalence of Hepatitis B Surface Antigen Carriage in an Endemic Area: A Review. Hepat Res Treat [Internet]. 2012 Jan [Cited 2014 Dec 28];2012:1–8. Available from: https://www.ncbi.nlm.nih.gov/pmc/articles/PMC3465960/?tool=pmcentrez.
11. Frambo A a B, Atashili J, Fon PN, Ndumbe PM. Prevalence of HBsAg and knowledge about hepatitis B in pregnancy in the Buea Health District, Cameroon: a cross-sectional study. BMC Res Notes [Internet]. Jan [Cited 2015 Jan 13];7(1):394. 2014; Available from: https://bmcresnotes.biomedcentral.com/articles/10.1186/1756-0500-7-394.
12. Malungu Ngaira JA, Kimotho J, Mirigi I, Osman S, Ng'ang'a Z, Lwembe R, et al. Prevalence, awareness and risk factors associated with Hepatitis B infection among pregnant women attending the antenatal clinic at Mbagathi District Hospital in Nairobi, Kenya. Pan Afr Med J [Internet]. 2016 [cited 2017 Jan 24;24. Available from: http://www.panafrican-med-journal.com/content/article/24/315/full/.
13. Adekanle O, Ndububa D a, Olowookere SA, Ijarotimi O, Ijadunola KT. Knowledge of Hepatitis B Virus Infection, Immunization with Hepatitis B Vaccine, Risk Perception, and Challenges to Control Hepatitis among Hospital Workers in a Nigerian Tertiary Hospital. Hepat Res Treat [Internet]. 2015 Dec [Cited 2015 Dec 20];2015 Available from: https://www.ncbi.nlm.nih.gov/pmc/articles/PMC4320901/?tool=pmcentrez.
14. Adeyemi a B, Enabor OO, Ugwu I a, Bello F a, Olayemi OO. Knowledge of hepatitis B virus infection, access to screening and vaccination among pregnant women in Ibadan, Nigeria. J Obstet Gynaecol (Lahore) [Internet]. 2013 Feb [cited 2014 Dec 28];33(2):155–9. Available from: https://www.ncbi.nlm.nih.gov/pubmed/23445138.
15. Ghana Statistical Service. Ghana Living Standard Survey Round 6 (GLSS 6) [Internet]. Accra, Ghana; 2014 Aug [cited 2015 Nov 9]. Available from:http://www.statsghana.gov.gh/docfiles/glss6/GLSS6_Main%20Report.pdf.
16. Wa Municipal Health Directorate. 2014 annual performance report. Wa Municipality; 2014.
17. Dirctorate LDH. LAWRA district annual performance report, 2014. UWR: Lawra; 2014.
18. Cochran GW. Sampling Techniques [Internet]. 2nd ed. New York: John Wiley and Sons, Inc.; 1963. 450–451 p. Available from: https://www.amazon.com/Sampling-Techniques-2nd-William-Cochran/dp/0471162388.
19. WHO, Noreen N, Kumar R, Shaikh BT. Knowledge about hepatitis B vaccination among women of childbearing age: a cross-sectional study from a rural district of Punjab, Pakistan. East Mediterr Heal J. 2015;21(2):129–133.
20. Afzali H, Momen Heravi M, Moravveji SA, Poorrahnama M. Prevalence of Hepatitis B Surface Antigen in Pregnant Women in Beheshti Hospital of Kashan, Isfahan. Iran Red Crescent Med J [Internet]. 22 [Cited 2015 Sep 12]; 17(7). 2015 Jul. Available from: http://ircmj.com/20598.abstract.
21. Kuta FA, Babatunde OE. Epidemiology of hepatitis B virus surface and core antigens among pregnant women visiting Ring Road Hospital for antenatal care in Ibadan South-West, Local Government Area, Oyo State, Nigeria. Brazilian J Biol Sci [Internet]. Jun [Cited 2015 Nov 10];2(3):13–6. 2015; Available from: http://revista.rebibio.net/v2n3/v02n03a02.html.
22. Anaedobe CG, Fowotade A, Omoruyi C, Bakare R. Prevalence, sociodemographic features and risk factors of Hepatitis B virus infection among pregnant women in Southwestern Nigeria. Pan Afr Med J [Internet]. 2015 Apr 24 [Cited 2015 Dec 17];20(406). Available from: http://www.panafrican-med-journal.com/content/article/20/406/full/.
23. Ghana Statistical Service. 2010 Population & Housing Census: Lawra District Analytical Report [Internet]. Accra, Ghana; 2014 Oct [cited 2015 Dec 21]. Available from: http://www.statsghana.gov.gh/docfiles/2010_District_Report/Upper%20West/LAWRA.pdf.
24. UNICEF. Statistics | At a glance: Ghana [Internet]. 2013 [cited. Nov 9. 2015; Available from: https://www.unicef.org/infobycountry/ghana_statistics.html.
25. Mywage.org/Ghana. Ghana - Living wages, Minimum Wages, National Poverty Line, Actual Salaries [Internet]. Mywage.org/Ghana. 2017 [cited 2015 Nov 9]. Available from: http://www.mywage.org/ghana/home/salary/wages-in-context.
26. Alison B. Comfort, Lauren A. Peterson LEH. Effect of Health Insurance on the Use and Provision of Maternal Health Services and Maternal and Neonatal Health Outcomes: A Systematic Review. J Health Popul Nutr [Internet]. 2013 Dec 1 [cited 2015 Nov 9];31(4 Suppl 2):S81. Available from: /pmc/articles/PMC4021700/?report=abstract.
27. Ugbebor O, Aigbirior M, Osazuwa F, Enabudoso E, Zabayo O. The prevalence of hepatitis B and C viral infections among pregnant women. N am J med Sci. 2011;3(5):238–41.
28. Brouard C, Gautier A, Saboni L, Jestin C, Semaille C, Beltzer N. Hepatitis B knowledge, perceptions and practices in the French general population: the room for improvement. BMC Public Health [Internet]. 2013 Jan [Cited 2015

Nov 22];13:576. Available from: https://www.ncbi.nlm.nih.gov/pmc/articles/PMC3849746/?tool=pmcentrez.

29. Kolawole OM, Wahab AA, Adekanle DA, Sibanda T, Okoh AI. Seroprevalence of hepatitis B surface antigenemia and its effects on hematological parameters in pregnant women in Osogbo, Nigeria. Virol J [Internet]. 2012 Jan [Cited 2015 Sep 12];9(1):317. Available from: https://virologyj.biomedcentral.com/articles/10.1186/1743-422X-9-317.
30. ul Haq N, Hassali MA, Shafie AA, Saleem F, Farooqui M, Haseeb A, et al. A cross-sectional assessment of knowledge, attitude and practice among Hepatitis-B patients in Quetta, Pakistan. BMC Public Health [Internet]. 2013 Jan 6 [Cited 2015 Dec 22];13(1):448. Available from: https://bmcpublichealth.biomedcentral.com/articles/10.1186/1471-2458-13-448.
31. Karaivazoglou K, Triantos C, Lagadinou M, Bikas C, Michailidou M, Kalafateli M, et al. Acceptance of hepatitis B vaccination among health care workers in Western Greece .Arch Environ Occup Health [Internet]. 2014 Jan [cited 2015 Dec 11];69(2):107–11. Available from: https://www.ncbi.nlm.nih.gov/pubmed/24205962.
32. Norman ul H, Mohammed AH, Asrul AS, Fahad S, Farooqui M, Alijadhey H, et al. Association between Hepatitis B-Related Knowledge and Health-Related Quality of Life. Trop J Pharm Res [Internet]. 2014 Jul [Cited 2015 Dec 17];13(7):1163–8. Available from: https://www.tjpr.org/vol13_no7/2014_13_7_22.pdf.

Comparison of hepatitis E virus seroprevalence between HBsAg-positive population and healthy controls in Shandong province, China

Li Zhang[1,2†], Zechun Jiang[3†], Jingjing Lv[2], Jiaye Liu[2], Bingyu Yan[2], Yi Feng[2], Li Li[4], Guomin Zhang[4], Fuzhen Wang[4] and Aiqiang Xu[1,2*]

Abstract

Background: Persons with chronic hepatitis B (CHB) infection were reported to suffer severe disease after hepatitis E virus (HEV) superinfection, but the studies regarding HEV seroprevalence in this population were limited. A recent study in Vietnam found higher HEV seroprevalence among CHB patients compared with healthy controls.

Methods: A community-based case-control study was conducted in two counties of Shandong province, China, where hepatitis E incidence was at the highest (Rushan) and lowest (Zhangqiu) in the province based on data from routine public health surveillance. Four townships were selected randomly from each county and all residents in these townships were tested for hepatitis B surface antigen (HBsAg). Those tested positive for HBsAg (CHB group) and the 1:1 age and sex-matched HBsAg-negative residents (control group) were included. Anti-HEV IgM and IgG were tested and positive rates of IgG and IgM were compared between the CHB group and the control group.

Results: In total, 2048 CHB participants and 2054 controls were included in the study. In the CHB group, HEV IgG seroprevalence was 9.16% (95% *CI*: 7.47–11.09) in Zhangqiue and 38.06% (95% *CI*: 35.07–41.19) in Rushan ($P < 0.001$); the corresponding rates of IgM were 0.1% (95% *CI*: 0.002–0.54) and 1.57% (95% *CI*: 0.90–2.53), respectively ($P < 0.001$). HEV IgG seroprevalence was similar between CHB group and the control group in both counties ($P = 0.21$, $P = 0.47$, respectively) and the same results were found for the positive rate of IgM ($P = 0.103$, $P = 0.262$, respectively). Multivariable analysis showed the status of HBsAg was not independently associated with the status of anti-HEV IgG in either Zhangqiu or Rushan [$P = 0.187$, $OR = 1.23$(95% *CI*: 0.90, 1.68); $P = 0.609$, $OR = 1.05$ (95% *CI*: 0.87, 1.26)].

Conclusions: The seroprevalence of HEV varies greatly in different geographic areas, but the seroprevalence is similar between populations with and without CHB. CHB patients residing in high HEV endemic areas might be at higher risk for HBV-HEV superinfection.

Keywords: Hepatitis E virus, Chronic hepatitis B, Seroprevlance, Superinfection

* Correspondence: aqxuepi@163.com
†Equal contributors
[1]Academy of Preventive Medicine, Shandong University, Jinan, China
[2]Shandong Provincial Key Laboratory of Infectious Disease Control and Prevention, Shandong Center for Disease Control and Prevention, Jinan, China
Full list of author information is available at the end of the article

Background

Hepatitis E virus (HEV) was discovered in 1980's and has been documented to be prevalent in many countries [1]. HEV seroprevalence among the general population was 1.95% in the Netherlands [2], 5.3% in Japan [3] and 21% in the United States [4]. HEV is among the leading causes of acute viral hepatitis in developing countries [5] and is responsible for approximately 56,600 deaths in the world annually [6]. HEV infection is often asymptomatic, however in some special populations including pregnant women, patients with chronic hepatitis and those who are immunosuppressed, it might cause severe disease or chronic infection [7–9].

Although HEV is primarily transmitted by the faecal-oral route, its transmission by transfusion has already been documented [5]. HEV RNA was detected in 0.001% to 0.33% of blood donors in Australian, the United States and Qatar [10–12], suggesting the risk of HEV infection through transfusion. It is well known that hepatitis B and C could also be transmitted by transfusion. The studies from Turkey and Sweden found the seroprevalence of HEV was significantly higher among chronic hepatitis C patients compared with the general population [13, 14]. A study in Vietnam found significantly higher seroprevalence of HEV among chronic hepatitis B (CHB) patients [15], while the study in France found no difference [16].

Both hepatitis B and hepatitis E are endemic in China. The seroprevalence of hepatitis B surface antigen (HBsAg) and anti-HEV IgG was 7.18% and 23.1%, respectively according to a national survey in 2006 [17, 18]. The estimated number of persons with CHB is up to 90 million in China [17]. Although the superinfection of HBV and HEV has been widely reported in China [19, 20], all available studies are hospital-based focusing on clinical outcomes after superinfection. HEV seroprevalence among persons with CHB is poorly understood in China.

We conducted this study to evaluate HEV seroprevalence among persons with and without CHB in Shandong province, China.

Methods

Study population

Shandong province is located in eastern China. The province has 140 counties and a population of 97 million. The average seroprevalence of anti-HEV IgG was 11% among the general population [21]. This study was conducted during April and July 2014. The study population was selected by two-stage sampling method. First, all counties were ranked by HEV incidence reported through China National Notifiable Disease Reporting System (NNDRS) in 2013 and the county with the highest (Rushan) and the lowest (Zhangqiu) HEV incidence were selected. Second, four townships were selected by simple random sampling from each county. All residents in these townships were tested for HBsAg. All HBsAg-positive inhabitants and 1:1 age and sex-matched inhabitants negative for HBsAg were included in the study. The study flow chart is shown in Fig. 1.

Questionnaire survey

A face-to-face interview was conducted by the staff from the county level Center for Disease Control and Prevention (CDC). The information was collected on age, gender, education attainment, special occupations (seafood cultivation, processing and selling; swine laughter or selling), health habits including washing hands before dining, drinking boiled water and not-eating out of home and the histories of chronic diseases such as hypertension, heart disease, stroke, etc.

Sample collection and testing

Blood samples of 5 ml were collected from each participant. HBsAg was detected using Xinchuang ELISA kits (Xinchuang Biology Co., Xiamen, China). Anti-HEV IgG and IgM were detected using the Wantai ELISA kits (Wantai Biology Co., Beijing, China). HEV RNA was tested by real-time PCR for the serum positive for anti-HEV IgM (Invitrogen, one step qRT-PCR system). All tests were performed following the manufacturers' instructions and were conducted by staff at Shandong Provincial CDC.

Medical examination for HBsAg-positive participants

Further medical examination was carried out for HBsAg-positive participants in local hospitals, including physical examination, Ultrasound examination of liver, testing of HBV serological markers including antibody against HBsAg (anti-HBs), antibody against hepatitis B core antigen (anti-HBc), hepatitis B e antigen (HBeAg) and antibody against hepatitis B e antigen (anti-HBe), and HBV DNA level and Alanine aminotransferase (ALT) level. The participants were classified into HBV carrier, CHB patients, cirrhosis and hepatocellular carcinoma (HCC) according to the above medical examination. HBV carrier was defined as: (1) Tested positive for HBsAg; (2) had no signs and symptoms suggestive of hepatitis; (3) ALT level was within normal limit (< 40 IU/ml) [22]; (4) B ultrasound examination did not find any abnormalities in the liver. A case of chronic hepatitis patient was defined as: (1) HBsAg seropositive status lasted for 6 months or beyond; (2) had signs and symptoms suggestive of hepatitis; (3) HBV DNA was positive and ALT level increased(≥40 IU/ml) and (4) B ultrasound examination showed chronic liver disease. Cirrhosis and HCC were diagnosed mainly according to ultrasound findings.

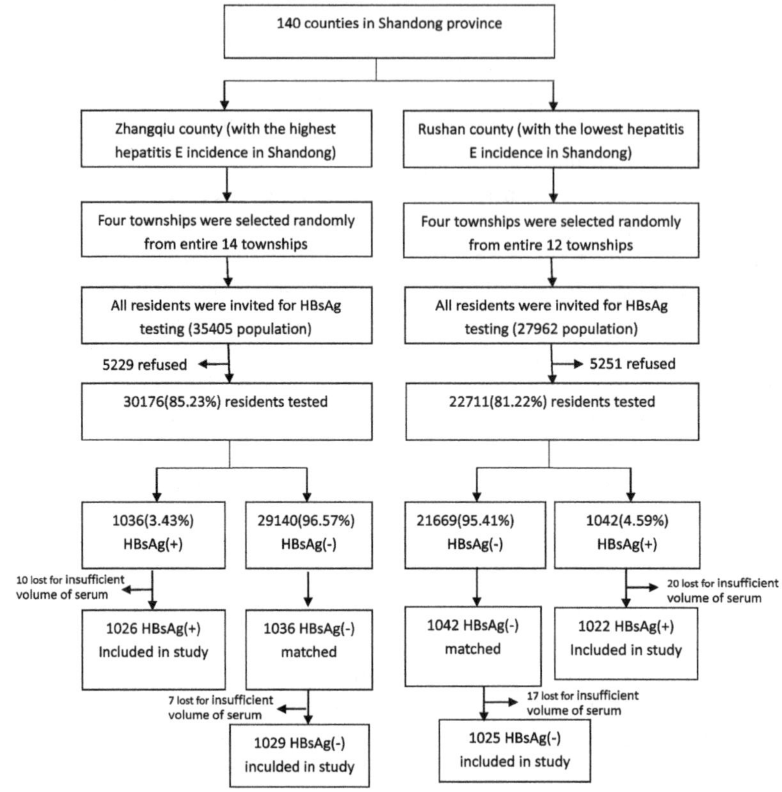

Fig. 1 Study participant flow chart

Statistical analyses

The seroprevalence of anti-HEV IgG and IgM across different groups was assessed with Pearson Chi-square test, trend Chi-square test and fisher's exact test as appropriate. Multivariable logistic regression model was built to estimate the independent association between status of anti-HEV IgG and HBsAg. The analyses were conducted with STATA 10.0 and the P value < 0.05 was considered to be statistically significant.

Ethical issues

This study was approved by Ethics Committee of Shandong Provincial CDC and a written informed consent form was signed by each participant.

Table 1 Demographic characteristics of HBsAg positive and negative participants in Zhangqiu and Rushan county, Shandong province, China

	Zhangqiu county			Rushan county		
	HBsAg-positive group (number, %)	HBsAg-negative group (number, %)	*P* value	HBsAg-positive group (number, %)	HBsAg-negative group (number, %)	*P* value
Total	1026 (100.00)	1029 (100.00)		1022 (100.00)	1025 (100.00)	
Age (yrs)						
Under 30	57 (5.56)	40 (3.89)	0.232	66 (6.46)	72 (7.02)	0.462
30–39	161(15.69)	170(16.52)		79(7.73)	79(7.71)	
40–49	284 (27.68)	275 (26.72)		242 (23.68)	237 (23.12)	
50–59	226 (22.03)	234 (22.74)		336 (32.88)	331 (32.29)	
60–69	196 (19.10)	200 (19.44)		211 (20.65)	222 (21.66)	
Above 70	102 (9.94)	110 (10.69)		88 (8.61)	84 (8.20)	
Gender						
Male	520 (50.68)	529 (51.41)	0.742	516 (50.49)	525 (51.22)	0.471
Female	506 (49.32)	500 (48.59)		506 (49.51)	500 (48.78)	

Results

Demographic characteristics of the participants

As shown in Tables 1, 1026 HBsAg-positive participants (age: 51.13 ± 13.42 years, age range: 6–85 years) and 1029 HBsAg-negative participants (51.62 ± 13.40 years, age range: 8–92 years) were included in the analysis in Zhangqiu. The corresponding numbers of participants were 1022 (52.11 ± 13.07 years, age range: 8–80 years) and 1025 (51.63 ± 13.65 years, age range: 5–86 years) in Rushan. No significant differences were found in age and gender between HBsAg-positive and HBsAg-negative group in both counties (Zhangqiu: $P = 0.232$, 0.742; Rushan: $P = 0.462$, 0.471). In Zhangqiu, the HBsAg-positive group was consisted of 658 HBV carriers, 102 chronic hepatitis, 22 cirrhotic cases, 1 HCC case and 243 participants with unknown clinical type. In Rushan, the corresponding numbers were 838, 74, 8, 3 and 99.

Anti-HEV IgG seroprevalence among HBsAg-positive individuals

HEV IgG seroprevalence was 9.16% (95% *CI* 7.47–11.09) in CHB group in Zhangqiu and was lower in comparison with that in Rushan (38.06%, $P < 0.001$). IgG seroprevalence increased with age in both counties ($P < 0.01$), although the seroprevalence was significantly higher in Rushan than in Zhangqiu in all age groups except those above 70 years ($P < 0.05$). IgG seroprevalnce was similar in males and females in Zhangqiu ($P = 0.938$), but was significantly different in Rushan ($P < 0.001$). The rate was much higher among HBV carriers in Rushan than in Zhangqiu ($P < 0.001$) and the same result was observed among hepatitis cases ($P < 0.001$). No significant difference in HEV IgG seroprevalence was found among different CHB groups in Zhangqiu ($P = 0.714$) and the same result was found in Rushan ($P = 0.267$). The details are shown in Tables 2, 3 and Fig. 2.

Table 2 Seroprevalence of hepatitis E IgG in HBsAg-positive group and HBsAg- negative group by age and gender in Zhangqiu and Rushan

	HBsAg-positive group		HBsAg-negative group		*P* value#*
	Number detected	Positive, *n* (%, 95% *CI*)	Number detected	Positive, *n* (%, 95% *CI*)	
Zhangqiu county					
Total	1026	94 (9.16,7.47–11.09)	1029	112 (10.88, 9.05–12.95)	0.21
Age (yrs)					
0-	53	0 (0.00, 0–6.72)	38	4 (10.53, 2.94–24.80)	0.03
30-	157	5 (3.18, 1.04–7.28)	167	7 (4.19, 1.70–8.44)	0.77
40-	275	18 (6.55, 3.92–10.15)	275	21 (7.64, 4.79–11.44)	0.74
50-	232	10 (4.31, 2.09–7.78)	237	24 (10.13, 6.60–14.69)	0.02
60-	217	33 (15.21, 10.70–20.69)	217	29 (13.36, 9.14–18.63)	0.68
70-	92	28 (30.43, 21.27–40.90)	95	27 (28.42, 1.96–38.60)	0.87
Gender					
Male	520	48 (9.23, 6.88–12.05)	500	52 (10.40, 7.86–13.41)	0.60
Female	506	46 (9.09, 6.73–11.94)	1029	112 (10.88, 9.05–12.95)	0.33
Rushan county					
Total	1022	389 (38.06, 35.07–41.19)	1025	407 (39.71, 36.70–42.78)	0.47
Age (yrs)					
0-	67	5 (7.46, 2.47–16.56)	73	15 (20.55, 11.98–31.62)	0.027
30-	74	25 (33.78, 23.19–45.18)	78	26 (33.33, 23.06–44.92)	1.00
40-	234	95 (40.60, 34.25–47.19)	234	94 (40.17, 33.84–46.76)	1.00
50-	337	132 (39.17, 33.92–44.60)	340	139 (40.88, 35.61–46.76)	0.70
60-	226	103 (45.58, 38.96–52.31)	225	100 (44.44, 37.84–51.20)	0.85
70-	84	29 (34.52, 24.48–45.69)	75	33 (44.00, 32.55–55.94)	0.26
Gender					
Male	516	216 (41.86, 37.56–46.25)	525	229 (43.62, 39.33–47.98)	0.57
Female	506	173 (34.19, 30.06–38.50)	500	178 (35.60, 31.40–39.97)	0.64

Comparison between HBsAg positive and negative participants

*Fisher exact test

Table 3 Prevalence of anti-HEV IgG among HBsAg-positive participants by clinical types in Rushan county and Zhangqiu county, Shandong province, China

County	Clinical type	Number detected	HEV IgG(+) Number (%, 95% *CI*)	*P* value
Zhangqiu	HBV carrier	658	53 (8.05, 6.09–10.40)	0.714
	Chronic case	102	9 (8.82, 4.11–16.09)	
	Cirrhosis case	22	0 (0.00, 0–15.44)	
	HCC case	1	0 (0.00, 0–97.5)	
Rushan	HBV carrier	838	314 (37.47, 34.18–40.85)	0.267
	Chronic case	74	30 (40.54, 29.27–52.59)	
	Cirrhosis case	8	3 (37.50, 8.52–75.51)	
	HCC case	3	3 (100.00, 29.24, 100.00)	

HBV hepatitis B virus, *HCC* hepatocellular carcinoma

In the CHB group, the positive rate of HBeAg among anti-HEV IgG (+) participants was significantly lower than the rate among anti-HEV IgG (–) participants (17.18% vs 24.54%, $P = 0.001$), and the same trend was found in the proportion of participants with HBV DNA > 10^3 copies/ml (32.92% vs 40.38%, $P = 0.011$). No significant difference was found between the participants positive for anti-HEV IgG and negative for anti-HEV IgG in the proportions of participants with elevated ALT level and the liver damage identified by ultrasound ($P > 0.05$). The details are shown in Table 4.

Anti-HEV IgM seroprevalence among HBsAg-positive individuals

Only one participant was positive for anti-HEV IgM in CHB group in Zhangqiu and the positive rate was 0.1% (95%*CI:* 0.002–0.54). The corresponding rate was 1.57% (16/1022, 95% *CI*: 0.90–2.53) in Rushan, which was much higher than the rate in Zhangqiu ($P < 0.001$). The positive rate of IgM in Rushan was not statistically significant by age, gender and clinical types ($P > 0.05$). HEV RNA has been tested for all serum positive for anti-HEV IgM, but none was positive. The details are shown in Table 5.

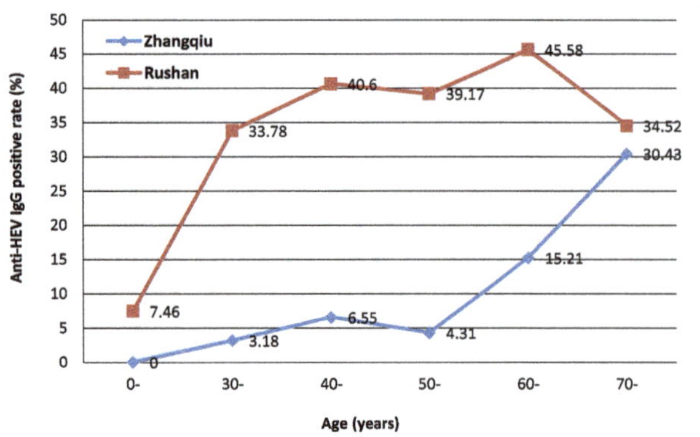

Fig. 2 Anti-HEV IgG seroprevalence by age among HBsAg-positive participants in Zhangqiu county and Rushan county, Shandong province, China

Comparison of HEV seroprevalence between CHB group and control group

HEV IgG seroprevalence was 9.16% and 10.88% in the CHB group and the control group, respectively, in Zhangqiu and the corresponding rates were 38.06% and 39.71% in Rushan. No significant difference between the two groups was found in either county ($P = 0.21$, $P = 0.47$, respectively). Age-specific and sex-specific seroprevalence of HEV IgG was similar between the CHB group and the control group except in age-groups of 0–29 years and 50–59 years in Zhangqiu and 0–29 years in Rushan. The positive rate of anti-HEV IgM was 0.1% and 0.48% respectively among CHB group and the control group in Zhangqiu ($P = 0.103$). The corresponding rates in Rushan were 1.57% and 2.24% and the difference was not significant too ($P = 0.262$).

Multivariable analysis showed that only age was independently associated with anti-HEV IgG in Zhangqiu ($P < 0.05$), and gender, age and education attainment were independently associated with anti-HEV IgG in Rushan ($P < 0.05$). The status of HBsAg was not independently associated with the status of anti-HEV IgG in either county ($P > 0.05$). The details are shown in Table 6.

Discussion

Our study showed similar HEV seroprevalence between HBsAg-positive and negative participants in areas with different HEV endemicity. This result is consistent with some previous studies [13, 23], but different from the study by Hoan NX [15]. The reason for the above difference might be due to differences in the participants in these studies. Our study is community-based and most HBsAg-positive participants are HBV carriers, while Hoan NX's study is hospital-based and most participants are chronic hepatitis patients. HEV genotype 4 is predominant in Shandong province [24, 25], and its epidemiology differs from other genotyopes [5, 26], so

Table 4 The results of medical examination in HBsAg-positive participants by anti-HEV IgG

	Anti-HEV IgG positive		Anti-HEV IgG negative		*P* value
	Number	%	Number	%	
Total	483	100.00	1565	100.00	
HBeAg					
Positive	83	17.18	384	24.54	0.001
Negative	400	82.82	1181	75.46	
Anti-HBe					
Positive	313	64.80	1022	65.30	0.840
Negative	170	35.20	543	34.70	
HBV DNA (IU/ml)					
$< 10^3$	324	67.08	933	59.62	0.011
10^3–10^6	97	20.08	404	25.81	
$\geq 10^6$	62	12.84	228	14.57	
ALT(U/L)					
Normal	440	91.10	1442	92.14	0.463
Elevated	43	8.90	123	7.86	
Liver abnormality[a]					
Yes	5	1.04	13	0.83	0.674
No	478	98.96	1552	99.17	

[a]Identified by B ultrasound

Table 5 Seroprevalence of anti-HEV IgM among population with chronic hepatitis B infection in Rushan county, Shandong province, China

	Number detected	Positive number	Positive rate (%, 95% *CI*)	*P* value
Total	1022	16	1.57 (0.90–2.53)	–
Age group (yrs)				
Under 30	66	0	0 (0–5.44)	0.768
30–39	79	1	1.26 (0.03–6.85)	
40–49	242	6	2.48 (0.92–5.32)	
50–59	336	5	1.49 (0.48–3.44)	
60–69	211	3	1.42 (0.29–4.10)	
Above 70	88	1	1.14 (0.03–6.17)	
Gender				
Male	516	8	1.55 (0.67–3.03)	0.969
Female	506	8	1.58 (0.68–3.09)	
Clinical type[a]				
HBV carrier	838	12	1.43 (0.74–2.49)	0.060#
Chronic cases	74	0	0 (0–4.86)	
Cirrhosis	8	0	0 (0–36.94)	
HCC	3	1	33.33 (0.84–90.57)	

HBV hepatitis B virus, *HCC* hepatic cellular cancer
Fisher's exact test
[a]Ninety nine participants with unknown clinical type were not involved in the analysis

our finding should be further studied in other areas with different HEV genotypes.

Our study has provided the preliminary evidence for high incidence of HBV-HEV superinfection, in HEV hyper-endemic areas. According to our study, positive results for anti-HEV IgG were found approximately among 40% of HBsAg-positive persons in Rushan. In China, most chronic HBV infections occur at birth or early childhood, while most HEV infections occur in adults [18]. So it is most likely that HEV infection in our study participants had occurred after HBV infection. Although the duration of the persistence of anti-HEV IgG is still unclear, it is sure not to be life-long [27, 28]. Given this fact, the real seroprevalence of HEV among HBsAg-positive participants might be higher than what we observed in the study.

The detection of anti-HEV IgM could give the direct evidence of acute hepatitis E infection among persons with chronic HBV infection. Although the positive rate of anti-HEV IgM was very low among HBsAg-positive participants in Rushan in our study (only 1%), it suggests a high risk to attack HEV acute infection among HBsAg-positive patients in the county because this result came from a cross-section study instead of a cohort study.

Some studies showed that HEV infection could result in severe disease in patients with underlying CHB even liver failure [8, 29–31], but the other obtained the opposite conclusion [32]. We did not find more active HBV replication and more severe live damage in HBsAg(+), anti-HEV IgG(+) participants than in HBsAg(+), anti-HEV IgG(−) participants in the present study. However, it must be noted that most participants were HBV carriers in our study, while most previous studies were conducted among patient with chronic hepatitis or in cirrhotic patients.

Hepatitis E vaccine was licensed in China in 2011 and is the unique commercially available hepatitis E vaccine in the world till now [33]. The immunogenicity and safety of hepatitis E vaccine has been documented in HBV carriers [34], but no similar studies are available among CHB, cirrhosis and HCC patients. Given the fact that most CHB patients develop from HBV carriers and the long-lasting anti-HEV IgG induced by hepatitis E vaccine has been documented [35], hepatitis E vaccine is recommended to HBV carriers to prevent HBV-HEV superinfection, especially in HEV hyperendemic areas.

Two counties with different HEV prevalent level were included in the study, giving the study more depth and improved the generalisability of the findings. However, due to the community-based design of the study, most HBsAg-positive participants were carriers in our study and the conclusions should be further documented in clinical cases.

Table 6 Multivariable analysis of the risk factors associated with anti-HEV IgG in Zhangqiu county and Rushan county, Shandong province, China

	Zhangqiu			Rushan		
	Participant number	*P*	*OR* (95% CI)	Participant number	*P*	*OR* (95% CI)
Gender						
Male	1049	Ref.	Ref.	1041	Ref.	Ref.
Female	1006	0.05	0.72 (0.52,0.98)	1006	< 0.001	0.71 (0.58,0.86)
Age (yrs)						
Under 30	97	Ref.	Ref.	138	Ref.	Ref.
30–39	331	0.54	0.71 (0.24,2.10)	158	< 0.001	3.38 (1.87,6.11)
40–49	559	0.46	1.45 (0.54,3.88)	479	< 0.001	4.64 (2.74,7.86)
50–59	460	0.41	1.53 (0.56,4.17)	667	< 0.001	4.17 (2.49,6.99)
60–69	396	0.02	3.22 (1.18,8.73)	433	< 0.001	5.47 (3.20,9.35)
Above 70	212	< 0.001	8.62 (3.08,24.15)	172	< 0.001	4.49 (2.45,8.22)
Education attainment						
Illiteracy	227	Ref.	Ref.	115	Ref.	Ref.
Primary school	739	0.246	1.32 (0.83,2.09)	560	0.025	1.66 (1.06,2.60)
Junior middle school	972	0.676	1.12 (0.64,1.96)	1121	0.037	1.63 (1.03,2.58)
Senior middle school and above	117	0.715	1.18 (0.48,2.92)	251	0.033	1.76 (1.04,2.96)
Occupation about swine laughter or selling						
Yes	11	Ref.	Ref.	61	Ref.	Ref.
No	2044	0.122	0.29 (0.06,1.39)	1986	0.654	1.13 (0.66,1.93)
Occupation about seafood cultivation, processing or selling						
Yes	0	–	–	43	Ref.	Ref.
No	2055	–	–	2004	0.103	0.59 (0.31,1.11)
Wash hands before dining						
≧2 times per day	2015	Ref.	Ref.	1877	Ref.	Ref.
≦one time per day	40	0.506	0.61 (0.14,2.63)	170	0.984	1.00 (0.72,1.39)
Drinking unboiled water						
≧3 times per week	51	Ref.	Ref.	143	Ref.	Ref.
1–2 times per week	417	0.637	1.32 (0.42, 4.12)	214	0.12	0.69 (0.44,1.09)
Less than once per week	1587	0.673	1.27 (0.42, 3.87)	1690	0.6	0.91 (0.63,1.31)
Eating outside						
≧3 times per week	94	Ref.	Ref.	98	Ref.	Ref.
1–2 times per week	611	0.926	1.04 (0.47,2.29)	140	0.924	0.97 (0.55,1.72)
Less than once per week	1350	0.644	0.83 (0.38,1.81)	1809	0.34	1.25 (0.79,1.96)
Chronic hepatitis B infection						
Yes	1026	Ref.	Ref.	1022	Ref.	Ref.
No	1029	0.187	1.23 (0.90,1.68)	1025	0.609	1.05 (0.87,1.26)

Conclusions

The HEV seroprevalence is similar between HBsAg-positive and HBsAg-negative participants in the same area. The risk of HBV-HEV superinfection could vary greatly in different areas and the HBsAg-positive persons living in HEV hyperendemic areas might be at higher risk for HBV-HEV superinfection. Further study should be conducted to determine the epidemiological characteristics and clinical outcome of HEV-HBV superinfection in HEV hyperendemic areas.

Abbreviations

Anti-HBs: antibody against HBsAg; CHB: Chronic hepatitis B; CI: Confidential interval; HBsAg: Hepatitis B surface antigen; HBV: Hepatitis B virus; HCC: Hepatocellular carcinoma; HEV: Hepatitis E virus

Acknowledgments

We thank our colleagues at Zhangqiu county CDC and Rushan county CDC for their help in questionnaire survey and blood collection.

Funding

This work was supported by the grants from the Major Project of National Science and Technology (No. 2013ZX10004902),a cooperation project of China Foundation for Hepatitis Prevention and Control, Chinese Center for Disease Control and Prevention and Shandong Provincial Center for Disease Control and Prevention (2014–32-R-019), Taishan Scholar Program of Shandong Province (No. ts20151105) and the Shandong Medical Health Science and Technology Development Programs (2011HD006, 2016ws0386). The funders had no role in study design, data collection and analysis, decision to publish, or preparation of the manuscript.

Author's contributions

LZ contributed to the study design, data collection and the manuscript draft. BY and YF contributed to the laboratory test. ZJ contributed to the study design, questionnaire investigation and blood sample collection. JLv and JLiu contributed to questionnaire investigation, data entry and analysis. LL, GZ, FW contributed to the study design and data collection. AX contributed to the study design and the manuscript revision. All authors have read and approved the manuscript.

Consent for publication

Not applicable.

Competing interests

The authors declare that they have no competing interests.

Author details

[1]Academy of Preventive Medicine, Shandong University, Jinan, China. [2]Shandong Provincial Key Laboratory of Infectious Disease Control and Prevention, Shandong Center for Disease Control and Prevention, Jinan, China. [3]Rushan Center for Disease Control and Prevention, Weihai, China. [4]Chinese Center for Disease Control and Prevention, Beijing, China.

References

1. Kamar N, Bendall R, Legrand-Abravanel F, Xia NS, Ijaz S, Izopet J, Dalton HR. Hepatitis E. Lancet. 2012;379(9835):2477–88.
2. Verhoef L, Koopmans M, Duizer E, Bakker J, Reimerink J, Van Pelt W. Seroprevalence of hepatitis E antibodies and risk profile of HEV seropositivity in The Netherlands, 2006-2007. Epidemiol Infect. 2012;140(10):1838–47.
3. Takahashi M, Tamura K, Hoshino Y, Nagashima S, Yazaki Y, Mizuo H, Iwamoto S, Okayama M, Nakamura Y, Kajii E, et al. A nationwide survey of hepatitis E virus infection in the general population of Japan. J Med Virol. 2010;82(2):271–81.
4. Kuniholm MH, Purcell RH, McQuillan GM, Engle RE, Wasley A, Nelson KE. Epidemiology of hepatitis E virus in the United States: results from the third National Health and nutrition examination survey, 1988-1994. J Infect Dis. 2009;200(1):48–56.
5. Hepatitis E vaccine: WHO position paper, May 2015. *Releve epidemiologique hebdomadaire* 2015, 90(18):185–200.
6. Holla RP, Ahmad I, Ahmad Z, Jameel S. Molecular virology of hepatitis E virus. Semin Liver Dis. 2013;33(1):3–14.
7. Kamar N, Selves J, Mansuy JM, Ouezzani L, Peron JM, Guitard J, Cointault O, Esposito L, Abravanel F, Danjoux M, et al. Hepatitis E virus and chronic hepatitis in organ-transplant recipients. N Engl J Med. 2008;358(8):811–7.
8. Ramachandran J, Eapen CE, Kang G, Abraham P, Hubert DD, Kurian G, Hephzibah J, Mukhopadhya A, Chandy GM. Hepatitis E superinfection produces severe decompensation in patients with chronic liver disease. J Gastroenterol Hepatol. 2004;19(2):134–8.
9. Centers for Disease C. Prevention: investigation of hepatitis E outbreak among refugees - upper Nile, South Sudan, 2012-2013. MMWR Morb Mortal Wkly Rep. 2013;62(29):581–6.
10. Hoad VC, Seed CR, Fryk JJ, Harley R, Flower RLP, Hogema BM, Kiely P, Faddy HM. Hepatitis E virus RNA in Australian blood donors: prevalence and risk assessment. Vox Sang. 2017;112(7):614–21.
11. Roth NJ, Schafer W, Alexander R, Elliott K, Elliott-Browne W, Knowles J, Wenzel JJ, Simon TL. Low hepatitis E virus RNA prevalence in a large-scale survey of United States source plasma donors. Transfusion. 2017;
12. Nasrallah GK, Al Absi ES, Ghandour R, Ali NH, Taleb S, Hedaya L, Ali F, Huwaidy M, Husseini A. Seroprevalence of hepatitis E virus among blood donors in Qatar (2013-2016). Transfusion. 2017;57(7):1801–7.
13. Bayram A, Eksi F, Mehli M, Sozen E. Prevalence of hepatitis E virus antibodies in patients with chronic hepatitis B and chronic hepatitis C. Intervirology. 2007;50(4):281–6.
14. Mellgren A, Karlsson M, Karlsson M, Lagging M, Wejstal R, Norder H. High seroprevalence against hepatitis E virus in patients with chronic hepatitis C virus infection. J Clin Virol. 2017;88:39–45.
15. Hoan NX, Tong HV, Hecht N, Sy BT, Marcinek P, Meyer CG, Song le H, Toan NL, Kurreck J, Kremsner PG, et al. Hepatitis E virus superinfection and clinical progression in hepatitis B patients. EBioMedicine. 2015;2(12):2080–6.
16. Roux P, Le Gall JM, Debrus M, Protopopescu C, Ndiaye K, Demoulin B, Lions C, Haas A, Mora M, Spire B et al. Innovative community-based educational face-to-face intervention to reduce HIV, hepatitis C virus and other blood-borne infectious risks in difficult-to-reach people who inject drugs: results from the ANRS-AERLI intervention study. Addiction 2016, 111(1):94–106.
17. Liang X, Bi S, Yang W, Wang L, Cui G, Cui F, Zhang Y, Liu J, Gong X, Chen Y, et al. Epidemiological serosurvey of hepatitis B in China–declining HBV prevalence due to hepatitis B vaccination. Vaccine. 2009;27(47):6550–7.
18. Jia Z, Yi Y, Liu J, Cao J, Zhang Y, Tian R, Yu T, Wang H, Wang X, Su Q, et al. Epidemiology of hepatitis E virus in China: results from the third National Viral Hepatitis Prevalence Survey, 2005-2006. PLoS One. 2014;9(10):e110837.
19. Shang Q, Yu J, Xiao D, Xu C, Chen C, Zhang G. The effects of hepatitis E virus superinfection on patients with chronic hepatitis B: a clinico-pathological study. Zhonghua nei ke za zhi. 2002;41(10):656–9.
20. Cheng SH, Mai L, Zhu FQ, Pan XF, Sun HX, Cao H, Shu X, Ke WM, Li G, Xu QH. Influence of chronic HBV infection on superimposed acute hepatitis E. World J Gastroenterol. 2013;19(35):5904–9.
21. Yan BYFY, Zhang L, Li MS, Song LZ, Xu Q, Xiao ZQ, Xu AQ. A seroepidemiological investigation on hepatitis E in Shandong Province. Zhong Hua Ji Bing Kong Zhi Za Zhi. 2013;17(9):785–8.
22. Omata M, Cheng AL, Kokudo N, Kudo M, Lee JM, Jia J, Tateishi R, Han KH, Chawla YK, Shiina S, et al. Asia-Pacific clinical practice guidelines on the management of hepatocellular carcinoma: a 2017 update. Hepatol Int. 2017;11(4):317–70.
23. Pischke S, Gisa A, Suneetha PV, Wiegand SB, Taubert R, Schlue J, Wursthorn K, Bantel H, Raupach R, Bremer B, et al. Increased HEV seroprevalence in patients with autoimmune hepatitis. PLoS One. 2014;9(1):e85330.
24. Zhang L, Yan B, Xu A. A hepatitis E outbreak by genotype 4 virus in Shandong province, China. Vaccine. 2016;34(33):3715–8.
25. Yang D, Jiang M, Jin M, Qiu ZG, Shen ZQ, Cui WH, Wang DN, Gong LF, Li B, Wang XW, et al. Seroprevalence and evolutionary dynamics of genotype 4 hepatitis E virus in Shandong Province, China. World J Gastroenterol. 2014;20(24):7955–63.
26. Teshale EH, Hu DJ. Hepatitis E: epidemiology and prevention. World J Hepatol. 2011;3(12):285–91.
27. Ke WM, Tan D, Li JG, Izumi S, Shinji Y, Hotta H, Yao JL. Consecutive evaluation of immunoglobulin M and G antibodies against hepatitis E virus. J Gastroenterol. 1996;31(6):818–22.
28. Khuroo MS, Kamili S, Dar MY, Moecklii R, Jameel S. Hepatitis E and long-term antibody status. Lancet. 1993;341(8856):1355.
29. Kumar M, Sharma BC, Sarin SK. Hepatitis E virus as an etiology of acute exacerbation of previously unrecognized asymptomatic patients with hepatitis B virus-related chronic liver disease. J Gastroenterol Hepatol. 2008;23(6):883–7.

30. Ke WM, Li XJ, Yu LN, Lai J, Li XH, Gao ZL, Chen PJ. Etiological investigation of fatal liver failure during the course of chronic hepatitis B in southeast China. J Gastroenterol. 2006;41(4):347–51.
31. Chow CW, Tsang SW, Tsang OT, Leung VK, Fung KS, Luk WK, Chau TN. Comparison of acute hepatitis E infection outcome in patients with and without chronic hepatitis B infection: a 10 year retrospective study in three regional hospitals in Hong Kong. J Clin Virol. 2014;60(1):4–10.
32. Blasco-Perrin H, Madden RG, Stanley A, Crossan C, Hunter JG, Vine L, Lane K, Devooght-Johnson N, McLaughlin C, Petrik J, et al. Hepatitis E virus in patients with decompensated chronic liver disease: a prospective UK/French study. Aliment Pharmacol Ther. 2015;42(5):574–81.
33. Li SW, Zhao Q, Wu T, Chen S, Zhang J, Xia NS. The development of a recombinant hepatitis E vaccine HEV 239. Human vaccines & immunotherapeutics. 2015;11(4):908–14.
34. Wu T, Huang SJ, Zhu FC, Zhang XF, Ai X, Yan Q, Wang ZZ, Yang CL, Jiang HM, Liu XH, et al. Immunogenicity and safety of hepatitis E vaccine in healthy hepatitis B surface antigen positive adults. Human vaccines & immunotherapeutics. 2013;9(11):2474–9.
35. Su YY, Huang SJ, Guo M, Zhao J, Yu H, He WG, Jiang HM, Wang YJ, Zhang XF, Cai JP, et al. Persistence of antibodies acquired by natural hepatitis E virus infection and effects of vaccination. Clin Microbiol Infect. 2017;23(5):336 e331–4.

Angiopoietin-like protein as a novel marker for liver fibrosis in chronic hepatitis B patients with normal to minimally raised ALT

Yongqiong Deng[1,2†], Hong Zhao[1†], Jiyuan Zhou[1], Linlin Yan[1], Guiqiang Wang[1,3,4*]
and China HepB-Related Fibrosis Assessment Research Group

Abstract

Background: For hepatitis B patients who do not meet the treatment criteria recommended by guidelines, therapy decisions depend on hepatic histology. Angiopoietin-like protein 2 (Angptl2) is a mediator of chronic inflammation that contributes to extracellular matrix remodeling. The aim of this study was to explore the predictive value of Angptl2 as a novel biomarker of liver histology.

Methods: Hepatitis B patients with normal to minimally raised ALT were recruited. Serum Angptl2 concentrations were detected using commercial ELISA kit. The fibrosis score were assessed according to Ishak criteria. Significant fibrosis was defined as ISHAK score ≥ 3.

Results: Of 460 patients, 223 cases served as training cohort and 237 ones as validation cohort. Serum Angptl2 concentration was significantly associated with fibrosis scores in both training and validation group. Angptl2 combined index (ACI) for assessing significant fibrosis was developed from training cohort, based on Angptl2 and conventional variables. ACI showed areas under receiver-operating characteristic curve (AUC) of 0.835 for predicting significant fibrosis, which was superior to APRI (AUC = 0.776, $P = 0.049$), FIB-4 (AUC = 0.750, $P = 0.010$), Hui model (AUC = 0.756, $P = 0.028$), and had a better trend than Forn's index (AUC = 0.796, $P = 0.083$) in training cohort. Finally, validation cohort revealed its robustness and reliability.

Conclusion: Higher Angptl2 level represents as a potential biomarker independently associated with fibrosis stages. Compared with APRI, Hui model, FIB-4, Forn's index, ACI did better in diagnosing significant fibrosis in hepatitis B patients.

Keywords: Angiopoietin-like protein, Hepatitis B, Liver fibrosis

* Correspondence: john131212@126.com
[†]Equal contributors
[1]Department of Infectious Disease, Center for Liver Disease, Peking University First Hospital, No. 8, Xishiku Street, Xicheng District, Beijing 100034, China
[3]The Collaborative Innovation Center for Diagnosis and Treatment of Infectious Diseases, Zhejiang University, Zhejiang, Hangzhou, China
Full list of author information is available at the end of the article

Background

Approximately 3.61% of the world's population (248 million individuals) is chronically infected with hepatitis B virus (HBV), and China, India, and Nigeria are the top three countries with the highest population of HBV surface antigen (HBsAg) positive patients [1]. At least 30% of cirrhosis and 50% of hepatocellular carcinoma (HCC) cases are associated with chronic HBV infection [2]. From an epidemiological survey conducted by the Chinese Center for Disease Control and Prevention in 2006, the weighted prevalence of HBsAg, anti-HBs, and hepatitis B core antigen antibody (anti-HBc) in Chinese individuals aged 1 to 59 years was 7.2, 50.1, and 34.1%, respectively [3]. An accurate initial evaluation of liver damage and the correct treatment decision for this population will not only decrease the future incidence of cirrhosis and HCC but also improve the quality of life and the survival rate. The 2015 APASL guidelines recommend immediately antiviral therapy for HBeAg-positive patients with HBV DNA levels ≥20,000 IU/ml or HBeAg-negative patients with HBV DNA levels ≥2000 IU/ml as well as patients with alanine aminotransferase (ALT) levels greater than 2 times the upper limit of normal (ULN); for patients with ALT <2 × ULN and HBV DNA below thresholds, treatment was suggested if moderate to severe inflammation or significant fibrosis (Ishak fibrosis score ≥ 3) [4]. Although liver biopsy was considered as the reference standard for staging inflammation and fibrosis, it was imperfect due to its invasiveness, sampling bias, inter-observer variations, intra-observer variations, risk of bile leakage, and hemorrhage [5–7]. In the last two decades, a variety of biomarkers and indexes has been developed for non-invasive diagnosis. But few of them were designed for hepatitis B patients with normal to minimally raised aminotransferases, for whom therapy decisions depend on hepatic histology.

Angptl2, a member of the angiopoietin-like protein family, has been recently shown to mediate chronic inflammation and subsequent pathological irreversible tissue remodeling [8]. Angptl2 increases matrix metalloproteinase (MMP) expression and activity through integrin a5ba-mediated activation of P38 mitogen-activated protein kinase (MAPK), thus promoting extracellular matrix (ECM) remodeling [9, 10]. Integrins, which act as functional receptors for Angptl2, are abundantly expressed on macrophages, endothelial cells, and adipocytes [8, 10]. Activated macrophages play a major role in chronic liver disease by synthesizing and releasing a battery of pro-fibrogenic and pro-inflammatory mediators [11]. It reported that angptl2 mRNA was expressed in liver and secreted by hepatocytes [12]. Additionally, higher level of Angptl2 in serum has been found in patients with non-small cell lung cancer, arteriosclerotic occlusion, gastric cancer [13–15], but whether the circulatory concentration of angtpl2 increased in liver disease was unknown. In this study, we hypothesized that Angptl2 participates in hepatic fibrogenesis in chronic liver disease and would be as a potential biomarker for diagnosis of liver fibrosis. The information presented herein might help to improve treatment decision making and avoid liver biopsy in patients with hepatitis.

Methods

Patients

Patients aged 18 – 65 years who showed HBsAg positivity for at least 6 months were recruited from 24 centers in Mainland China between October 2013 and May 2016. All patients were treatment naive. Exclusion criteria for this study included concomitant infection with hepatitis C virus (HCV) or human immunodeficiency virus (HIV) and other chronic liver diseases, such as alcoholic liver disease, autoimmune liver disease, heretic liver disease, drug-induced liver disease, and nonalcoholic liver disease. Patients with HCC or decompensate cirrhosis were also excluded. Clinical data, including age, gender, and body mass index (BMI), were recorded at the time of liver biopsy. There were 30 healthy people recruited as control subjects.

Laboratory tests

Serum hematological and biochemical parameters, such as platelet counts (PLT), ALT, aspartate aminotransferase (AST), albumin, gamma-glutamyltransferase (GGT), prothrombin time (PT), Total bilirubin (TBil) and cholesterol, were routinely obtained within 4 weeks of liver biopsy using standard methodologies in local hospitals. In this study, we are using ALT of 40 IU/ml as the upper limit of the normal [4].

Serum HBsAg levels were quantified using the Roche Elecsys® HBsAg II assay (Roche Diagnostics, Penzberg, Germany), and serum HBV-DNA (dynamic range 2.0×10^{1}–1.7×10^{8} IU/ml) was measured with the COBAS AmpliPrep/COBAS TaqMan method as previously described [16]. The qualitative detection of HBeAg and anti-HBe was also performed using relevant Roche Elecsys® assays according to the manufacturer's instructions.

The serum concentrations of Collagen IV, laminin (LN), hyaluronic acid, procollagen type III N-terminal peptide (PIIINP) were detected as previously described [17].

Non-invasive indexes for fibrosis, such as APRI, FIB-4, AAR, and Forns' index, were calculated as follows: $\text{APRI} = ([\text{AST}/\text{ULN}]/\text{platelet count}[\times 10^9/\text{L}]) \times 100$; $\text{FIB-4} = (\text{age} \times \text{AST})/(\text{platelet count})[\times 10^9/\text{L}] \times \text{ALT}^{1/2})$; $\text{Forns' index} = 7.811 - 3.131 \times \text{LN}(\text{Platelet count}) + 0.781 \times \text{LN}(\text{GGT}) + 3.467 \times \text{LN}(\text{Age}) - 0.014 \times \text{LN}(\text{cholesterol})$; Hui model: $gx = 1.23 + 0.167 \times \text{BMI} + 1.191 \times (\text{ALP}/135) + 0.081 \times \text{TBi} - 0.139 \times \text{Albumin} - 0.017 \times \text{PLT}$, $\text{Hui model} = \exp(gx)/(1 + \exp(gx))$ [18–21].

Serum Angptl2 concentration

Serum Angptl2 concentrations were determined using the Human ANGPTL2 Assay kit (Immuno-Biological Laboratories Co., Ltd., Japan) according to the manufacturer's instructions. To ensure that all samples underwent only one freeze-thaw cycle, the blood samples obtained were used to generate small volume aliquots, which were stored at −80 °C. All Angptl2 tests were performed within 2 weeks. The samples were retested if the coefficient of variation between the duplicate wells was less than 10% or if the R squared value of the standard curve was less than 0.99. In this study, we detected angptl2 concentration in both patients with hepatitis B and 30 healthy people as control.

Hepatic histological assessment

Ultrasonographic-guided liver biopsies were routinely processed at each institute according to a standardized protocol after receiving the patient's written informed consent. Specimens were fixed, paraffin-embedded, and stained with hematoxylin-eosin and Masson's trichrome. A minimum of 2.0 cm of liver tissue with at least 11 portal tracts was required for diagnosis. Pathological interpretations were conducted in the Department of Pathology at the You An Hospital affiliated with Capital Medical University. Each section was blindly and independently assessed by 2 pathologists. When discrepancies occurred, the samples were reviewed by experienced pathologists who were also responsible for reassessment in 10% of randomly selected samples. The strength of concordance was defined by the kappa value. To minimize inter- and intra-observer discrepancies, pre-reading was conducted, and a kappa value 0.81 was required. The histological fibrosis stage were assessed according to Ishak criteria [22].

Statistical analysis

Statistical analyses were performed using SPSS 17.0. Quantitative variables were expressed as the mean ± standard deviation (SD) unless otherwise specified. Categorical variables were compared using Chi-squared tests, and continuous variables were compared using the Kruskal-Wallis and Mann-Whitney U-tests. Spearman's rank tests were used to study associations between variables and histological scores. Spearman's correlation coefficient was used as necessary. To determine the independent factors of liver fibrosis, a binary backward stepwise logistic regression analysis was conducted with ISHAK fibrosis stage as the dependent and variables as explanatory variables. Meanwhile the regression coefficient of each independent factors was output at the last step of the binary logistic regression analysis. We calculated a new index gx based on the independent factors and their coefficients, then the model ACI was developed by the formula exp.(gx)/(1 + exp.(gx)). Receiver-operating characteristic (ROC) curves were created for the assessment of variables for staging fibrosis. The performance of variables for predicting the severity of liver damage, expressed as AUC, sensitivity, specificity, positive predictive value (PPV), and negative predictive value (NPV), was calculated. Comparison of ROC curves was performed by MedCalc. All p values reported are two sided, and $p < 0.05$ was considered statistically significant.

Results

Clinical characteristics of study population

Although there were 685 hepatitis B patients collected, only 460 patients with ALT <2× ULN and qualified biopsy were analyzed in this study. According to the order into the project, 223 cases served as training cohort and 237 ones as validation cohort. Among total patients with normal to minimally raised ALT, one hundred and sixty nine ones showed significant/severe fibrosis (F ≥ 3, 36.8%) (Table 1). In patients with low normal (<0.5 × ULN, $n = 51$), high normal(between 0.5 and 1 × ULN, $n = 145$) and minimally raised ALT (between ULN and 2 × ULN, $n = 264$), Ishak fibrosis score ≥ 3 diagnosed in 13 (25.5%), 55 (37.9%), 100 (38.9%) cases respectively, the data was not shown. Although serum level of AST, Albumin, TBil, PT, Hyaluronic and HBV DNA indicated statistically different between training and validation cohort, fibrosis stages equally distributed in the two sets ($P = 0.835$).

The 30 healthy people aged 18 to 65 years (≥40 year, $n = 13$) were recruited as control subjects, of whom the normal ALT, AST, ALP, GGT, Albumin, TBil, PT and serum HBsAg, HBeAg, HBeAb negativity were required. The HBVDNA level in the control subjects were less than 20 IU/ML. Seventy percent of them were male, and all of them had BMI within 24 kg/m^2.

Serum Angptl2 concentration independently associated with significant fibrosis in training group

In 30 healthy people, we detected the Angptl2 concentration of 3.92 ± 1.53 (ng/ml) in serum, which was not different from that in patients with no/moderate fibrosis. However, serum Angptl2 concentration was closely associated with Ishak fibrosis scores for patients in training group, higher the fibrosis stages resulted in higher serum Angptl2 concentrations ($p < 0.001$) (Fig. 1). In patients with normal ALT ($n = 88$), the higher Angptl2 concentration of 6.05 ± 3.94 (ng/ml) was found in 27 (30.7%) patients with significant fibrosis, compared to those with no/moderate fibrosis, who had the Angptl2 level of 4.16 ± 1.66 (ng/ml).

Apart from the higher serum concentrations of Angptl2 in the patients with significant fibrosis, higher levels of Age, AST, ALP, GGT, albumin, PT, hyaluronic, LN, PIIINP, and Collagen IV, as well as lower HBsAg titers and PLT were also found when compared to the other ones with nil/moderate fibrosis. Finally, BMI, age, gender which has been reported to be associated with liver fibrosis and other

Table 1 Baseline Characteristics: Comparison Between the Training and the Validation cohort

Parameter	Training cohort (*n* = 223)	Validation cohort (*n* = 237)	Total (*n* = 460)	*P* value
Age (≥40 year, %)	98 (43.9%)	107 (45.1%)	205 (44.6%)	0.851
Gender (Male, %)	170 (76.2%)	175 (73.8%)	345 (75.0%)	0.591
BMI (≥24 kg/m^2, %)	82 (36.8%)	84 (35.4%)	166 (36.1%)	0.772
Platelet count (× 10^9/L)	173.57 ± 56.23	172.42 ± 60.38	172.33 ± 59.08	0.526
ALT (U/L)	44.28 ± 17.13	41.93 ± 17.02	43.07 ± 17.10	0.163
AST (U/L)	35.04 ± 14.58	33.81 ± 16.19	35.50 ± 17.84	0.02
ALP (U/L)	76.06 ± 21.71	78.67 ± 29.75	77.31 ± 26.07	0.736
GGT (U/L)	39.13 ± 43.35	42.76 ± 45.72	41.50 ± 47.42	0.622
Albumin (g/L)	44.45 ± 5.32	44.60 ± 4.98	44.48 ± 5.26	0.039
TBil (μmol/L)	15.65 ± 16.36	19.00 ± 29.98	16.94 ± 22.78	0.037
PT (S)	12.74 ± 1.25	12.36 ± 1.72	12.56 ± 1.49	0.001
HBsAg (log$_{10}$IU/ML)	3.56 ± 0.94	3.57 ± 0.81	3.56 ± 0.88	0.583
Collagen IV (Pg/ML)	936.82 ± 610.24	866.57 ± 472.39	869.97 ± 540.96	0.401
Hyaluronic (μg/L)	124.20 ± 73.76	107.49 ± 68.30	115.26 ± 71.14	0.001
Laminin (μg/L)	94.56 ± 206.58	75.71 ± 145.84	84.24 ± 177.79	0.661
PIIINP (μg/L)	3.59 ± 5.31	3.75 ± 4.86	3.65 ± 5.04	0.442
HBeAg (positive, %)	136 (61.0%)	131 (55.3%)	267 (58.7%)	0.221
HBV DNA (log$_{10}$IU/ML)	6.14 ± 1.93	5.69 ± 2.08	5.89 ± 2.03	0.034
Fibrosis stages (n, %)				0.835
F0	9 (4%)	11 (4.6)	20 (4.3%)	
F1	70 (31.4%)	66 (27.8)	136 (29.6%)	
F2	62 (27.8%)	73 (30.8%)	135 (29.3%)	
F3	40 (17.9%)	45 (19%)	85 (18.5%)	
F4	34 (15.2%)	34 (14.3%)	68 (14.8%)	
F5-6	8 (3.6%)	8 (3.4%)	16 (3.5)	

BMI body mass index, *ALT* alanine transaminase, *AST* aspartate transaminase, *ALP* alkaline phosphatase, *GGT* gamma-glutamyltransgerase, *PT* prothrombin time, *HBV*, hepatitis B virus, *HBsAg* HBV surface antigen, *LN* laminin, *PIIINP* Procollagen III N-terminal Peptide

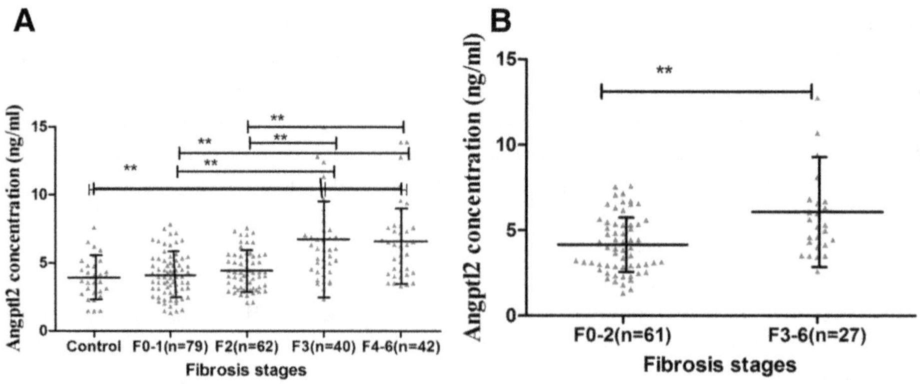

Fig. 1 Boxplot of the serum Angptl2 concentrations in relation to fibrosis score in the training cohort all patients (**a**) and patients with normal ALT (**b**) .The above and below lines indicate the SD. The middle line represents the medians. *** $p < 0.001$, **$p < 0.01$, and *$p < 0.05$. For all patients in the training cohort, $p < 0.001$. For patients with normal ALT in the training cohort, $p = 0.003$

parameters which showed significantly higher or lower in patients with significant/severe fibrosis (F ≥ 3) were included in multivariate analysis (Table 2). It indicated that serum Angptl2 concentration (p = 0.007), PLT (p = 0.040), AST (p = 0.005), hyaluronic (p = 0.002), and LN (p = 0.007) were independently associated with Ishak fibrosis score ≥ 3.

Based on the variables above, we developed an ACI by binary logistic regression.

$$Gx = -1.774 + 0.027 \times AST - 0.01 \times PLT + 0.144 \times Angptl2 + 0.004 \times Laminin + 0.009 \times Hyaluronic.$$

$$ACI = \exp.(gx)/(1 + \exp.(gx)).$$

ACI was compared with APRI, FIB-4, Forn's index and Hui model for predicting significant fibrosis in training cohort

To assess the efficiency of models in predicting significant fibrosis, ROC curves were created (Fig. 2). In the training cohort (223 patients), the AUC of ACI for distinguishing patients who showed significant fibrosis (F ≥ 3) from patients who have no significant fibrosis (F0–2) was 0.835 (95% CI: 0.781, 0.889). Using a cutoff value of ≥0.2, ≥0.3, ≥0.5, patients who need immediate anti-HBV therapy could be correctly identified with a sensitivity of 93.8`, 85.2%, 55.6%, a specificity of 44.0%, 67.2%, 85.8%, a of 50.3%, 61.1%, 70.3%, and a NPV of 92.2%, 88.2%, 76.2% respectively.

Compared to the existing non-invasive assessments, ACI was superior to APRI (AUC = 0.776 (95% CI: 0.713, 0.840)) (P = 0.049, Z = 1.962), FIB-4 (AUC = 0.750 (95% CI: 0.684, 0.816)) (P = 0.010, Z = 2.571), Hui model (AUC = 0.756 (95% CI: 0.685, 0.827)) (P = 0.028, Z = 2.191), and had a better trend than Forn's index (AUC = 0.796 (95% CI: 0.732, 0.860)) (P = 0.083, Z = 1.732) for predicting significant fibrosis (F ≥ 3) in the training group (Fig. 2 A).

Furthermore, predicting value of models for patients with normal ALT were also compared (Fig. 2 B). Similarly, ACI produced AUC of 0.861 (95% CI: 0.778, 0.944) for significant fibrosis, superior to the AUCs of APRI (P = 0.063, Z = 1.863), Forn's index (P = 0.023, Z = 2.280), Hui model (P = 0.044, Z = 2.016) with 0.811 (95% CI: 0.706, 0.918), 0.792 (95% CI: 0.678, 0.905) and 0.798 (95% CI: 0.685, 0.912), and had a better trend than the AUC of FIB-4 (P = 0.089, Z = 1.697) with 0.813 (95% CI: 0.717, 0.909).

Assessment of noninvasive predictive models in the validation cohort

Serum Angptl2 concentration showed closely association with Ishak fibrosis scores for patients in training group (Additional file 1: Fig. S1). Diagnostic value of ACI was further assessed together with APRI, FIB-4, Forn's index,

Table 2 Variables Association with the Presence of Significant Fibrosis in the Training cohort by Univariate and Multivariate Analyses

Parameters	Univariate analysis			Multivariate analysis	
	F0–2 (n = 141)	F ≥ 3 (n = 82)	P	Exp (B) (95%CI)	P
Gender (Male, %)	113 (80.1%)	57 (69.5%)	0.076	1.219 (0.637, 2.332)	0.550
Age (≥35 year, %)	51 (36.2%)	47 (57.3%)	0.03	1.029 (0.988, 1.072)	0.165
BMI (≥24 kg/m^2, %)	51 (36.2%)	31 (37.8%)	0.886		
Platelet count (× 10^9/L)	190.68 ± 53.07	142.49 ± 49.17	<0.001	0.990 (0.985, 0.995)	0.001
ALT (IU/L)	42.99 ± 17.28	46.18 ± 16.68	0.159	0.987 (0.969, 1.005)	0.158
AST (IU/L)	31.46 ± 10.24	41.34 ± 18.53	<0.001	1.027 (1.008, 1.047)	0.005
ALP (IU/L)	72.03 ± 19.22	83.55 ± 24.05	0.001	1.006 (0.994, 1.017)	0.339
GGT (IU/L)	27.70 ± 21.92	59.06 ± 61.50	<0.001	1.005 (0.996, 1.013)	0.28
Albumin (g/L)	45.04 ± 4.97	43.27 ± 5.78	0.001	1.027 (0.973, 1.084)	0.334
TBil (μmol/L)	15.41 ± 19.93	16.01 ± 8.11	0.182		
PT (s)	12.54 ± 1.14	13.10 ± 1.38	<0.001	1.067 (0.879, 1.296)	0.509
HBeAg (positive, %)	89 (63.1%)	47 (57.3%)	0.397		
HBV DNA (log$_{10}$IU/ML)	6.43 ± 1.97	5.64 ± 1.77	<0.001	0.782 (0.603, 1.013)	0.063
Collagen IV (Pg/ML)	774.30 ± 302.67	1175.98 ± 887.97	<0.001	1.000 (0.999, 1.002)	0.472
Hyaluronic (μg/L)	97.83 ± 37.96	155.78 ± 86.27	<0.001	1.010 (1.004, 1.016)	0.002
Laminin (μg/L)	32.36 ± 50.72	196.10 ± 312.13	<0.001	1.004 (1.001, 1.006)	0.007
PIIINP (μg/L)	2.97 ± 5.79	4.85 ± 4.98	<0.001	0.968 (0.908, 1.103)	0.312
HBV DNA/HBeAg (n, %)	6.43 ± 1.97	5.64 ± 1.77	<0.001	0.782 (0.603, 1.013)	0.063
Angptl2 (ng/ml)	4.54 ± 1.96	6.07 ± 3.23	0.008	1.152 (1.039, 1.278)	0.007

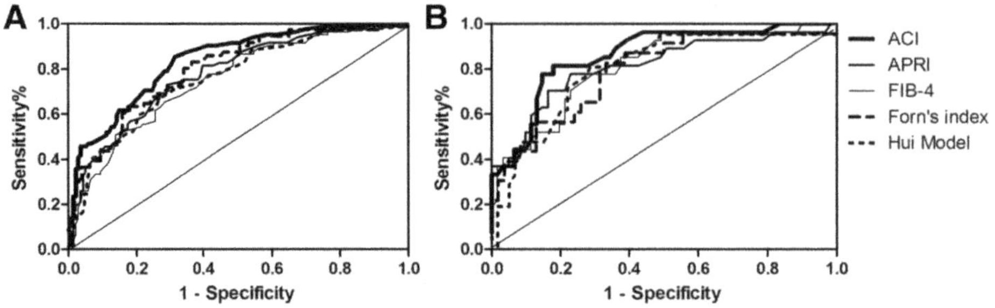

Fig. 2 Receiver operating characteristics (ROC) cures of the Angptl2 combined index (ACI), APRI, FIB-4, Forns' index to distinguish patients with and without significant fibrosis in the Training cohort. **a** Area under the ROC curves (AUC) of above models in the training set. **b** AUC for above models in patients with Normal ALT in the training set

and Hui model (Fig. 3). For predicting significant fibrosis in validation group, the AUROCs were 0.795 (95% CI: 0.730, 0.851) for ACI, 0.715 (95% CI: 0.647, 0.783) for APRI, 0.730 (95% CI: 0.661, 0.799) for FIB-4, 0.735 (95% CI: 0.658, 0.811) for Forn's index, and 0.719 (95% CI: 0.646, 0.791) for Hui model (Fig. 3A). For patients with normal ALT, the AUC of ACI for predicting significant fibrosis, the indication of urgent anti-HBV therapy was 0.810 (95% CI: 0.727, 0.893), and the AUCs of APRI, FIB-4, Forns' index and Hui model were 0.766 (95% CI: 0.675, 0.858), 0.717 (95% CI: 0.608, 0.826), 0.732 (95% CI: 0.607, 0.856), 0.721 (95% CI: 0.610, 0.832), respectively (Fig. 3B).

In total 460 patients, predictive accuracy of the models for diagnosing significant fibrosis were calculated, data was shown in Table 3.

Discussion

The indications for antiviral treatment of hepatitis B were at a long time generally based mainly on the combination of three criteria: serum HBV DNA levels, serum ALT levels and severity of liver disease. According to the treatment criteria of the APASL guideline [4], this 460 patients with ALT <2 × ULN should monitor ALT level every 3 months, biopsy was considered if ALT was persistently elevated, noninvasive tests suggested evidence of significant fibrosis, age > 35 years or family h/o HCC or cirrhosis. In the guideline, although the additional factors were taken into account, the antiviral treatment decision for patients with ALT <2 × ULN still depended on hepatic histology, which is a significantly invasive process.

To date, many publications have demonstrated the growing interest in non-invasive biomarkers and indexes to overcome the limitations of liver biopsy. Individual markers, such as hyaluronate [23], type IV collagen [24], MMPs [25], and CD163 [26, 27], as well as indexes, such as APRI, AAR, FIB-4, Forns' index and Hui model, have been the most extensively studied. However, the majority of studies investigating non-invasive markers have focused only patients with ALT ≥2 × ULN.

Although ALT levels reflect liver inflammation to some degree, Recent data has increasingly shown that patients with normal or mildly elevated serum ALT levels are not guaranteed to be free from liver damage and liver-related mortality [28]. Twenty eight to thirty seven percent of patients with normal ALT levels were reported to exhibit histologically advanced fibrosis [29–31]. However, few existed serum markers were available that exhibited efficacy for diagnosing significant fibrosis or that aid in treatment decision making in clinical practice, for patients

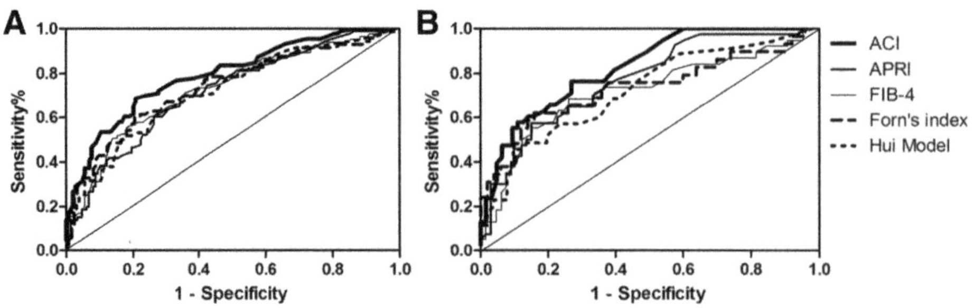

Fig. 3 Receiver-operating characteristic curve (ROC) cures of the ACI, APRI, FIB-4, Forns' index to distinguish patients with and without significant fibrosis in the Validation cohort. (**a**) AUC of above models in the validation set. (**b**) AUC for above models in patients with normal ALT in validation set

Table 3 Predictive accuracy of ACI and other index for diagnosing significant fibrosis in total patients

Index	Patients	AUC (95% CI)	Cut-off	Sensiti -vity (%)	Speci-ficit (%)	PPV (%)	NPV (%)	LR
ACI	ALT <2 × ULN (*n* = 460)	0.813 (95% CI: 0.772, 0.854)	≥0.2	88.0	50.9	51.3	90.8	1.6
			≥0.3	76.1	74.4	64.0	84.0	2.97
			≥0.5	50.9	90.0	66.7	74.9	4.80
	Normal ALT (*n* = 196)	0.824 (95% CI: 0.763, 0.884)	≥0.2	81.8	63.7	54.0	87.5	2.25
			≥0.3	65.2	86.3	66.1	84.0	4.75
			≥0.5	40.0	94.4	75.7	75.9	6.98
APRI	ALT <2 × ULN (*n* = 460)	0.742 (95%CI: 0.695, 0.789)	≥0.5	70.0	63.6	53.9	78.8	2.07
			≥1.0	26.4	94.4	73.8	68.9	4.71
	Normal ALT (*n* = 196)	0.780 (95% CI: 0.710, 0.849)	≥0.5	55.2	85.8	58.9	78.3	3.90
			≥1.0	16.4	98.4	84.6	69.1	10.43
FIB-4	ALT <2 ULN (*n* = 460)	0.741 (95% CI: 0.693, 0.788)	≥1.0	89.6	34.2	43.9	66.4	1.42
			≥1.5	17.7	96.4	75.6	67.1	4.97
	Normal ALT (*n* = 196)	0.763 (95% CI: 0.689, 0.830)	≥1.0	90.8	31.8	40.4	86.7	1.33
			≥1.5	21.5	96.8	77.8	70.5	6.78
Forns' index	ALT <2 × ULN (*n* = 460)	0.766 (95% CI: 0.717, 0.816)	≥6.0	90.1	37.5	44.9	86.8	1.44
			≥8.0	54.6	83.5	64.7	75.8	3.3
	Normal ALT (*n* = 196)	0.762 (95% CI: 0.689, 0.847)	≥6.0	86.54	40.38	41.3	85.1	1.43
			≥8.0	50.0	87.5	67.5	78.4	4.00
Hui Model	ALT <2 × ULN (*n* = 460)	0.736 (95% CI: 0.686, 0.787)	≥0.15	60.1	74.4	58.1	76.5	2.55
			≥0.3	38.5	90.9	71.3	71.7	4.25
	Normal ALT (*n* = 196)	0.745 (95% CI: 0.664, 0.825)	≥0.15	51.8	81.8	58.8	77.4	2.85
			≥0.3	33.9	91.8	66.7	72.7	4.15
			≥0.3	33.9	91.8	66.7	72.7	4.15

with normal or minimally elevated ALT.In our study, 36.8% of 460 patients who needed biopsies to determine treatment decisions had significant fibrosis. Therefore, non-invasive markers for predicting fibrosis in patients with normal ALT are needed.

This study demonstrated that Angptl2 was significantly associated with fibrosis in patients with normal and minimally elevated ALT. Furthermore, multivariate analysis identified Angptl2 concentration as an independent predictive factor, together with PLT, LN, AST and hyaluronic and developed a model, ACI. To investigate the efficiency of ACI a Angptl2 based model for diagnosing significant fibrosis, we performed further ROC analyses and found it superior to the other 4 existing fibrosis models (APRI, FIB-4, Forns' index and Hui model). Additionally, validation cohort revealed its robustness and reliability. There was also some problem about standard detection method of angptl2. The circulatory level of Angptl2 in healthy people of different articles changed [13–15], it would be due to measurement by different commercial kit. In this study, the normal level of ANGPTL2 in 30 healthy people was 3.92 ± 1.53 (ng/ml). In the further, the standard kit for testing ANGPTL2 was needed for clinic application.

Normal Angptl2 signaling functions in angiogenesis and tissue repair, whereas excess Angptl2 signaling leads to chronic inflammation and subsequent pathological irreversible tissue remodeling [8]. It was reported that expression of Angptl2 induced by mechanical stress in LF fibroblasts promotes ligamentum flavum (LF) tissue degeneration by activation of TGF-β1/Smad signaling, which resulted in LF hypertrophy in patients with lumbar spinal canal stenosis [32]. Additionally, high levels of Angptl2 protein positively was correlated with histological grade, and liver cirrhosis HCC patients [33]. In this study, Angptl2 exhibited association with liver fibrosis in hepatitis B patients. As discussed above, this may suggests that Angptl2 promote liver fibrogenesis through TGF-β1/Smad signaling, the most potent factor in stimulating collagen gene transcription. The mechanistic studies will be required to clarify the issue.

The current study has limitations that are presented below. First, it is a cross-sectional study. Although a longitudinal study is more powerful in an observational study, most study refer to noninvasive assessment of liver fibrosis are cross-sectional and our multi-center data could be the offset. Second, in this study, normal and minimally elevated ALT is defined within one test and without monitoring it every 3 months. However ALT is just the marker for assessing liver inflammation, but not a marker for diagnosing hepatic fibrosis. Additionally, ALT monitoring always takes time in clinical practice, noninvasive marker superior to ALT to diagnose fibrosis stages could benefit to treatment decision making. The third limitation of our study is clinical research and no mechanism exploration. The basic research of the relationship between Angptl2 and liver fibrosis is currently in progress. Of course, missing imaging examination is also the drawback of this study. The last limitation was that the Angptl2 levels in patients with F3–6 were overlapped with those in patients with F0–2, suggesting the difficulties to set up a cut-off level to estimate the fibrosis stages in chronic hepatitis B patients. So, we developed the ACI model based on Angptl2 together with conventional markers to avoid this problem.

Conclusion

Although serum Angptl2 concentration needs more extensive validation in the future, the results from this multicenter, prospective study was sufficient to suggest serum Angptl2 concentration as a potentially novel biomarker for predicting the severity of liver injury. In addition, the angptl2 combined index ACI did better in diagnosing significant fibrosis in hepatitis B patients, compared with APRI, Hui model, FIB-4, Forn's index.

Abbreviations

AASLD: American Association for the Study of Liver Diseases; ALT: Alanine aminotransferase; Angptl2: Angiopoietin-like protein 2; APASL: the Asian Pacific Association for the Study of Liver; AST: Aspartate aminotransferase; AUC: Area under the curve; BMI: Body mass index; ECM: Extracellular matrix; GGT: Gamma-glutamyltransferase; HAI: Histological activity index; HBsAg: HBV surface antigen; HBV: Hepatitis B virus; HCC: Hepatocellular carcinoma; HCV: Hepatitis C virus; HIV: Human immunodeficiency virus; LN: Laminin; MAPK: Mitogen-activated protein kinase; MMP: Matrix metalloproteinase; NPV: Negative predictive value; PIIINP: Procollagen type III N-terminal peptide; PPV: Positive predictive value; PT: Prothrombin time; ROC: Receiver-operating characteristic curves; SD: Standard deviation; TBil: Total bilirubin; ULN: upper limit of normal

Acknowledgements

Additional group members of China HepB Related Fibrosis Assessment Research Group: An-Lin Ma, from departments of Infectious Disease, China-Japan Friendship Hospital, Beijing; Shi-Bin Xie, from departments of Infectious Disease, The Third Affiliated Hospital Sun Yat-Sen University, Guangzhou, Guangdong; Xu-Qing Zhang, from department of Infectious Diseases, South West Hospital affiliated to Third Military Medical University, Chongqing; Da-Zhi Zhang, from department of Infectious Diseases, Second Affiliated Hospital Of Chongqing Medical University, Chongqing; Qing Xie, from department of Infectious Diseases, Rui Jin Hospital Shanghai Jiao Tong University School of Medicine, Shanghai; Guo Zhang, from department of Infectious Diseases, The People's Hospital Of Guang Xi Zhuang Autonomous Region, Nanning, Guangxi; Jia Shang, from department of Infectious Diseases, The People's Hospital Of He Nan province, Zheng zhou, Henan; Jun Chen, from department of Infectious Diseases, Di Tan Hospital affiliated to Capital Medical University, Beijing; Wei-Feng Zhao, MM, from department of Infectious Diseases, Xinxiang Medical University Third Hospital, Xinxiang, Henan; Zhi-Qiang Zhou, from department of Infectious Diseases, Yantai City Hospital for Infectious Disease, Yantai, Shandong; Ying-Xia Liu, from department of Infectious Diseases, Shenzhen Third People's hospital of, Shenzhen; Zhan-Qin Zhang, from department of Infectious Diseases,Public Health Clinical Center Affiliated to Fudan University, Shanghai; Xun Peng, Xie-Wen Sun, from department of Infectious Diseases, Third Hospital Of Qin Huang Dao, Qin Huang Dao, Hebei; Ming-Xiang Zhang, from department of Infectious Diseases, Shenyang Sixth People's Hospital, Shenyang, Liaoning; Fu-Dong Lv, from department of pathology, You An Hospital affiliated to Capital Medical University, Beijing; Jun Li, from department of Infectious Diseases, Jiang Su Province Hospital, Nanjing, Jiangsu; Wan-Li Sun, from department of Infectious Diseases, Dailian Sixth People's Hospital, Dalian, Shandong; Lang Bai, from department of Infectious Diseases, West China School of Medicine/West China Hospital Sichuan University, Chengdu, Sichuan; Li-Ming Chen, from department of Infectious Diseases; Dan Liu, Hong-Li Xi, Yi-Hang Zhou, Min Yu, from department of Infectious Disease, Center for Liver Disease, Peking University First Hospital, Beijing.
We thank Professor Xin Xu (Nanfang Medical University) for his guidance with the statistics.

Funding

This study was supported by China Mega-Project for Infectious Diseases (grant number 2013ZX10002005, 2012ZX10002006), Project of Beijing science and technology committee (grant number D121100003912002) and National Key Clinical Program of the Ministry of Health.

Author's contributions

YD: completing experimental detection, analysis and interpretation of data; drafting of the manuscript; critical revision of the manuscript for important intellectual content; statistical analysis. HZ: study concept and design; acquisition of data; analysis and interpretation of data; critical revision of the manuscript for important intellectual content; technical and material support. JZ, LY: acquisition of data; analysis and interpretation of data. GW: study concept and design; analysis and interpretation of data; critical revision of the manuscript for important intellectual content; obtained funding; study supervision. YD, HZ, JZ, LY, and GW read, commented and approved the final manuscript.

Consent for publication

Not applicable.

Competing interests

The authors declare that they have no competing interests.

Author details
[1]Department of Infectious Disease, Center for Liver Disease, Peking University First Hospital, No. 8, Xishiku Street, Xicheng District, Beijing 100034, China. [2]The Department of dermatology, The Affiliated Hospital of Southwest Medical University, Luzhou, Sichuan, China. [3]The Collaborative Innovation Center for Diagnosis and Treatment of Infectious Diseases, Zhejiang University, Zhejiang, Hangzhou, China. [4]The coordination innovation centerMinistry of education, Beijing, China.

References

1. Schweitzer A, Horn J, Mikolajczyk RT, Krause G, Ott JJ. Estimations of worldwide prevalence of chronic hepatitis B virus infection: a systematic review of data published between 1965 and 2013. Lancet. 2015;386:1546–55.
2. Perz JF, Armstrong GL, Farrington LA, Hutin YJ, Bell BP. The contributions of hepatitis B virus and hepatitis C virus infections to cirrhosis and primary liver cancer worldwide. J Hepatol. 2006;45:529–38.
3. Liang X, Bi S, Yang W, Wang L, Cui G, Cui F, et al. Epidemiological serosurvey of hepatitis B in China–declining HBV prevalence due to hepatitis B vaccination. Vaccine. 2009;27:6550–7.
4. Sarin SK, Kumar M, Lau GK, Abbas Z, Chan HL, Chen CJ, et al. Asian-Pacific clinical practice guidelines on the management of hepatitis B: a 2015 update. Hepatol Int. 2016;10:1–98.
5. Colloredo G, Guido M, Sonzogni A, Leandro G. Impact of liver biopsy size on histological evaluation of chronic viral hepatitis: the smaller the sample, the milder the disease. J Hepatol. 2003;39:239–44.
6. Bedossa P, Dargère D, Paradis V. Sampling variability of liver fibrosis in chronic hepatitis C. Hepatology. 2003;38:1449–57.
7. Regev A, Berho M, Jeffers LJ, Milikowski C, Molina EG, Pyrsopoulos NT, et al. Sampling error and intraobserver variation in liver biopsy in patients with chronic HCV infection. Am J Gastroenterol. 2002;97:2614–8.
8. Kadomatsu T, Endo M, Miyata K, Oike Y. Diverse roles of ANGPTL2 in physiology and pathophysiology. Trends Endocrinol Metab. 2014;25:245–54.
9. Odagiri H, Kadomatsu T, Endo M, Masuda T, Morioka MS, Fukuhara S, et al. The secreted protein ANGPTL2 promotes metastasis of osteosarcoma cells through integrin α5β1, p38 MAPK, and matrix metalloproteinases. Sci Signal. 2014;7:ra7.
10. Tazume H, Miyata K, Tian Z, Endo M, Horiguchi H, Takahashi O, et al. Macrophage-derived angiopoietin-like protein 2 accelerates development of abdominal aortic aneurysm. Arterioscler Thromb Vasc Biol. 2012;32:1400–9.
11. Novo E, Cannito S, Paternostro C, Bocca C, Miglietta A, Parola M. Cellular and molecular mechanisms in liver fibrogenesis. Arch Biochem Biophys. 2014;548:20–37.
12. Kim I, Kim HG, Kim H, Kim HH, Park SK, Uhm CS, et al. Hepatic expression, synthesis and secretion of a novel fibrinogen/angiopoietin related protein that prevents endothelial-cell apoptosis. Biochem J. 2000;346:603–10.
13. Yoshinaga T, Shigemitsu T, Nishimata H, Kitazono M, Hori E, Tomiyoshi A, et al. Angiopoietin-like protein 2 as a potential biomarker for colorectal cancer. Mol Clin Oncol. 2015;3:1080–4.
14. Chen Y, Jiang H, Zhu L, Wang P, Liu S, Xiao X, et al. Diagnostic and prognostic value of serum Angiopoietin-like protein 2 in patients with non-small cell lung cancer. Clin Lab. 2017;63:59–65.
15. Liang Y, Nie H, Ren H, Li F, Tian C, Li H, et al. Change of serum Angiopoietin-like protein 2 and its significance in patients with arteriosclerotic occlusion. Zhong guo Yi Xue Ke Xue Yuan Xue Bao. 2017;39:188–95.
16. Jia W, Song LW, Fang YQ, Wu XF, Liu DY, Xu C, et al. Antibody to hepatitis B core antigen levels in the natural history of chronic hepatitis B: a prospective observational study. Medicine (Baltimore). 2014;93:e322.
17. Deng Y, Zhao H, Zhou J, Yan L, Wang G. China HepB-related fibrosis assessment research group. Complement 5a is an indicator of significant fibrosis and earlier cirrhosis in patients chronically infected with hepatitis B virus. Infection. 2017;45:75–81.
18. Wai CT, Greenson JK, Fontana RJ, Kalbfleisch JD, Marrero JA, Conjeevaram HS, et al. A simple noninvasive index can predict both significant fibrosis and cirrhosis in patients with chronic hepatitis C. Hepatology. 2003;38:518–26.
19. Hui AY, Chan HL, Wong VW, Liew CT, Chim AM, Chan FK, et al. Identification of chronic hepatitis B patients without significant liver fibrosis by a simple noninvasivepredictive model. Am J Gastroenterol. 2005;100:616–23.
20. Vallet-Pichard A, Mallet V, Nalpas B, Verkarre V, Nalpas A, Dhalluin-Venier V, et al. FIB-4: an inexpensive and accurate marker of fibrosis in HCV infection comparison with liver biopsy and fibrotest. Hepatology. 2007;46:32–6.
21. Forns X, Ampurdanès S, Llovet JM, Aponte J, Quintó L, Martínez-Bauer E, et al. Identification of chronic hepatitis C patients without hepatic fibrosis by a simple predictive model. Hepatology. 2002;36:986–92.
22. Ishak K, Baptista A, Bianchi L, Callea F, De Groote J, Gudat F, et al. Histological grading and staging of chronic hepatitis. J Hepatol. 1995;22:696–9.
23. Walsh KM, Fletcher A, MacSween RN, Morris AJ. Basement membrane peptides as markers of liver disease in chronic hepatitis C. J Hepatol. 2000; 32:325–30.
24. Murawaki Y, Koda M, Okamoto K, Mimura K, Kawasaki H. Diagnostic value of serum type IV collagen test in comparison with platelet count for predicting the fibrotic stage in patients withchronic hepatitis C. J Gastroenterol Hepatol. 2001;16:777–81.
25. Murawaki Y, Ikuta Y, Idobe Y, Kawasaki H. Serum matrix metalloproteinase-1 in patients with chronic viral hepatitis. J Gastroenterol Hepatol. 1999;14:138–45.
26. Kazankov K, Barrera F, Møller HJ, Bibby BM, Vilstrup H, George J, et al. Soluble CD163, a macrophage activation marker, is independently associated with fibrosis in patients with chronic viral hepatitis B and C. Hepatology. 2014;60:521–30.
27. Grønbaek H, Sandahl TD, Mortensen C, Vilstrup H, Møller HJ, Møller S. Soluble CD163, a marker of Kupffer cell activation, is related to portal hypertension in patients with liver cirrhosis. Aliment Pharmacol Ther. 2012;36:173–80.
28. Kim WR, Flamm SL. Di Bisceglie AM, Bodenheimer HC, public policy Committee of the American Association for the study of liver disease. Serum activity of alanine aminotransferase (ALT) as an indicator of health and disease. Hepatology. 2008;47:1363–70.
29. Kumar M, Sarin SK, Hissar S, Pande C, Sakhuja P, Sharma BC, et al. Virologic and histologic features of chronic hepatitis B virus-infected asymptomatic patients with persistently normal ALT. Gastroenterol. 2008;134:1376–84.
30. Lai M, Hyatt BJ, Nasser I, Curry M, Afdhal NH. The clinical significance of persistently normal ALT in chronic hepatitis B infection. J Hepatol. 2007;47:760–7.
31. Tsang PS, Trinh H, Garcia RT, Phan JT, Ha NB, Nguyen H, et al. Significant prevalence of histologic disease in patients with chronic hepatitis B and mildly elevated serum alanine aminotransferase levels. Clin Gastroenterol Hepatol. 2008;6:569–74.
32. Nakamura T, Okada T, Endo M, Kadomatsu T, Taniwaki T, Sei A, et al. Angiopoietin-like protein 2 induced by mechanical stress accelerates degeneration and hypertrophy of the Ligamentum Flavum in lumbar Spinal Canal Stenosis. PLoS One. 2014;17(9):e85542.
33. Gao L, Ge C, Fang T, Zhao F, Chen T, Yao M, et al. ANGPTL2 promotes tumor metastasis in Hepatocellular carcinoma. J Gastroenterol Hepatol. 2015;30:396–404.

Clinical characteristics of acute hepatitis A outbreak in Taiwan, 2015–2016: observations from a tertiary medical center

Nan-Yu Chen[1], Zhuo-Hao Liu[2], Shian-Sen Shie[1], Tsung-Hsing Chen[3] and Ting-Shu Wu[1*]

Abstract

Background: Acute hepatitis A is a fecal-oral transmitted disease related to inadequate sanitary conditions. In addition to its traditional classification, several outbreaks in the men who have sex with men (MSM) population have resulted in acute hepatitis A being recognized as a sexually transmitted disease. However, few studies have clarified the clinical manifestations in these outbreaks involving the MSM population.

Methods: Beginning in June 2015, there was an outbreak of acute hepatitis A involving the MSM population in Northern Taiwan. We conducted a 15-year retrospective study by recruiting 207 patients with the diagnosis of acute hepatitis A that included the pre-outbreak (January 2001 to May 2015) and outbreak (June 2015 to August 2016) periods in a tertiary medical center in Northern Taiwan. Using risk factors, comorbidities, presenting symptoms, laboratory test results and imaging data, we aimed to evaluate the clinical significance of acute hepatitis A in the MSM population, where human immunodeficiency virus (HIV) coinfection is common.

Results: There was a higher prevalence of reported MSM ($p < 0.001$), HIV ($p < 0.001$) and recent syphilis ($p < 0.05$) coinfection with acute hepatitis A during the outbreak period. The outbreak population had more prominent systemic symptoms, was more icteric with a higher total bilirubin level ($p < 0.05$) and had a 7-times higher tendency ($p < 0.05$) to have a hepatitis A relapse.

Conclusions: The clinical course of acute hepatitis A during an outbreak involving the MSM and HIV-positive population is more symptomatic and protracted than in the general population.

Keywords: Acute hepatitis A, HIV infection, Men who have sex with men, Male homosexual, Outbreak

Background

Acute hepatitis A is a fecal-oral transmitted disease related to inadequate hygienic and sanitary conditions. In developed countries, through the elevation of public health standards, hepatitis A has become an imported disease related to travel to endemic countries. Thus, studies have shown decreases in antibody seroprevalence against hepatitis A in developed countries [1], which may also suggest that a large portion of the population is at risk should a hepatitis A outbreak occur. In addition to the traditional transmission route, the role of acute hepatitis A as a sexually transmitted disease (STD) has been recognized due to several reported outbreaks among men who have sex with men (MSM) since the 1990s [2–5]. Previous studies have linked acute hepatitis A to certain risk factors [2, 6–8], including oral-anal sexual practices and intravenous drug use. However, the impact of acute hepatitis A on high-risk populations, particularly the MSM population and those with preexisting human immunodeficiency virus (HIV) infections, has not yet been clarified.

Acute hepatitis A was endemic in Taiwan before 1995 and has been a notifiable disease according to the Centers of Disease Control (CDC), Taiwan, since 1999 [9]. Since June 1995, when efforts in public health and the free vaccination program for children in 30 indigenous townships were initiated, annual hepatitis A cases have declined from 2.96/100,000 in 1995 to 0.9/100,000

* Correspondence: 2626@cgmh.org.tw
[1]Division of Infectious Diseases, Department of Internal Medicine, Chang Gung Memorial Hospital, Chang Gung University College of Medicine, 5 Fuhsing Street, Kueishan, Taoyuan 333, Taiwan
Full list of author information is available at the end of the article

in 2003–2008 [9]. Since then, acute hepatitis A has become a disease mainly related to international travel, and the estimated seroprevalence against hepatitis A has decreased to less than 10% in those under the age of 20 according to the 2011 epidemiologic surveillance [10]. This population is particularly vulnerable to an acute hepatitis A outbreak. According to the CDC, Taiwan, there has been an acute hepatitis A outbreak (serotype IA) in Northern Taiwan since June 2015, notably involving the MSM population, with half of the cases also being infected with HIV [11]. According to the literature, only a few studies have attempted to describe acute hepatitis A in MSM or HIV-infected populations [12, 13]. By the time this manuscript is submitted, more acute hepatitis A cases will have been reported. The aim of this study was to explore the risk differential between the outbreak and sporadic cases in the pre-outbreak period, which may contribute to our understanding of acute hepatitis A involving the MSM and HIV-positive populations.

Methods

This retrospective study was approved by the Institutional Review Board at Chang Gung Medical Foundation in Taiwan (approval number: 201600805A3). We conducted a 15-year retrospective, single-center study at Chang Gung Memorial Hospital, a tertiary hospital in Northern Taiwan. All patients with a positive or equivocal hepatitis A virus (HAV) immunoglobulin M (IgM) level detected by either an enzyme-linked immunosorbent assay (ELISA) or a radioisotope assay between January 2001 through August 2016 were reviewed for the presence of elevated liver enzymes and symptoms/signs of hepatitis. A case was defined as having acute hepatitis A when there was positive/equivocal HAV IgM together with elevated liver enzymes. Two hundred and sixty-four cases were collected. Twenty-four cases with unavailable/incomplete medical records and 10 cases that came for a health re-check after an acute hepatitis A episode treated elsewhere were excluded. Twenty-three patients with an alternative diagnosis or severe clinically confronting diseases were further excluded (Additional file 1).

A total of 207 acute hepatitis A cases were collected and divided into the following two groups: 163 cases in the pre-outbreak period (January 2001 to May 2015) and 44 cases in the outbreak period (June 2015 to August 2016), as the first case of this national acute hepatitis A outbreak was reported in June 2015 according to a statement by the CDC, Taiwan. Clinical manifestations, laboratory abnormalities, image findings and treatment outcomes were compared between these two groups. The HIV infection status was defined by standard ELISA and Western blotting methods or if the patient was already on combination antiretroviral therapy (cART). Recent travel was defined by domestic or international visits within 2 months before the diagnosis of acute hepatitis A was made. Close contact was defined as living with a confirmed acute hepatitis A case or a person having symptoms or signs of acute hepatitis A in the same household/dormitory or working/studying/in a relationship with a symptomatic person or a confirmed acute hepatitis A case. A recently active syphilis infection was defined as a 4X rise in rapid plasma reagin (RPR)/venereal disease research laboratory (VDRL) test titer or if the patient received benzathine penicillin treatment for syphilis within 6 months of the acute hepatitis A event. In this study, a relapse was arbitrarily defined as a more than 0.5X normal upper limit elevation of either aspartate aminotransferase (AST) or alanine aminotransferase (ALT) during the convalescence phase before liver function normalized.

Statistical analyses

Analyses were conducted using SigmaPlot 12.0 (Systat Software, Inc., San Jose, California, USA). The differences between groups (before the outbreak and during the outbreak) were tested for significance using the Mann-Whitney Rank Sum test and Pearson's chi-square test for numerical variables and categorical variables, respectively. Values were reported as the median and ranges, and p value of less than 0.05 was considered significant for all statistical tests.

Results

Between June 2015 and August 2016, while Northern Taiwan was experiencing a hepatitis A outbreak, a similar trend was detected at Chang Gung Memorial Hospital (Fig. 1). The number of acute hepatitis A cases increased from 2 to 18 cases/year to 36 cases in 2016 (until Aug 2016). Throughout these 15 years, males often had a stronger association with acute hepatitis A (male/total cases ratio ranging from 36.4 to 84.6%), with a female predominance observed only in 2001 and 2006. The male predominance in acute hepatitis A was further exaggerated during the outbreak (male/total cases ratio of 85.7% in 2015 and 91.7% in 2016), reaching statistical significance ($p < 0.001$, Table 1). As shown in the patient demographic and risk factor analysis (Table 1), recent travel (56/207, 29.4%), particularly international travelling (37/56, 66%), was the most often reported factor among pre-outbreak cases. Conversely, the most frequently reported risk factor for outbreak cases was MSM or HIV infection (40.9%), although recent travel was still reported in a minority of cases (18.2%). Notably, during the outbreak, there were also more cases reported to have close contact to a confirmed acute hepatitis A case or a person having symptoms or signs of acute hepatitis A. The average age of acute hepatitis A cases was quite

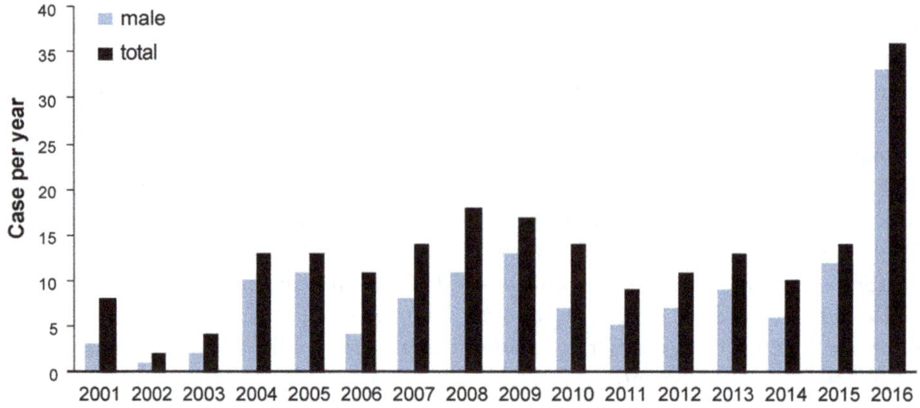

	2001	2002	2003	2004	2005	2006	2007	2008	2009	2010	2011	2012	2013	2014	2015	2016
Male	3	1	2	10	11	4	8	11	13	7	5	7	9	6	12	33
Female	5	1	2	3	2	7	6	7	4	7	4	4	4	4	2	3
Total	8	2	4	13	13	11	14	18	17	14	9	11	13	10	14	36
M/T(%)	37.5	50.0	50.0	76.9	84.6	36.4	57.1	61.1	76.5	50.0	55.6	63.6	69.2	60.0	85.7	91.7

Fig. 1 Annual case numbers of acute hepatitis A in the study center from January 2001 to August 2016. M/T: male/total case number ratio. There was an outbreak of acute hepatitis A in the male population in 2015 and 2016

young (33 and 31 years in the pre-outbreak and outbreak groups, respectively). The prevalence of both HIV (31.8%, $p < 0.001$) and active syphilis infections within 6 months (9.1%, $p = 0.002$) was higher in the outbreak group, suggesting a nature of sexually transmitted hepatitis A during this outbreak. The prevalence of positive hepatitis B surface antigen (HBsAg) was 20.2 and 9.1% in the pre-outbreak and outbreak groups, respectively, and the prevalence of a positive anti-hepatitis C virus (anti-HCV) antibody was 1.2% in the pre-outbreak group and 4.5% in the outbreak group. The difference between the two groups in the underlying viral hepatitis did not reach statistical significance.

Table 1 Patient characteristics and demographics

	Total	2001/1–2015/5	2015/6–2016/8	*P* value
Case number	207	163	44	
Gender (M/F[a])	142/65	102/61	40/4	< 0.001*
Age (median, range)	32 (4–89)	33 (4–89)	31 (10–68)	0.006*
HIV[b] (n, %)	14 (6.8%)	0	14 (31.8)	< 0.001*
Hospitalization (n, %)	139 (67.1)	110 (67.5)	29 (66.0%)	0.843
Risk factor (n, %)				
Travel	56 (27.1)	48 (29.4)	8 (18.2)	0.136
MSM[c]	14 (6.8)	0	14 (31.8)	< 0.001*
MSM/HIV	18 (8.7)	0	18 (40.9)	< 0.001*
Close contact	8 (3.9)	4 (2.5)	4 (9.1)	0.043*
Foreign workers/ indigenous townships	6 (2.9)	4 (2.5)	2 (4.5)	0.463
Positive HBsAg (n, %)	37 (17.9)	33 (20.2)	4 (9.1)	0.087
Positive anti-HCV (n, %)	4 (1.9)	2 (1.2)	2 (4.5)	0.156
Recent syphilis (n, %)	4 (1.9)	0	4 (9.1)	0.002*

Note: [a]M: male, F: female. [b]HIV: human immunodeficiency virus, [c]MSM: men who sex with men, MSM/HIV: MSM or HIV infection
* denotes a significant post hoc comparison between two groups

Considering the clinical manifestations of these cases (Table 2), the duration of the prodromal period was generally about 1 week, with a median of 6 days, and the most common symptoms (>50%) were fever, malaise, nausea/vomiting, poor appetite, abdominal discomfort and jaundice/tea-colored urine. Other symptoms (in order from high to low frequency) included chills (18.4%), arthralgia/myalgia (15.5%), upper respiratory symptoms (14.5%), diarrhea (11.6%), light colored stool (10.1%), headache (8.2%), sore throat (3.9%), hepatic encephalopathy (3.9%), pruritus (2.4%), hiccups (1.5%) and skin rash (0.97%).

Table 3 shows the laboratory abnormalities of all cases. The white blood cells were generally within normal limits, with a median of 6.0 X 10^9/L (range 1.5–21.2 X 10^9/L). The median hemoglobin (Hb) level was 145 g/L (range 76–186 g/L). Although the platelet count was normal in most cases (median 173 X 10^9/L, range 57–481 X 10^9/L), thrombocytopenia was observed in 32.4% of patients (platelet <150 X 10^9/L). Renal function impairment in acute hepatitis A was more relevant to the patient's underlying renal disease, with the median serum creatinine level being 74.3 μmol/L (range 26.5–1674.3 μmol/L). Upon comparison of the two study groups, the outbreak group was more likely to have jaundice/tea-colored urine ($p = 0.032$) with a higher total

Table 2 Symptoms and signs of acute hepatitis A

	Total (207)	2001/1–2015/5 (163)	2015/6–2016/8 (44)	*P* value
Prodromal period (median, range)	6 (1–21)	6 (1–21)	6 (2–14)	0.981
Fever (n, %)	116 (56)	86 (52.8)	30 (68.2)	0.050
Chills	38 (18.4)	31 (19)	7 (15.9)	0.668
Malaise	115 (55.6)	85 (52.1)	30 (68.2)	0.042*
Headache	17 (8.2)	15 (9.2)	2 (4.5)	0.532
Nausea/Vomiting	121 (58.5)	93 (57.1)	28 (63.6)	0.361
Poor appetite	108 (52.2)	82 (50.3)	26 (59.1)	0.250
Sore throat	8 (3.9)	6 (3.7)	2 (4.5)	0.675
URI symptoms	30 (14.5)	26 (16)	4 (9.1)	0.272
Arthralgia/myalgia	32 (15.5)	26 (16)	6 (13.6)	0.736
Rash	2 (0.97)	2 (1.2)	0	1.000
Pruritus	5 (2.4)	4 (2.5)	1 (2.3)	0.957
Jaundice or tea-colored urine	139 (67.1)	104 (63.8)	35 (79.5)	0.032*
Jaundice	98 (47.3)	74 (45.4)	24 (54.5)	0.251
Tea-colored urine	104 (50.2)	75 (46)	29 (65.9)	0.014*
Diarrhea	24 (11.6)	16 (9.8)	8 (18.2)	0.114
Abdominal discomfort	106 (51.2)	81 (49.7)	25 (56.8)	0.342
Hiccup	3 (1.5)	3 (1.8)	0	1.000
Light color stool	21 (10.1)	14 (8.6)	7 (15.9)	0.159
Hepatic encephalopathy	8 (3.9)	7 (4.3)	1 (2.3)	1.000

* denotes a significant post hoc comparison between two groups

bilirubin level (p = 0.009) and a trend of more patients with fever.

The most common imaging analysis performed was abdominal sonography (87%) (Table 3), with gallbladder wall thickening/edema being the most common finding (42%). We found that gallbladder wall edema may not be a purely benign sign in acute hepatitis A, as there was one case reported in our study to have gallbladder rupture necessitating surgical intervention. Nevertheless, most cases with gallbladder changes underwent a smooth course, and it did not take long for the edema to resolve (in one case the edema resolved in 3 days). Other common imaging abnormalities were splenomegaly (27.1%), hepatomegaly (15.5%), ascites (7.2%) and lymphadenopathy (1.9%). There were no significant differences in these image abnormalities between the two study groups.

With respect to disease outcome (Table 4), there was an overall complications rate of 6.8% and a mortality rate of 3.9% in the 207 cases. Renal complications were the most common (9/14) and, in some cases, required transient hemodialysis. Two cases exhibited complications with spontaneous bacterial peritonitis, one case had deep vein thrombosis, one case had pulmonary embolism and one case had gallbladder rupture. Mortality and complication rates were not significantly different between the two study groups; however, more hepatitis A relapses during the convalescence phase were observed in the outbreak group (p = 0.019). Among these six cases with hepatitis A relapse, two cases were HIV-positive (ages 34 and 36 years), one case had thalassemia (age 33 years), one case had newly diagnosed diabetes mellitus (age 35 years), one case had pre-existing congestive heart failure and chronic renal insufficiency (age 68 years) and one case had underlying hepatitis B virus (HBV)-related liver cirrhosis and hepatocellular carcinoma (age 61 years). Together, these observations suggest

Table 3 Laboratory and imaging abnormalities of acute hepatitis A

	Total	2001/1–2015/5	2015/6–2016/8	*P* value
WBC count (× 10^9/L) (median, range)	6.0 (1.5–21.2)	6.1 (1.5–21.2)	5.7 (1.9–13.8)	0.438
Hemoglobin (g/L)	145 (76–186)	141 (76–185)	150 (106–186)	0.079
Platelet count (X 10^9/L)	173 (57–481)	172 (57–464)	176 (76–481)	0.668
ALT (U/L)	1904 (40–8378)	1849 (40–8378)	2006 (49–5428)	0.595
ALK-P (U/L)	177 (44–933)	171 (44–638)	187 (58–933)	0.216
Total bilirubin (μmol/L)	106.0 (6.9–1145.7)	100.9 (6.8–1145.7)	118.0 (63.3–489.1)	0.009*
Creatinine (μmol/L)	74.3 (26.5–1674.3)	75.1 (26.5–1674.3)	72.9 (38–385.4)	0.240
CT, MRI or Sonography (n, %)	183 (88.4)	145 (89)	38 (86.4)	0.633
Sonography	180 (87)	143 (87.7)	37 (84)	0.525
CT	16 (7.7)	11 (6.7)	5 (11.4)	0.341
Hepatomegaly	32 (15.5)	28 (17.2)	4 (9.1)	0.251
Splenomegaly	56 (27.1)	40 (24.5)	16 (36.4)	0.060
Lymphadenopathy	4 (1.9)	4 (2.5)	0	0.582
Gallbladder wall thickening/ edema	87 (42)	74 (45.4)	13 (29.5)	0.070
Ascites	15 (7.2)	14 (8.6)	1 (2.3)	0.314

Note: *WBC* white blood cells, *ALT* alanine aminotransferase, *ALK-P* alkaline phosphatase, *CT* computed tomography, *MRI* Magnetic resonance imaging
* denotes a significant post hoc comparison between two groups

Table 4 Outcome comparison

	Total (207)	2001/1–2015/5 (163)	2015/6–2016/8 (44)	*P* value
Mortality (n, %)	8 (3.9)	7 (4.3)	1 (2.3)	1.000
Complications	14 (6.8)	13 (8)	1 (2.3)	0.310
Hepatitis A relapse	6 (2.9)	2 (1.2)	4 (9.1)	0.019*

* denotes a significant post hoc comparison between two groups

a role for the underlying immune status in the course of acute hepatitis A, which was more prominently observed during the outbreak.

Considering the cases of mortality (Additional file 1), none of the mortality cases were HIV-positive. Seventy-five percent (6/8) of mortality cases had underlying positive HBsAg, 12.5% (1/8) had underlying positive anti-HCV, 37.5% (3/8) had pre-existing heart diseases and 25% (2/8) had chronic renal diseases. Of note, younger cases of mortality were specifically associated with an underlying HBV infection. In these younger cases, there were issues of multiple substance abuse and poor socioeconomic support, concurrent spontaneous bacterial peritonitis, unstable hemodynamics caused by acute renal failure and upper gastrointestinal bleeding, which deterred the possibility of prompt liver transplantation. There were two young mortality cases with positive cytomegalovirus IgM, although the clinical significance is questionable. In our study, hepatic encephalopathy was an indicator of a grave prognosis, as none of the patients who developed hepatic encephalopathy survived. In contrast, HIV infection did not seem to contribute to mortality in this study.

Discussion

Acute hepatitis A is an infectious disease whose transmission route, clinical manifestations and risk factors have long been well-characterized. However, the ever-changing population characteristics and the increasing prevalence of people living with HIV have brought clinicians new challenges and insights regarding this disease. The high HIV infection rate during this acute hepatitis A outbreak has drawn our attention, particularly when considering that the prevalence of HIV infection in the general population is as low as 0.1% in Taiwan. Previous studies by Ida et al. showed that HIV-infected patients have a higher HAV viral load, a longer viremia stage and that some HIV-1-infected patients may have HAV viremia even when the clinical symptoms have disappeared and the aminotransferase levels return to normal [14]. Their study may explain why several outbreaks occurred at such frequency among the MSM population or HIV-infected patients, which restates the vulnerability of this population to acute hepatitis A [2–5]. In Taiwan, the low levels of immunity in the young population created the fundamentals for the hepatitis A outbreak, where the seroprevalence of anti-HAV is less than 10% in the general population [10, 15, 16]. We examined acute hepatitis A in 207 patients who received contemporary standard-of-care treatment. The distinct patient demographics before and during the hepatitis A outbreak between June 2015 and August 2016 echo the emerging role of hepatitis A as an STD in the MSM population [17]. The average age of acute hepatitis A cases was quite young in our study, which may reflect the lack of immunity to HAV in young people and recapitulate the infectiousness of HAV in a sensitive otherwise healthy population. The pre-existing male predominance during the pre-outbreak period may reflect the fact that more males are engaged in international business/travel in this society, which was also observed (62%) in a recently published report based on the Taiwan National Health Insurance Research Database [18]. Previous reviews on relapsing hepatitis A have suggested an association between continuing viremia as well as shedding of the virus in stools during the relapse and an interaction between viral infection and immune mechanisms [19]. Our analysis found that acute hepatitis A in the outbreak population had a tendency toward a more icteric and relapsing disease course, which may reflect the frequent existence of immunodeficiency in this population. Previous studies attempting to assess the influence of MSM or HIV infections on acute hepatitis A were mostly limited by the study size. To our knowledge, this is the first study to suggest an impact of MSM or HIV infection on the clinical manifestations of acute hepatitis A.

There are several limitations to this study: 1. This was a single-center study in which the studied population may not represent the entire population of the country. This difference can be observed by the higher positive HBsAg prevalence (17.9%) in the studied population compared to the estimated number of HBV carriers in the entire population (10–13%, between 2.5 and 3 million people in Taiwan [20]) and a higher mortality rate (3.9%) compared to previous reports (1.68% [18], 0.3–0.6% [21]). This is, in part, related to the study center, which was a tertiary referral hospital with patients potentially bearing more co-morbidities. 2. Although we observed a significant increase in the number of MSM and HIV infections during the outbreak, the prevalences of both MSM and HIV infection were underestimated in this study. Before the acute hepatitis A outbreak onset in mid-2015, according to the CDC's statement on surveillance using phylogenic analysis (information from a CDC public talk held in Taipei on September 10th, 2016), there were only two sporadic HAV/HIV coinfection cases in the past 10 years in the entire population. Therefore, the whole society was not aware of the correlation between HAV/HIV and also HAV/MSM until mid-2015. The percentage of cases that have been tested for their HIV status before the outbreak was only 12.9% (21/163) in our study. During the outbreak, this percentage was increased to 77.3% (34/44), however, there were still cases that were not checked for HIV status either due to a low awareness of HIV/HAV association by the clinicians or a refusal of the test by the patient. Among HIV-positive cases, there were also 21% (3/14) that did not disclose their sexual orientation in our study. Taken together, the data suggested there may be an underestimation of HIV infections in this study, nevertheless, this effect is considered minimal in the pre-outbreak period and in favor of our conclusion in the outbreak period. 3. Because of the nature of retrospective studies and a smaller sample size of HIV-infected patients, we were unable to compare acute hepatitis A head-to-head between HIV-infected and non-HIV-infected patients. Therefore, we are planning to organize a case-controlled study recruiting larger sample sizes in the future in order to better clarify the effects of HIV infection and different cART regiments on the clinical manifestations and outcomes of acute hepatitis A. However, we believe that emphasizing the importance of hepatitis A vaccination among a high-risk population should not be delayed because we have observed a more protracted and symptomatic disease in this population.

The risks of mortality and complications of acute hepatitis A increase with age, pre-existing chronic liver disease and medical co-morbidities [18, 22, 23]. Our study reports that MSM and HIV-positive populations are also at increased risk of developing a more icteric and protracted course. Acute hepatitis A may cause considerable loss to both people and society. In light of outbreak preventions, study by Regan et al. suggested that the critical point of achieving herd immunity to prevent hepatitis A outbreaks is when the immune population to HAV is greater than ~70% [24]. Because viral interactions are not rare [25, 26] and our study described the likely detrimental effects of HIV infection on acute hepatitis A in a sensitive MSM population, these results call for public health awareness and encourage approaches, particularly HAV vaccination, in the MSM/HIV-positive population. This issue may be particularly important in low anti-HAV seroprevalence countries. During the preparation of this manuscript, a new HAV vaccination program targeting HIV-positive population and those recently diagnosed to have other sexually transmitted diseases was launched in October 2016 in Taiwan with an aim to stop this outbreak. Our results offer clinical evidence to recapitulate the importance of preventing a hepatitis A outbreak in the MSM/HIV-positive population.

Conclusions

In order to achieve control over an acute hepatitis A outbreak, clinical evidence is crucial to persuade high-risk populations into accepting the vaccination policy. MSM and HIV infection are risk factors of acute hepatitis A infection. This study recognized that the clinical course of acute hepatitis A during an outbreak involving the MSM/HIV-positive population is more symptomatic and protracted than the sporadic cases in general population. The result suggests the need to improve the anti-HAV seroprevalence in the MSM/HIV-positive population to reduce the incidence of acute hepatitis A and may be an important reference for developing public health policies.

Abbreviations

ALT: Alanine aminotransferase; AST: Aspartate aminotransferase; cART: Combination antiretroviral therapy; CDC: Centers of Disease Control; ELISA: Enzyme-linked immunosorbent assay; HAV: Hepatitis A virus; Hb: Hemoglobin; HBsAg: Hepatitis B surface antigen; HBV: Hepatitis B virus; HCV: Hepatitis C virus; HIV: Human immunodeficiency virus; IgM: Immunoglobulin M; MSM: Men who have sex with men; RPR/VDRL test: Rapid plasma regain/venereal disease research laboratory test; STD: Sexually transmitted disease

Acknowledgements

The authors wish to acknowledge the support of the Maintenance Project for Center for Big Data Analytics and Statistics (Grant CLRPG3D0043) from Chang Gung Memorial Hospital for data analysis. We also wish to thank Dr. Poyen Huang for his helpful discussions on this topic.

Funding

Not applicable

Authors' contributions

NYC and TSW contributed to the study concept and design. NYC drafted the manuscript. TSW supervised the study. ZHL performed the statistical analysis and interpretation of the data. THC and SSS provided important intellectual suggestions. SSS also contributed to the acquisition of the data. All authors read and approved the final manuscript.

Competing interests

The authors declare that they have no competing interests.

Consent for publication

Not applicable

Author details

[1]Division of Infectious Diseases, Department of Internal Medicine, Chang Gung Memorial Hospital, Chang Gung University College of Medicine, 5 Fuhsing Street, Kueishan, Taoyuan 333, Taiwan. [2]Department of Neurosurgery, Chang Gung Memorial Hospital, Chang Gung Medical College and University, 5 FuSing Street, Kueishan, Taoyuan, Taiwan. [3]Division of Gastroenterology and Hepatology, Department of Internal Medicine, Chang Gung Memorial Hospital, Chang Gung Medical College and University, 5 FuSing Street, Kueishan, Taoyuan, Taiwan.

References

1. Klevens RM, Denniston MM, Jiles-Chapman RB, Murphy TV. Decreasing immunity to hepatitis a virus infection among US adults: findings from the National Health and nutrition examination survey (NHANES), 1999-2012. Vaccine. 2015;33(46):6192–8.
2. From the Centers for Disease Control. Hepatitis A among homosexual men–United States, Canada, and Australia. JAMA. 1992;267(12):1587–8.
3. Bialek SR, Barry V, Bell BP, Valleroy LA, Behel S, Mackellar DA, et al. Seroprevalence and correlates of hepatitis a among HIV-negative American men who have sex with men. Sex Health. 2011;8(3):343–8.
4. Bordi L, Rozera G, Scognamiglio P, Minosse C, Loffredo M, Antinori A, et al. Monophyletic outbreak of hepatitis a involving HIV-infected men who have sex with men, Rome, Italy 2008-2009. J Clin Virol. 2012;54(1):26–9.
5. Sfetcu O, Irvine N, Ngui SL, Emerson C, McCaughey C, Donaghy P. Hepatitis A outbreak predominantly affecting men who have sex with men in Northern Ireland, October 2008 to July 2009. Euro Surveill. 2011;16(9):19808.
6. Mazick A, Howitz M, Rex S, Jensen IP, Weis N, Katzenstein TL, et al. Hepatitis A outbreak among MSM linked to casual sex and gay saunas in Copenhagen. Denmark Euro Surveill. 2005;10(5):111–4.
7. (CDC) CfDC. Hepatitis a among drug abusers. MMWR Morb Mortal Wkly Rep. 1988;37(19):297–300. 5
8. Henning KJ, Bell E, Braun J, Barker ND. A community-wide outbreak of hepatitis a: risk factors for infection among homosexual and bisexual men. Am J Med. 1995;99(2):132–6.
9. Tsou TP, Liu CC, Huang JJ, Tsai KJ, Chang HF. Change in hepatitis a epidemiology after vaccinating high risk children in Taiwan, 1995-2008. Vaccine. 2011;29(16):2956–61.
10. Tsai CF, Lin DB, Chen SC, Chang YH, Chen CY, Lin JB. Seroepidemiology of hepatitis a virus infection among schoolchildren in Taiwan. J Med Virol. 2011;83(2):196–200.
11. Centers of Diseases Control T. Taiwan national infectious diseases statistics system 2016 [Available from: http://nidss.cdc.gov.tw/en/SingleDisease.aspx?dc=1&dt=2&disease=0701.
12. Fonquernie L, Meynard JL, Charrois A, Delamare C, Meyohas MC, Frottier J. Occurrence of acute hepatitis a in patients infected with human immunodeficiency virus. Clin Infect Dis. 2001;32(2):297–9.
13. Gallego M, Robles M, Palacios R, Ruiz J, Nuño E, Márquez M, et al. Impact of acute hepatitis a virus (HAV) infection on HIV viral load in HIV-infected patients and influence of HIV infection on acute HAV infection. J Int Assoc Physicians AIDS Care (Chic). 2011;10(1):40–2.
14. Ida S, Tachikawa N, Nakajima A, Daikoku M, Yano M, Kikuchi Y, et al. Influence of human immunodeficiency virus type 1 infection on acute hepatitis a virus infection. Clin Infect Dis. 2002;34(3):379–85.
15. Tseng YT, Sun HY, Chang SY, Wu CH, Liu WC, Wu PY, et al. Seroprevalence of hepatitis virus infection in men who have sex with men aged 18-40 years in Taiwan. J Formos Med Assoc. 2012;111(8):431–8.
16. Sun HY, Kung HC, Ho YC, Chien YF, Chen MY, Sheng WH, et al. Seroprevalence of hepatitis a virus infection in persons with HIV infection in Taiwan: implications for hepatitis a vaccination. Int J Infect Dis. 2009;13(5):e199–205.
17. Chan PC. Reemerging threat of hepatitis a among men who have sex with men in Taiwan. J Formos Med Assoc. 2014;113(12):985–6.
18. Chen CM, Chen SC, Yang HY, Yang ST, Wang CM. Hospitalization and mortality due to hepatitis a in Taiwan: a 15-year nationwide cohort study. J Viral Hepat. 2016;23(11):940–5.
19. Glikson M, Galun E, Oren R, Tur-Kaspa R, Shouval D. Relapsing hepatitis A. Review of 14 cases and literature survey. Medicine (Baltimore). 1992;71(1):14–23.
20. Wait S, Chen DS. Towards the eradication of hepatitis B in Taiwan. Kaohsiung J Med Sci. 2012;28(1):1–9.
21. Fiore AE, Wasley A, Bell BP, (ACIP) ACoIP. Prevention of hepatitis A through active or passive immunization: recommendations of the Advisory Committee on Immunization Practices (ACIP). MMWR Recomm Rep. 2006;55(RR-7):1–23.
22. Brown GR, Persley K. Hepatitis a epidemic in the elderly. South Med J. 2002;95(8):826–33.
23. Lefilliatre P, Villeneuve JP. Fulminant hepatitis a in patients with chronic liver disease. Can J Public Health. 2000;91(3):168–70.
24. Regan DG, Wood JG, Benevent C, Ali H, Smith LW, Robertson PW, et al. Estimating the critical immunity threshold for preventing hepatitis A outbreaks in men who have sex with men. Epidemiol Infect. 2016;144(7):1528–37.
25. Coppola N, Marrocco C, Di Caprio D, Coviello G, Scolastico C, Filippini P, et al. Acute hepatitis B and C virus coinfection: a virological and clinical study of 3 cases. Clin Infect Dis. 2003;36(4):528–32.
26. Coppola N, Genovese D, Pisaturo M, Taffon S, Argentini C, Pasquale G, et al. Acute hepatitis with severe cholestasis and prolonged clinical course due to hepatitis A virus Ia and Ib coinfection. Clin Infect Dis. 2007;44(9):e73–7.

15

Estimating the scale of chronic hepatitis B virus infection among migrants in EU/EEA countries

Amena A. Ahmad[1,2*†], Abby M. Falla[3,4†], Erika Duffell[5], Teymur Noori[5], Angela Bechini[6], Ralf Reintjes[1] and Irene K. Veldhuijzen[4,7]

Abstract

Background: Chronic hepatitis B (CHB) related morbidity and mortality can be reduced through risk group screening, linkage to care and anti-viral treatment. This study estimates the number of CHB cases among foreign-born (migrants) in the European Union and European Economic Area (EU/EEA) countries in order to identify the most affected migrant populations.

Methods: The CHB burden was estimated by combining: demographic data on migrant population size by country of birth in the EU/EEA, extracted from European statistical databases; and CHB prevalence in migrants' countries of birth and in EU/EEA countries, derived from a systematic literature search. The relative contribution of migrants from endemic countries to the total CHB burden in each country was also estimated. The reliability of using country of birth prevalence as a proxy for prevalence among migrants was assessed by comparing it to the prevalence found in studies among migrants in Europe.

Results: An estimated 1–1.9 million CHB-infected migrants from endemic countries (prevalence ≥2%) reside in the EU/EEA. Migrants from endemic countries comprise 10.3% of the total EU/EEA population but account for 25% (15%–35%) of all CHB cases. Migrants born in China and Romania contribute the largest number of infections, with over 100,000 estimated CHB cases each, followed by migrants from Turkey, Albania and Russia, in descending order, with over 50,000 estimated CHB cases each. The CHB prevalence reported in studies among migrants in EU/EEA countries was lower than the country of birth prevalence in 9 of 14 studies.

Conclusions: Migrants from endemic countries are disproportionately affected by CHB; their contribution however varies between EU/EEA countries. Migrant focused screening strategies would be most effective in countries with a high relative contribution of migrants and a low general population prevalence. In countries with a higher general population prevalence and a lower relative contribution of migrants, screening specific birth cohorts may be a more effective use of scarce resources. Quantifying the number of CHB infections among 50 different migrant groups residing in each of the 31 EU/EEA host countries helps to identify the most affected migrant communities who would benefit from targeted screening and linkage to care.

Keywords: Hepatitis B, Chronic viral hepatitis, Migrants, Epidemiology, Europe

* Correspondence: amenaalmes.ahmad@haw-hamburg.de
[†]Equal contributors
[1]Faculty Life Sciences, Department of Health Sciences, Hamburg University of Applied Sciences, Ulmenliet 20, 21033 Hamburg, Germany
[2]Department of Internal Medicine, University Medical Center Hamburg-Eppendorf, Martinistr. 52, 20246 Hamburg, Germany
Full list of author information is available at the end of the article

Background

Migration flows in the first half of the twentieth century were predominantly from Europe towards America. Since the Second World War, economic and geopolitical factors such as decolonisation, labour migration, the collapse of communism, air travel, economic growth and political crisis have changed this and migration to Europe has increased [1]. Much of this migration has been from low- and middle-income countries in Asia and Africa, many of which have a high prevalence of hepatitis B and C [2, 3]. Existing case-based surveillance systems such as the European hepatitis B and C surveillance system managed by the European Centre for Disease Prevention and Control are unable to accurately quantify the number of chronic viral hepatitis cases among migrants on account of different reporting, testing and screening practices among member states. Additional information sources and epidemiologic research are needed to estimate the scale of chronic hepatitis B virus infection in this population [4].

Hepatitis B virus (HBV) infection primarily affects the liver. It usually has an insidious onset and can remain undetected for many years. Up to 5% of HBV infections in adults (up to 90% in young children) can progress to become chronic and up to 30% of chronic cases may develop liver cirrhosis [5].

Public health measures, including antenatal screening, childhood HBV vaccination, stringent testing of blood products, improved infection control practices and harm reduction programmes, have led to a significant reduction of viral hepatitis transmission and a decline in the number of acute HBV cases reported in many European Union/European Economic Area (EU/EEA) countries [6]. Limited or more recent implementation of these primary prevention measures explains the high prevalence of viral hepatitis seen in many parts of the world, but especially in South East Asia, Sub-Saharan Africa and Eastern Europe [7]. Vertical transmission from mother to child and nosocomial transmission are considered to be the main routes in intermediate (2–8%) and high (>8%) HBsAg prevalence countries [5, 7].

Worldwide viral hepatitis related mortality in absolute terms increased by 63% between 1990 and 2013, while the associated disability adjusted life years increased by 34% during this time [8]. This global increase is largely the result of inadequate prevention measures combined with population growth in hepatitis endemic areas [8]. An estimated 13 to 14 million people in the WHO European region are chronically infected with hepatitis B [9, 10] and about 36,000 people die every year as a consequence [9]. In Europe, chronic HBV infection is a major cause of liver cirrhosis and 10–15% of hepatocellular carcinoma (HCC), cases are attributed to chronic hepatitis B (CHB) [10].

Antiviral treatment with nucleot(s)ides such as tenofovir or entecavir can prevent the development of cirrhosis and HCC and can suppress viral replication in a very high proportion of cases [3]. However, because of the largely asymptomatic nature of the infection until late stages, it is estimated that between 40% and 80% of people infected are unaware of their infection and many are not diagnosed until after liver damage has occurred [10, 11]. The population health benefits of effective treatment can only be realised by improving early detection of infection through targeted testing among risk groups.

The WHO recently ratified the strategic goal to eliminate chronic viral hepatitis as a health threat in Europe by 2030. The strategy and action plan published to support countries and the region to achieve this goal highlight 'the who' and 'the where' as the first two strategic pillars of elimination [12, 13]. Whilst it is suspected that a large proportion of migrants to the EU come from hepatitis B (HBsAg) intermediate (2%–8%) and high (>8%) endemicity countries [2, 3], little is known about the epidemiology of CHB among migrants. Specifically lacking are robust estimates of the number of infections among migrants and knowledge about which groups are most affected. Estimates of which migrant groups are most affected and would therefore benefit most from (linguistically/culturally/specifically) targeted screening programmes, early detection and treatment are required if Europe is to achieve this ambitious elimination goal.

The aims of this study are: 1) to estimate the number of CHB cases among the foreign-born population originating from intermediate and high HBV endemicity countries residing in the 31 countries of the EU/EEA; 2) to estimate the relative contribution of migrants to the overall burden of CHB in Europe; and 3) to identify the migrant groups among whom the largest number of cases are found so as to help direct more effective screening programmes. In a sister paper (INFD-D-17-00468) [14], we conduct a similar analysis for chronic hepatitis C among migrants from endemic countries.

Methods

The data retrieval and analysis process are described in detail below and in a schematic representation (Fig. 1). To estimate the number of CHB cases among migrants in each EU/EEA country, demographic data on the number of foreign-born migrants by country of birth living, in EU/EEA countries were extracted from statistical databases. Country of birth-specific and EU/EEA country-specific general population Hepatitis B surface antigen (HBsAg) prevalence estimates were derived from a systematic literature search (Part 1). To assess the reliability of using country of birth-derived HBsAg prevalence as a proxy for the prevalence among migrants, a systematic

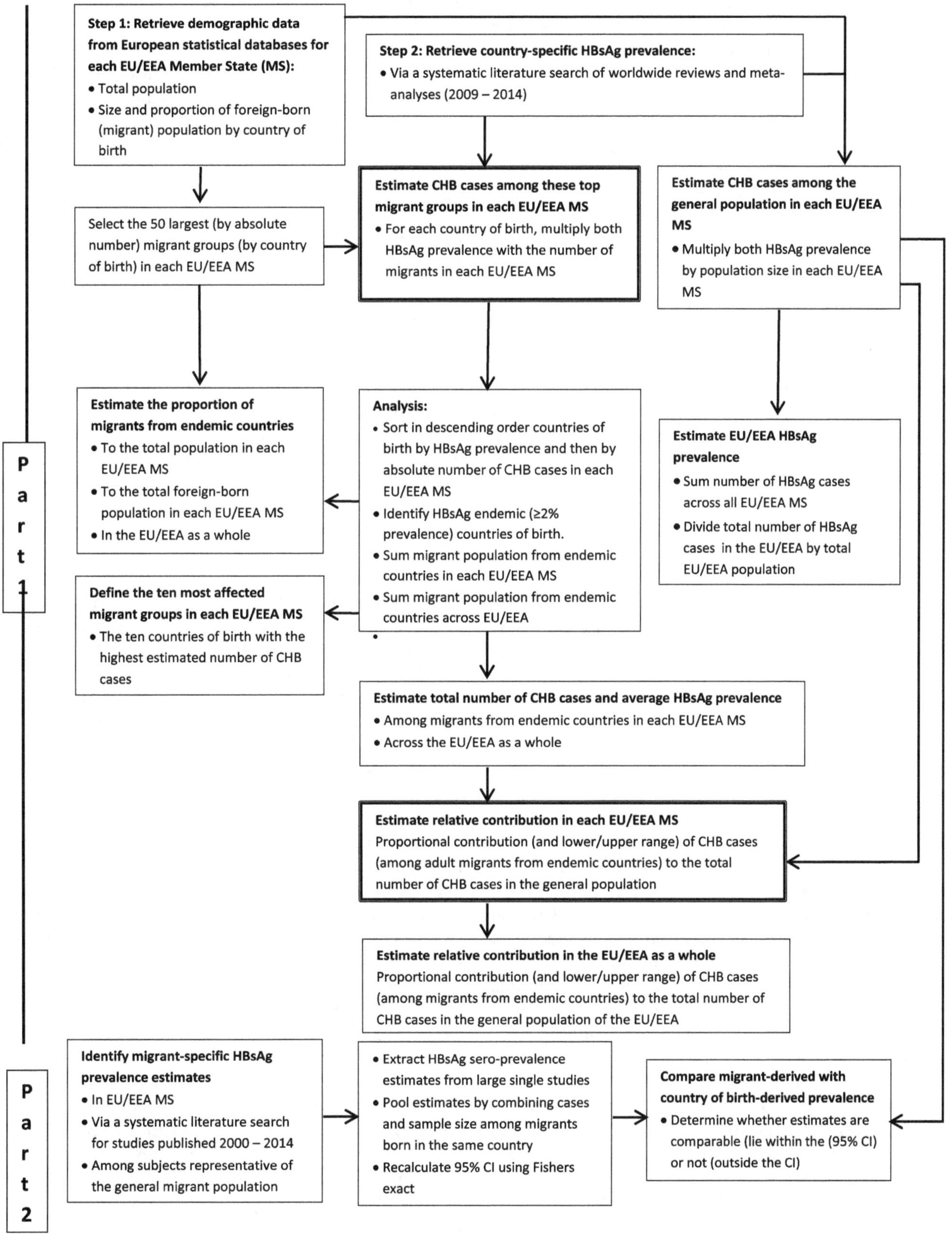

Fig. 1 Schematic representation of the methodological process to estimating the burden of chronic hepatitis B among migrants in the EU/EEA

literature search was conducted to identify prevalence estimates among migrants in Europe and to compare these with country of birth-derived prevalence (Part 2).

Definitions

Migrant (foreign-born population): includes all persons who were born outside their current country of residence (and listed in the demographic registration databases used in this study). This includes within-EU/EEA migrants, i.e. persons born in another EU/EEA country, as well as those born outside the EU. It does not include undocumented migrants.

Chronic hepatitis B (CHB): refers to a positive hepatitis B surface antigen (HBsAg) test Note: According to the WHO and EU (2012) case definition, detection of HBsAg on two occasions at least 6 months apart is classified as CHB. In this study, as in the seroprevalence and screening studies from which prevalence data for this study were extracted, the presence of HBsAg is taken as the standard proxy for chronic infection. The lack of regular screening for HBV and the reduction in incidence of acute HBV infections in most countries justify the assumption that the overwhelming majority of HBsAg positive cases are chronic.

Hepatitis B endemic country: countries with a ≥ 2% HBsAg prevalence in the general population. This follows from the WHO classification of low (<2%), intermediate (2% to 8%) and high (>8%) endemic countries.

Part 1: The contribution of migrants from endemic countries to the burden of CHB in the EU/EEA

Demographic data

The size and country of birth of the foreign-born migrant population was obtained for the 31 EU/EEA countries from Eurostat for 2013, if available [15]. Where Eurostat data by country of birth were missing (Croatia, Cyprus, France, Germany, Malta, Portugal and the UK), data from the EU 2011 – Housing and Population Census were used [16]. The most recent demographic data for Greece (2012) and Luxembourg (2010) were only available from the Organisation for Economic Co--operation and Development' (OECD) Stats website [17]. No demographic data were available from the above sources for Lithuania. Data were thus obtained from the Lithuanian National Statistics Service (2013) [18]. The data source is indicated in footnotes in Table 1. For each EU/EEA country, the countries of birth of foreign-born migrants were arranged in descending order of magnitude by the number of migrants. The top 50 countries of birth by size of migrant population were selected for estimating the CHB burden.

Systematic literature search to estimate country- specific HBsAg prevalence

The online databases Medline, Embase, the Cochrane library, Web of Science, Scopus, PubMed publisher and Google Scholar were searched in January 2015 for reviews, systematic reviews and meta-analyses in English about the prevalence of hepatitis B in the general population at national level. The search terms (described in full in Annex 1 of the Additional file 1) consisted of a combination of disease-related (hepatitis B), outcome-related (prevalence), population-related (general population, worldwide), and study design-related (reviews) terms. Since the aim was to identify recent reviews, the search was restricted to papers published between 2009 and 2014. The titles and abstracts of retrieved articles were assessed for relevance using exclusion criteria. Key exclusion criteria included studies about hepatitis other than type B; focusing on natural history, clinical features or complications of hepatitis; about medical treatment; focusing on high risk groups e.g. people who inject drugs; and single case studies and cost effectiveness analyses. Full texts of the selected abstracts were retrieved and assessed, decisions to exclude were recorded and a PRISMA flowchart (described in Annex 2 of the Additional file 1) was prepared.

From included reviews, country-specific HBsAg prevalence estimates and confidence intervals (CI) were extracted into a Microsoft Excel database. Where a country-specific estimate was unavailable, the relevant Global Burden of Disease region estimate was used, if available. If a meta-analysis reported a statistically significant time trend, the estimate from the most recent period was selected. When multiple estimates for a country were available from different reviews, the most robust or relevant review was selected based on the following criteria: sampling method; representativeness of population studied; geographical coverage; sample size; quality of included studies and data collection timeframe. Decisions were made jointly by two reviewers (AF and IV) with the rationale recorded for each decision about a chosen estimate. This rationale, together with the search strategy, the inclusion and exclusion criteria and the PRISMA flowchart are described in annexs 1, 2, 3 and 5 of the Additional file 1 to this article.

Estimating the number of CHB cases among foreign-born migrants from endemic countries in each EU/EEA country

The retrieved HBsAg general population prevalence estimate in the countries of origin were multiplied by the number of migrants from that respective country in each EU/EEA country. The number of migrants born in endemic countries (≥2%) was summed to determine the total and proportional contribution of migrants from intermediate/high hepatitis B endemicity countries to the overall number of migrants residing in the host country. The ten migrant populations originating from intermediate and high endemicity countries with the highest number of HBsAg infected cases in the EU/EEA were determined.

Relative contribution

To estimate the relative contribution of migrants born in endemic countries to the overall number of people infected with CHB in the respective EU host country, the estimated number of infected cases among migrants was divided by the number of infected persons in that country based on the general population prevalence. Given the uncertainty in the size of migrant population and the CHB prevalence estimates in the countries of birth, the range of the relative contribution with a lower and a higher limit was calculated using the Delta method [19].

EU/EEA-level estimates

The population of the EU/EEA was derived by summing up the population of all 31 EU/EEA countries as extracted from demographic sources. To estimate the HBsAg prevalence in the EU/EEA, the number of estimated HBsAg positive cases in all 31 EU/EEA countries was summed up and divided by the total EU/EEA population. To derive the lower and upper prevalence range, the lower and upper estimates of the number of cases across the 31 countries were summed up. To estimate the number of cases among migrants to and within the EU/EEA, the number of cases among migrants from endemic countries (≥2%) across all 31 countries was summed up. This was then divided by the number of cases in the EU/EEA to derive the relative contribution of migrants from endemic countries to the burden of CHB infection in the EU/EEA.

Part 2: Systematic literature search for HBsAg prevalence in migrant populations in Europe

The online databases Medline, Embase, the Cochrane library, Web of Science, Scopus, PubMed publisher and Google Scholar were searched in November 2014 for studies in English that estimate the prevalence of hepatitis B among migrants in any of the 31 EU/EEA countries. The search consisted of a combination of disease-related (hepatitis B), outcome-related (prevalence), population-related (migrants) and geographical area (EU/EEA countries) terms and was limited to studies published between 2000 and 2014. Only studies about the prevalence in migrants who were considered to be representative of the general migrant population (i.e. not refugees or asylum seekers, hospital patients or other higher risk groups and not lower risk groups like pregnant women or children) were compared with in-country of birth derived prevalence estimates. The full search strategy, inclusion and exclusion criteria and PRISMA flowchart can be found in annexs 3, 4 and 6 of the Additional file 1.

Country-level HBsAg prevalence estimates among migrants residing in different European countries were extracted from the included studies and entered into Microsoft Excel. Pooled estimates for countries of birth were produced by combining the numbers tested and the number of cases. A 95% CI was re-calculated using the Fisher's exact method. Both pooled and large single study (>25 subjects from a single country of birth) estimates were compared with the in-country estimates extracted in Part 1 to determine whether in-country estimates reflect the prevalence found in migrants. When the point estimate from a study in migrants (Part 2) fell within the CI of the in-country estimate (from Part 1), the estimate was considered to be comparable; when it fell below the lower CI limit, it was considered lower than the in-country prevalence; and when it was higher than the upper CI limit the prevalence in migrants was considered to be higher.

Results

Estimated CHB prevalence and number of infected cases in 31 EU/EEA countries

Chronic hepatitis B (HBsAg) prevalence differs considerably among EU/EEA countries, ranging from 0.1% in Ireland and the Netherlands to 5.5% in Romania. The average prevalence in the general population of the EU/EEA is estimated at 1.1%, corresponding to an estimated 5.7 million cases (range 4.0 to 7.5 million). These estimates, together with the total number of infected cases, are listed in Table 1. Italy and Romania are the EU/EEA countries with the highest estimated number of CHB cases, both above 1 million.

The distribution of migrants in the EU/EEA based on HBV endemicity in country of birth

The top 50 foreign-born populations in each EU/EEA country included in our analysis make up at least 95% of the total migrant population in 19 of 31 EU/EEA countries and at least 90% in all but three EU/EEA countries (Denmark, Sweden and the UK where it is at least 85%). These migrant populations account for approximately 9.5% of the population in the EU/EEA. The proportion, however, ranges from 0.9% in Romania and 1.3% in Bulgaria to more than 40% in Luxembourg and 62% in Liechtenstein (Fig. 2). Just over half of the EU/EEA migrant population were born in HBV endemic (≥2% prevalence) countries. EU/EEA countries with the highest proportion of migrants from endemic countries among their foreign-born population are Croatia,

Table 1 Chronic hepatitis B prevalence in the general population of 31 EU/EEA countries and the estimated number of infected cases

Country	Total Population	HBsAg prevalence			Estimated no. of CHB cases		
		%	Low 95% CI	High 95% CI	Central estimate	Lower estimate	Upper estimate
Austria	8,451,149	0.55	0.34	0.71	46,481	28,734	60,003
Belgium	11,161,642	0.7	0.4	1.2	78,131	44,647	133,940
Bulgaria	7,284,552	4.25	2.80	5.70	309,593	203,967	415,219
Croatia	4284,889[a]	1.47	0.84	2.10	62,988	35,993	89,983
Cyprus	840,407[a]	0.9	0.3	2	7564	2521	16,808
Czech Republic	10,516,125	0.70	0.43	0.98	73,613	45,219	103,058
Denmark	5,602,628	0.55	0.34	0.71	30,814	19,049	39,779
Estonia	1,320,174	0.58	0.42	0.74	7657	5545	9769
Finland	5,426,674	0.2	0.1	0.4	10,853	5427	21,707
France	64,932,339[a]	0.68	0.44	1.05	441,540	285,702	681,790
Germany	80,219,695[a]	0.6	0.4	0.8	481,318	320,879	641,758
Greece	11,090,000[b]	2.33	1.54	3.11	258,397	170,786	344,899
Hungary	9,908,798	1.08	0.04	2.11	107,015	3964	209,076
Iceland	321,857	0.55	0.34	0.71	1770	1094	2285
Ireland	4591,087	0.1	0	0.3	4591	0	13,773
Italy	59,685,227	1.89	1.26	2.52	1,128,051	752,034	1,504,068
Latvia	2,023,825	1.39	1.10	1.67	28,131	22,262	33,798
Liechtenstein	36,838	0.55	0.34	0.71	203	125	262
Lithuania	2,971,905 [d]	2.03	1.37	2.69	60,330	40,715	79,944
Luxembourg	506,953[c]	0.55	0.34	0.71	2788	1724	3599
Malta	417,432	0.55	0.34	0.71	2296	1419	2964
Netherlands	16,779,575	0.1	0	0.2	16,780	0	33,559
Norway	5,049,223	0.55	0.34	0.71	27,771	17,167	35,849
Poland	38,533,299	1.44	1.16	1.72	554,880	446,986	662,773
Portugal	10,562,178[a]	1.35	0.66	2.04	142,589	69,710	215,468
Romania	20,020,074	5.49	5.24	5.73	1,099,102	1,049,052	1,147,150
Slovakia	5,410,836	0.70	0.43	0.98	37,876	23,267	53,026
Slovenia	2,058,821	3.29	2.33	4.24	67,735	47,971	87,294
Spain	46,727,890	0.66	0.34	0.97	308,404	158,875	453,261
Sweden	9,555,893	0.2	0.1	0.4	19,112	9556	38,224
United Kingdom	63,182,180[a]	0.54	0.30	0.60	341,184	189,547	379,093
EU/EEA[e]	509,474,165	1.12	0.79[e]	1.47[e]	5,705,260	4,003,937	7,514,179

[*]Source is EUROSTAT 2013 unless indicated by the following symbol:
[a]ESS 2011 Census
[b]OECD 2012
[c]OECDC 2010
[d]http:///www.euras.lt (Lithuanian National Statistics Agency
[e]For the 31 EU/EEA countries the cumulative HBsAg prevalence and the upper and lower CI were estimated from the sum of the estimated number of CHB cases (central, lower and upper estimate), hence these should be considered as upper and lower prevalence ranges and not CI

Estonia and Latvia (>90%), and those with the lowest proportion are Liechtenstein, Luxembourg and Slovakia (<16%) (Fig. 2). The foreign-born population and the number and proportion from endemic countries in the EU/EEA and by country are shown in Table 2.

Country-specific HBsAg prevalence estimates

The most comprehensive systematic global review of country-specific prevalence in the general population identified by the systematic literature search was a review by Kowdley et al. published in 2012 [20]. This

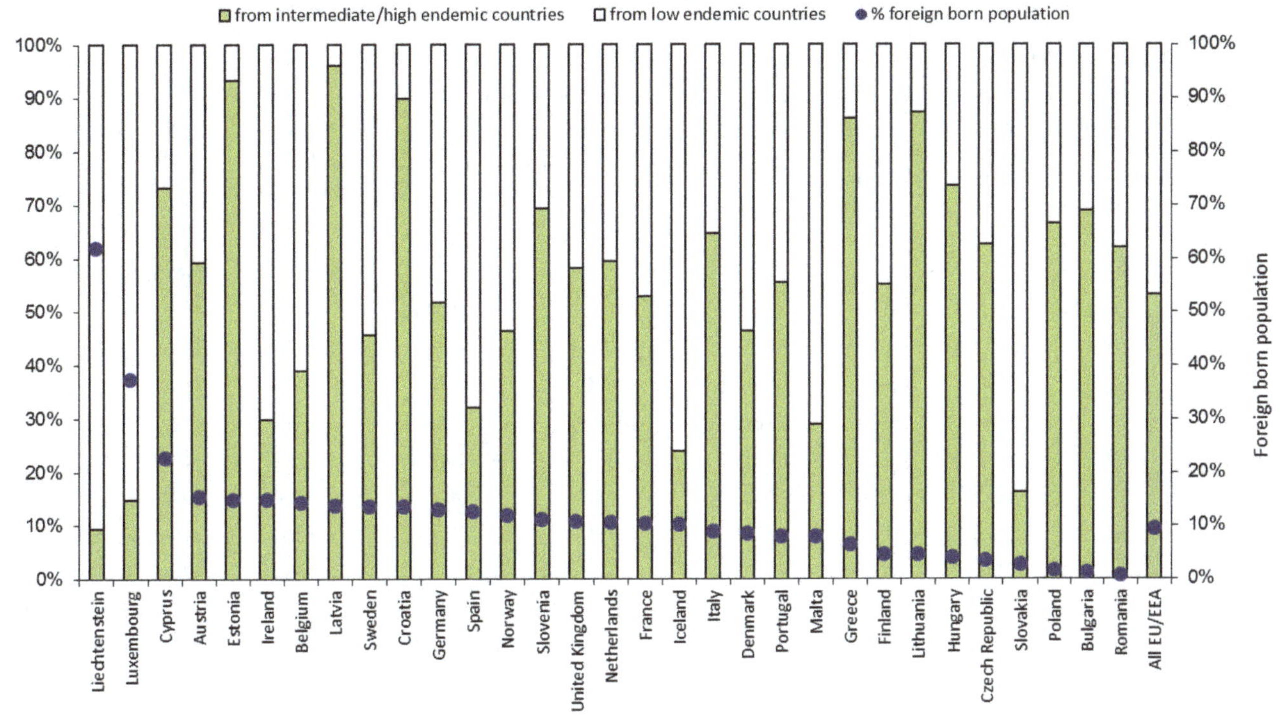

Fig. 2 Total (%) of foreign born population (blue dots) in each EU/EEA country and of those the proportion originating from HBsAg endemic countries (≥2%)

provided CHB prevalence estimates for 102 countries, based on studies published between 1980 and July 2010 using population-based surveys and studies of groups considered representative of the general population, such as pregnant women, school children, military recruits and healthy controls from cohort studies. Studies in emigrants to the United States, Europe, Australia and elsewhere were also included. Studies in blood donors and in higher risk populations were excluded. The Kowdley et al. review used meta-analytic methods to estimate country- and region-specific pooled HBsAg seroprevalence and corresponding 95% CI [20].

Since the Kowdley review did not include a prevalence estimate for the United States, this was taken from the most recent nationally representative survey in 2011 [21]. For 11 countries (China, Egypt, Ethiopia, Greece, Italy, Romania, Saudi Arabia, South Korea, Spain, Thailand and Turkey), Kowdley [20] reported a statistically significant decrease in prevalence over time and therefore the post-2000 estimate was taken. Estimates from other studies were considered more robust or relevant than this review for 11 countries (Albania, Algeria, Belgium, Cyprus, Finland, Ireland, Libya, Morocco, the Netherlands, Sweden and Tunisia) [9, 11, 22], and the reasons for this are listed in annex 7 of the Additional file 1. For the 44 countries and territories where no country estimate was available, the relevant regional estimate calculated by Kowdley was used. All country-specific prevalence estimates used can be seen in annex 8 of the Additional file 1, to this article.

Estimated prevalence and number of CHB infections among migrants

In the EU/EEA overall, between 1 million and 1.9 million migrants born in endemic countries are estimated to have CHB infection, which corresponds to an estimated prevalence of 5.5%. The estimated cumulative number and range of CHB cases among the top 50 migrant populations from intermediate and high endemicity countries in each EU/EEA country is listed in Table 2. The average HBsAg prevalence among migrants from intermediate and high endemicity countries is also available for each EU/EEA country, and ranges from 3% in Estonia, Latvia, Lithuania and Poland to 9% in Portugal.

Migrants originating from China and Romania contribute the largest number of infections, with over 100,000 CHB cases each, followed by migrants from Turkey, Albania and Russia, in descending order, with over 50,000 CHB cases each. Table 3 lists the ten migrant populations with the highest estimated number of CHB cases, adding up to over 680,000 cases and corresponding to 48% of CHB cases among migrants from endemic countries in the EU/EEA. Table 3 lists the EU host countries with the largest populations of migrants born in these countries. Estimates for the 50 migrant

Table 2 Foreign-born population and proportion of foreign-born population (from endemic (HBsAg ≥2%) countries), residing in the 31 EU/EEA host countries and the estimated number and range of CHB cases among migrants in these countries as well as the estimated relative contribution to the total number of cases in the EU/EEA host country

Country	Population of foreign-born migrants			Foreign-born migrants from endemic countries				
	Number from top 50 countries	Number from HBV endemic countries	Proportion from HBV endemic countries	Estimated number of CHB cases: Central estimate	Lower estimate	Upper estimate	Average CHB prevalence	Estimated relative contribution (and range) of CHB cases among migrants to the total number of CHB cases in the host country
Austria	1,298,945	768,773	9.1%	33,456	25,757	41,040	4.4%	72% (43% - >100%[a])
Belgium	1,596,848	622,206	5.6%	42,530	32,218	54,309	6.8%	54% (20% - 89%)
Bulgaria	90,990	62,755	0.9%	2436	1860	3039	3.9%	1% (0% - 1%)
Croatia	582,271	523,470	12.2%	18,673	11,966	25,376	3.6%	30% (13% - 46%)
Cyprus	190,568	139,689	16.6%	6770	5141	8445	4.8%	90% (2% - >100%[a])
Czech Republic	374,296	234,291	2.2%	12,185	9637	14,752	5.2%	17% (9% - 24%)
Denmark	484,139	224,384	4.0%	12,352	9605	15,152	5.5%	40% (24% - 56%)
Estonia	197,744	184,642	14.0%	5432	3822	7038	2.9%	71% (42% - 100%)
Finland	257,044	141,953	2.6%	8136	6206	10,067	5.7%	75% (16% - >100%[a])
France	6,775,948	3,591,002	5.5%	212,538	131,238	380,923	5.9%	48% (13% - 84%)
Germany	10,426,860	5,398,700	6.7%	234,792	180,867	288,066	4.3%	49% (29% - 68%)
Greece	713,471	615,986	5.6%	43,163	36,636	49,346	7.0%	17% (11% - 23%)
Hungary	411,403	302,781	3.1%	15,286	13,649	16,940	5.0%	14% (1% - 28%)
Iceland	32,910	7857	2.4%	421	349	494	5.4%	24% (15% - 33%)
Ireland	687,462	205,071	4.5%	13,196	10,935	15,574	6.4%	>100% (<0% - >100%[a])
Italy	5,319,754	3,443,409	5.8%	213,063	174,632	251,539	6.2%	19% (12% - 26%)
Latvia	278,243	267,617	13.2%	7866	5269	10,454	2.9%	28% (17% - 39%)
Liechtenstein	22,806	2140	5.8%	97	74	119	4.5%	48% (28% - 67%)
Lithuania	139,712	121,992	4.1%	3765	2469	5057	3.1%	6% (3% - 9%)
Luxembourg	189,858	28,085	5.5%	1450	913	2019	5.2%	52% (26% - 78%)
Malta	33,301	9629	2.3%	637	429	860	6.6%	28% (15% - 41%)
Netherlands	1,772,756	1,052,695	6.3%	56,650	40,335	73,016	5.4%	>100% (<0% - >100%[a])
Norway	597,316	277,047	5.5%	17,021	12,125	21,979	6.1%	61% (34% - 88%)
Poland	659,657	438,446	1.1%	11,679	7018	16,342	2.7%	2% (1% - 3%)
Portugal	854,830	475,155	4.5%	42,688	29,595	55,795	9.0%	30% (12% - 48%)
Romania	166,973	103,740	0.5%	7531	5453	9581	7.3%	1% (0% - 1%)
Slovakia	155,346	25,170	0.5%	1073	846	1301	4.3%	3% (2% - 4%)
Slovenia	231,276	160,220	7.8%	5713	3756	7663	3.6%	8% (5% - 12%)
Spain	5,930,170	1,909,343	4.1%	118,316	92,282	148,318	6.2%	38% (18% - 59%)
Sweden	1,304,130	596,303	6.2%	33,850	23,728	44,011	5.7%	>100% (34% - >100%[a])
United Kingdom	6,845,805	3,976,870	6.3%	244,409	195,342	294,417	6.1%	72% (47% - 96%)
EU/EEA	48,622,832	25.911.421	5.1%	1,427,174	1,074,152	1,873,032	5.5%	25% (15% - 35%)

[a]The Delta method does not give a reliable confidence interval around the relative contribution as the relative contribution is close to 100% and the distribution of cases in the general population is extremely skewed

groups in each EU/EEA country can be found in annex 9 of the Additional file 1 to this article.

Migrants from China, Romania and Russia are among the top ten migrant populations with the highest estimated number of CHB cases in 28, 19 and 18 respectively of the 31 EU/EEA countries as listed in Table 4.

At least three of the ten migrant populations most affected by CHB in the Czech Republic, Denmark,

Table 3 The ten migrant groups (from HBsAg endemic countries) with the highest estimated number of CHB cases (rounded) and the main host EU/EEA countries

Migrant country of origin	Total migrant population in Europe	HBsAg prevalence	Cumulative number of CHB cases	Host countries (first 6 with largest populations)[a]
Romania	2,817,458	5.5	154,679	Italy, Spain, Germany, Hungary, UK, Austria
China	1,012,550	10.2	103,585	UK, Italy, Spain, France, Germany, Netherlands
Turkey	2,266,977	4.3	97,255	Germany, France, Netherlands, Austria, Belgium, UK
Albania	804,570	9.0	72,412	Italy, Greece, Belgium, Austria, Bulgaria
Russia	1,810,197	2.9	52,315	Germany, Latvia, Estonia, Italy, Spain, Lithuania
Vietnam	365,048	12.5	45,557	France, Germany, Czech Republic, UK, Sweden, Norway
Nigeria	336,155	13.3	44,741	UK, Italy, Spain, Ireland, Netherlands, Austria
Kazakhstan	828,526	5.0	41,013	Germany, Latvia, Czech Republic, Poland, Lithuania, Estonia
Algeria	1,482,465	2.6	38,544	France, Spain, Belgium, Italy, Ireland
India	1,120,352	3.2	36.188	UK, Italy, Germany, France, Spain, Ireland
Total			686,289[b]	

[a]if migrant population is at least 1000
[b]The sum of CHB cases among the ten migrant groups with the largest number of CHB cases (686,289) corresponds to 48% of the total number of CHB cases among migrants from endemic countries (1,427,174)

Table 4 Countries of birth of foreign-born migrants found amongst the ten migrant groups most affected by chronic hepatitis B in 10 or more of the 31 EU/EEA countries[a]

Country of birth of migrants	Number of EU/EEA countries (of 31)	EU/EEA Countries
China	28	AUT, BEL, BLG, HR, CZ, DK, DE, FIN, FR, EE, HU, IRL, ISL, IT, LIE, LT, LUX, MT, NL, NO, PL, PT, RO, SK, SI, ES, SE, UK
Romania	19	AUT, BEL, BLG, HR, CY, CZ, DK, DE, GRC, HU, IRL, ISL, IT, LUX, MT, PL, PT, SK, ES,
Russia	18	AT, BLG, HR, CY, CZ, DE, FIN, EE, GRC, HU, ISL, LT, LV, MT, PL, RO, SK, SI
Ukraine	14	BLG, HR, CZ, DE, EE, HU, IT, LT, LV, PL, PT, RO, SK, SI
Vietnam	14	BLG, CY, CZ, DK, DE, FIN, FR, HU, ISL, NL, NO, PL, SK, SE
Turkey	12	AUT, BEL, BLG, DK, DE, FIN, FR, GRC, LIE, NL, RO, SE
Moldova	11	BLG, CY, CZ, EE, IRL, IT, LT, LV, PT, RO, SI
Philippines	11	AUT, CY, DK, GRC, IRL, ISL, IT, MT, NO, ES, UK
Afghanistan	10	AUT, BEL, DK, DE, FIN, HU, NL, NO, SK, SE
Bosnia and Herzegovina	10	AUT, HR, DK, DE, LIE, LUX, NO, PL, SI, SE

[a]selected from the ten largest CHB affected migrant groups from intermediate/high endemicity countries in the EU/EEA countries

Finland, Hungary, Iceland, Liechtenstein, Norway, the Netherlands and Sweden were born in South-East or East Asian countries including China, Vietnam, the Philippines and Thailand. People born in Yugoslavia before 1992 or in one of the former Yugoslav Republics since 1992 are represented among three or more of the top ten migrant populations with the highest number of infected cases in Austria, Liechtenstein and Luxembourg as well as in Croatia and Slovenia. Similarly, people born in the Soviet Union before 1991 or in one of the former Soviet Republics since 1991 are represented among three or more of the top ten migrant populations most affected by CHB in Bulgaria, Cyprus, the Czech Republic, Germany, Hungary, Poland, Romania and Slovenia as well as in the Baltic states of Estonia, Latvia and Lithuania (see annex 9 of the Additional file 1).

In the UK, migrants from India, Pakistan and Bangladesh are among the top ten migrant populations with the highest number of infected cases. Migrants from Maghreb countries such as Algeria and Tunisia are represented in the top ten in France. Across the EU/EEA, African countries of origin that contribute a large number of estimated cases include Eritrea, Ghana, Nigeria, Senegal, Somalia and South Africa. In Belgium, France, Luxembourg, Malta, Portugal and the UK, four or more of the ten migrant populations most affected by CHB are from African countries.

Relative contribution of migrants from endemic countries to the overall CHB burden in EU/EEA countries

The relative proportion of infected migrants from endemic countries among the overall number of CHB cases in EU/EEA countries is shown in Table 2 and Fig. 3. Migrants from intermediate and high endemicity countries contribute more than 90% and, in some instances, up to 100% of the total estimated number of CHB cases in Cyprus, Ireland, the Netherlands and Sweden. Conversely, in Bulgaria, Poland, Romania and Slovakia, migrants contribute less than 4% of the total.

Comparing migrant-derived HBsAg prevalence with country of origin estimates

Sixteen HBsAg prevalence studies in migrants residing in Europe were identified from the literature search for comparison with the in-country estimates derived in Part 1 (Table 5). Prevalence figures for migrants from Suriname and the Dutch Antilles could only be compared with a regional estimate, since in-country data were not available from the review studies in Part 1.

In nine of the remaining 14 studies in migrants, HBsAg prevalence figures were lower than the derived in-country estimate. Prevalence among migrants was comparable with the in-country or region estimate for four migrant populations. HBsAg prevalence among migrants from Albania was higher than the in-country estimate.

Discussion

The number of CHB cases in the general population of the 31 EU/EEA countries is estimated at between 4 million and 7.5 million cases, with a disproportionately high number of these cases found among migrants. Although migrants from endemic countries make up only one in 20 EU/EEA citizens, they account for one in four of all CHB infections. Migrants from ten countries account for 48% of all CHB cases among migrants in the EU/EEA.

The data suggest that the relative contribution of migrants to the overall CHB burden is higher in Western and Northern European countries than in Southern and Eastern European countries. The relative contribution of migrants to the overall burden of CHB is lowest (<4%) in EU/EEA countries with a higher HBsAg prevalence and a lower proportion of migrants such as Romania, Bulgaria, Slovakia and Poland. Conversely, the relative contribution is very high (>100%) in EU/EEA countries with a very low HBsAg prevalence such as Ireland, the Netherlands and Sweden. The estimate of over 100% is a result of the prevalence in the general population of the host country likely to be underestimated (because migrants and other higher risk, harder to reach populations are underrepresented in the samples used to determine this prevalence) or because the prevalence in countries of birth of migrants is an over-estimation of the actual prevalence among migrants.

To assess whether the country of birth prevalence estimates used are over-estimates, we compared these estimates to the prevalence reported in migrant studies in Europe and found evidence indicating an over-estimation. Based on the epidemiologic features of HBV, the lower than in-country prevalence among migrants from 9 of 14 countries was surprising, since the infection is often acquired at birth or in early childhood in countries where HBV is endemic. One explanation could be an age or cohort effect, since the estimates of in-country prevalence include older data from the 1980s and 1990s, while most of the migrant studies in Europe used for comparison were conducted after 2000. A recent study estimating hepatitis B prevalence by region showed a decrease in most regions between 1990 and 2005 [6]. This decrease is largely explained by the widespread introduction of antenatal HBV screening together with risk group and infant HBV vaccination programmes [23] and the

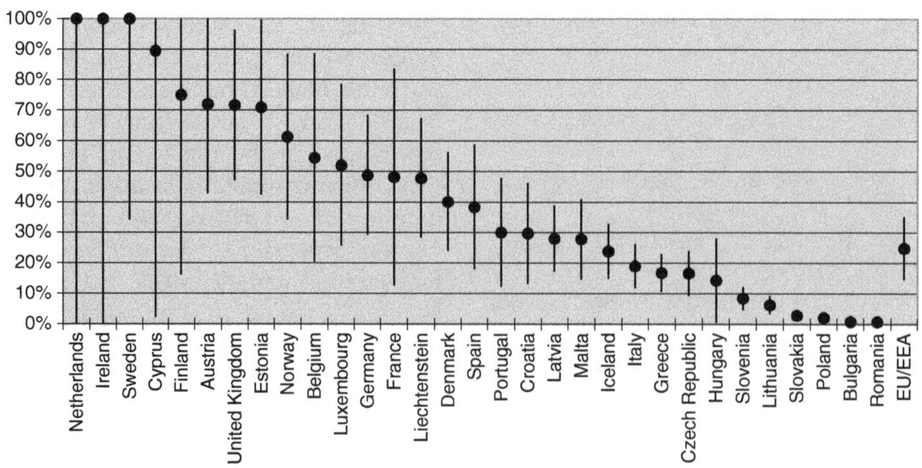

Fig. 3 Relative contribution of migrants to the total number of CHB cases per EU/EEA country

Table 5 HBsAg prevalence derived from studies among general migrant populations resident in Europe compared to in-country prevalence estimates derived from worldwide systematic reviews

Country	Migrants				In-country of origin			Comparison
	N tested	Prevalence	95% CI	Reference	Prevalence	95% CI	Reference	
Afghanistan	293	2.1	0.8–4.4	[30]	10.5	5.9–15.1	[20]	Lower
Albania	504[a]	11.7	9.0–14.8	[31]	9.0	8.1–9.8	[9]	Higher
Bangladesh	934	1.3	0.7–2.2	[32, 33]	4.8	4.0–5.6	[20]	Lower
China[b]	1319	9.4	7.9–11.1	[33, 34]	10.2 [c]	9.4–11.2	[20]	Comparable
Dutch Antilles	38	2.6	0.1–13.8	[35]	4.5[d]	2.5–6.6	[20]	Comparable
Egypt	465	1.1	0.4–2.5	[36]	4.2 [c]	1.9–6.5	[20]	Lower
Former USSR	675	4.7	3.3–6.6	[30, 37]	3.8	2.7–4.9	[20]	Comparable
India	1334	0.1	0–0.4	[32, 38]	3.2	2.9–3.6	[20]	Lower
Iran	153	0.7	0.1–2.5	[30]	3.1	2.7–3.5	[20]	Lower
Iraq	290	0.7	0–3.6	[30]	1.3	0–2.9	[20]	Comparable
Morocco	305	0.3	0–1.8	[35, 39]	1.8	1.5–5.9	[20, 22]	Lower
Pakistan	3786	1.6	1.2–2.1	[32, 33, 38, 40]	4.2	3.6–4.8	[20]	Lower
Somalia	317	7.3	4.6–10.7	[41]	12.4	8.9–15.9	[20]	Lower
Suriname	56	0	0–6.4	[35]	4.5[d]	2.5–6.6	[20]	Lower
Turkey	902	3.7	2.5–5.1	[30, 35, 39]	4.3[c]	3.7–4.9	[20]	Comparable
Vietnam	149	10.7	6.3–16.9	[30, 33]	12.5	11.5–13.5	[20]	Lower

Notes:
[a]age range of participants 10–23 years
[b]including Hong Kong
[c]statistically significant decline over time reported therefore the latest estimate (from year 2000 onwards) selected
[d]regional estimate for Caribbean only

resulting decline in incidence. The healthy migrant effect, the hypothesis that migrants are often younger and healthier than the general population in their countries of birth, may also be a factor [24]. Study design should also be considered. The figures for prevalence among migrants living in EU/EEA countries tend to be based on data from small-scale, local studies that mostly use convenience sampling, such as screening studies (Table 5). These may under-estimate the true prevalence because people who have already been diagnosed may not participate. Nevertheless, although prevalence among migrants from intermediate and high endemicity countries may not be as high as in the country of birth, the evidence strongly suggests that it is still considerably higher than among the host population in EU/EEA countries and high enough for screening of affected migrant groups to be cost-effective [11, 25].

This study seeks to inform national screening efforts. The results suggests that an approach focused solely on migrants would have limited impact in most Eastern European countries, specifically Bulgaria, Lithuania, Poland, Romania, Slovakia and Slovenia, where the relative contribution of migrants to the overall national burden of CHB is low (between 1% and 8%) and the proportion of migrants from endemic countries is also low (<5%). In addition, Bulgaria, Lithuania, Romania and Slovenia are HBV-endemic countries with an HBsAg prevalence of >2.0% to 5.5%. A more effective approach would be to screen sub-groups of the general population, i.e. birth cohorts born before antenatal screening, childhood HBV vaccination and the regular screening of blood/blood products were introduced. Screening individuals potentially exposed to HBV through transfusions, transplants and dental or surgical procedures may also help to identify cases.

In contrast, targeted migrant screening approaches would be of value in countries such as Austria, Cyprus, Estonia, Finland, Ireland, the Netherlands, Sweden and UK, where more than 70% of CHB cases are estimated to be among migrants from endemic countries. To optimise cost-effectiveness, screening should target those migrant populations that are most at risk of chronic viral hepatitis infection where the likelihood of detecting cases is higher.

Screening and subsequent contact tracing increases the diagnosis rate and, together with effective linkage to and retention in care and antiviral treatment, are the key to effective secondary prevention. The asymptomatic nature of the disease until its late stages and the lack of awareness of risk among migrants and often also among health care providers limit early detection. Other barriers to screening include language, health care access and entitlement issues, high work-load among health care staff, and the potential stigma or fear associated with being diagnosed positive [26, 27]. The EU-funded HEPscreen project describes four different screening approaches: (i) outreach screening (e.g. through awareness raising and screening sessions in communities or workplaces); (ii) extension of existing screening programmes (e.g. expanding tuberculosis screening to include other diseases); (iii) opportunistic screening (e.g. offering viral hepatitis screening when patients attend for other health care services); and (iv) invitation-based screening (e.g. using municipal or general practice registers). Summaries of screening studies conducted using these different methods, practical guides on how to implement different screening approaches among migrants and resource and logistical considerations are available on the website http://www.hepscreen.eu/ and present a useful resource for public health practitioners [28].

Undocumented migrants are also an important and vulnerable group. Lack of robust demographic data and the diversity in size and country of birth of undocumented migrants [29] hinder effective planning, resourcing and evaluation of screening interventions for this population. In addition, undocumented migrants face specific access and entitlement challenges when accessing public health services. Promoting voluntary screening for this vulnerable group would have public health benefits, but would require national policies that allow undocumented migrants to receive treatment without adverse consequences.

The systematic approach to estimation of the burden of CHB among migrant populations in the EU/EEA overall and in each of the 31 EU/EEA countries is a strength of this study. The data that underpin these estimates are derived from a common demographic data source (Eurostat 2013) for most countries and from published meta-analytic studies. A potential limitation is that, for some countries, demographic data from earlier years and other sources had to be used. In addition, there are differences in population registration and reporting systems between EU/EEA countries. However, using data from 2013 or earlier has the advantage of limiting the effect of reporting delays with respect to accurate numbers of migrants and their countries of birth.

Using country of birth prevalence data to estimate the CHB burden among migrants may have resulted in a degree of over-estimation for some countries, because of differences in the age structure, risk profile and socio-economic status between different migrant groups. Migrants sharing the same country of birth but residing in different EU/EEA countries may also differ in terms of risk profile as a result of differences in host country pull factors and reasons for migration. Data allowing a comparison of prevalence figures between the general population in the migrants' countries of birth and from studies among migrants in Europe were however only available for 14 countries. An additional strength of this study is that, even if the absolute number of estimated CHB cases lies closer to the lower estimate, it identifies which migrant populations would benefit most from targeted screening programs and linkage to care.

Conclusions

Today, anti-viral treatments for CHB can benefit most patients, offering the prospect of significant public health gains through secondary prevention. Expanded access to screening, linkage to care and treatment, together with the continued implementation of existing primary prevention measures such as vaccinaiton and antenatal screening, are the cornerstones of eliminating viral hepatitis as a global public health threat in the next few decades.

This study confirms that migrant populations are a key risk group for CHB in specific EU/EEA countries. It details the number of CHB cases among migrants by country of birth in each EU/EEA country, identifies the migrant populations that would benefit most from screening and treatment, and highlights which EU/EEA countries would benefit from a migrant-targeted screening approach. The findings in this study about which migrant groups are at highest risk is also useful for developing linguistically-specific and culturally-sensitive screening programmes and raising awareness among physicians so that they offer screening. Efficient and innovative public health approaches to increase access to screening and to screen high-risk populations are needed. Experience from a migrant-specific screening project conducted at the EU/EEA level [28] can help to inform the design of screening programmes that can successfully reach migrant communities. Planners and practitioners can also use the results presented here and those from the HEPscreen project to develop evidence-based screening interventions that target the most affected migrant populations.

Further research is required to inform the development and assessment of effective and cost-effective screening interventions and long-term patient follow up, as well as to improve linkage to and retention in treatment and care among hard to reach risk populations, if we are to realise the vision of a world free of viral hepatitis.

Additional file

Additional file 1: Estimating the scale of chronic hepatitis B virus infection among migrants in EU/EEA countries. The 'Chronic Hepatitis B (CHB) Additional file 1' includes 9 annexes. Annexs 1, 2, 5 and 7 present data on the search strategy, the PRISMA flow chart, the inclusion and exclusion criteria of global/worldwide systematic reviews and meta-analyses and the rationale for the selected country specific hepatitis B and C prevalence figures. (ii) Annexs 3, 4 and 6 present data on the search strategy, the PRISMA flow chart and the inclusion and exclusion criteria for chronic hepatitis B/C prevalence studies among migrants in the EU/EEA. (iii) Annex 8 presents a list of the country specific HBsAg prevalence estimates selected along with the corresponding source. (iv) Annex 9 presents country tables which list the estimated number of Chronic Hepatitis B (CHB) cases among the 50 largest migrant populations residing in the individual EU/EEA host countries. (DOCX 487 kb)

Abbreviations

CHB: Chronic hepatitis B; CI: Confidence intervals; EU/EEA: European Union and European Economic Area; HBsAg: Hepatitis B surface antigen; HBV: Hepatitis B virus; HCC: Hepatocellular carcinoma; Migrants: Foreign-born population; OECD: Organisation for Economic Co-operation and Development; PRISMA: Preferred Reporting Items for Systematic Reviews and Meta Analyses; UK: United Kingdom; WHO: World Health Organisation

Acknowledgements

This study was funded by the European Centre for Disease Prevention and Control (ECDC). We would like to thank Wichor Bramer (librarian Erasmus MC) for assistance with the systematic literature search. We also acknowledge the assistance of Annika Krueger (masters student, Hamburg University of Applied Sciences) in the demographic data collection process. Jelle Koopson (RIVM), Daan Nieboer (Statistician, Department of Public Health, Erasmus MC) and Dr. Luc Coffeng (Assistant Professor, Department of Public Health, Erasmus MC) for statistical advice regarding the comparison of in-country with migrant derived prevalence estimates. Dr. Jan van de Kassteele (Statistician, RIVM) for assistance with the Delta method to derive the relative contribution range.

Funding

This study was funded by the European Centre for Disease Prevention and Control (ECDC) under contract number ECD.4999.

Availability of data and materials

Data generated or analysed during this study are included in this published article and in an extensive Additional file 1to this manuscript. The Additional file 1 includes: (i) Annexs 1, 2, 5 and 7 which describe the search strategy, the PRISMA flow chart, the inclusion and exclusion criteria for selection of global/worldwide systematic reviews and meta-analyses and the rationale for the selected country specific hepatitis B and C prevalence figures. (ii) Annexs 3, 4 and 6 which provide information on the search strategy, the PRISMA flow chart and the inclusion and exclusion criteria for chronic hepatitis B/C prevalence studies among migrants in the EU/EEA. (iii) Annex 8 which presents a list of the country specific HBsAg prevalence estimates selected along with the corresponding source. (iv) Annex 9 includes 31 EU/EEA country tables each including a list of the estimated number of Chronic Hepatitis B cases among the 50 largest migrant populations residing in the individual EU/EEA host countries. Other datasets used and/or analysed during the current study are available from the corresponding author on reasonable request.

Authors' contributions

AAA: study concept and design, literature search, acquisition of data, analysis and interpretation of data, drafting of the manuscript. AMF: study concept and design, literature search, acquisition of data, analysis and interpretation of data, critical revision of the manuscript for important intellectual content. ED: study concept and design, interpretation of data, critical revision of the manuscript for important intellectual content, supervised the study, obtained funding. TN: study concept and design, interpretation of data, critical revision of the manuscript for important intellectual content, supervised the study, obtained funding. AB: interpretation of data, critical revision of the manuscript for important intellectual content. RR: interpretation of data, critical revision of the manuscript for important intellectual content. IKV: study concept and design, literature search, analysis and interpretation of data, critical revision of the manuscript for important intellectual content, supervised the study.
All authors read and approved the final manuscript.

Consent for publication

Not applicable.

Competing interests

None of the authors have any competing interests to declare.

Author details

[1]Faculty Life Sciences, Department of Health Sciences, Hamburg University of Applied Sciences, Ulmenliet 20, 21033 Hamburg, Germany. [2]Department of Internal Medicine, University Medical Center Hamburg-Eppendorf, Martinistr. 52, 20246 Hamburg, Germany. [3]Department of Public Health, Erasmus MC, University Medical Center Rotterdam, Wytemaweg 80, 3015 Rotterdam, CN, Netherlands. [4]Division of Infectious Disease Control, Municipal Public Health Service Rotterdam-Rijnmond, Schiedamsedijk 95, 3011 Rotterdam, EN, Netherlands. [5]European Centre for Disease Prevention and Control, Granits väg 8, 171 65 Solna, Stockholm, Sweden. [6]Department of Health Sciences, University of Florence, Viale G.B. Morgagni, 48, 50134 Florence, Italy. [7]Center for Infectious Disease Control, National Institute for Public Health and the Environment, Antonie van Leeuwenhoeklaan 9, 3721 Bilthoven, MA, Netherlands.

References

1. Rica S, Glitz A and Ortega F. Immigration in Europe: trends, policies and empirical evidence. Discussion paper series, IZA discussion paper no. 7778. Institute for the Study of labor, 2013. Available from: http://ftp.iza.org/dp7778.pdf
2. Sharma S, Carballo M, Feld JJ, Janssen HL. Immigration and viral hepatitis. J Hepatol. 2015; Epub 2015/05/13
3. Niederau C. Chronic hepatitis B in 2014: great therapeutic progress, large diagnostic deficit. World Journal of Gastroenterology : WJG. 2014;20(33): 11595–617.
4. European Centre for Disease Prevention and Control. Hepatitis B and C surveillance in Europe. Stockholm: ECDC; 2012. p. 2014. Available from: https://ecdc.europa.eu/sites/portal/files/media/en/publications/Publications/hepatitis-b-c-surveillance-europe-2012-july-2014.pdf
5. World Health Organisation. Hepatitis B fact sheet no. 204, 2015. Available from: http://www.who.int/mediacentre/factsheets/fs204/en/index.html
6. Ott JJ, Stevens GA, Groeger J, Wiersma ST. Global epidemiology of hepatitis B virus infection: new estimates of age-specific HBsAg seroprevalence and endemicity. Vaccine. 2012;30(12):2212–9.
7. Franco E, Bagnato B, Marino MG, Meleleo C, Serino L, Zaratti L, Hepatitis B. Epidemiology and prevention in developing countries. World J Hepatol. 2012;4(3):74–80.
8. Stanaway JD, Flaxman AD, Naghavi M, Fitzmaurice C, Vos T, Abubakar I, et al. The global burden of viral hepatitis from 1990 to 2013: findings from the global burden of disease study 2013. Lancet. 2016;388(10049):1081–8.
9. Hope VD, Eramova I, Capurro D, Donoghoe MC. Prevalence and estimation of hepatitis B and C infections in the WHO European region: a review of data focusing on the countries outside the European Union and the European free trade association. Epidemiol Infect. 2014;142(2):270–86.
10. Hatzakis A, Wait S, Bruix J, et al. The state of hepatitis B and C in Europe: report from the hepatitis B and C summit conference. J Viral Hepat. 2011;18:1–16.
11. Hahne SJM, Veldhuijzen IK, Wiessing L, Lim TA, Salminen M, Laar MVD. Infection with hepatitis B and C virus in Europe: a systematic review of prevalence and cost-effectiveness of screening. BMC Infect Dis. 2013;13(1):181.
12. World Health Organisation (WHO) (2016). Action plan for the health sector response to viral hepatitis in the WHO European region.
13. World Health Organisation (WHO) (2016). Global Health sector strategy on viral hepatitis 2016–2021: towards ending viral hepatitis.
14. Falla AM, Ahmad AA, Duffell E, Noori T and Veldhuijzen IK. Estimating the scale of chronic hepatitis C virus infection in the EU/EEA: a focus on migrants from anti-HCV endemic countries. BMC Infect Dis. 2018. https://doi.org/10.1186/s12879-017-2908-5.
15. Eurostat. Immigration by five-year age group, sex and country of birth [migr_imm3ctb]. 2013 [cited 2015]; Available from: http://appsso.eurostat.ec.europa.eu/nui/show.do?dataset=migr_imm3ctb&lang=en.
16. European Statistical System. EU 2011 - housing and Polulation census. 2011; Available from: https://ec.europa.eu/CensusHub2/.

17. Organisation for Economic Cooperation and Development (OECD). International migration database. 2013; Available from: http://stats.oecd.org/Index.aspx?DatasetCode=MIG
18. Lithuanian National Statistics Service. International migration flows. 2013; Available from: http://osp.stat.gov.lt/en/temines-lenteles1
19. Casella, G. and R.L. Berger, Statistical inference 2002.
20. Kowdley KV, Wang CC, Welch S, Roberts H, Brosgart CL. Prevalence of chronic hepatitis B among foreign-born persons living in the United States by country of origin. Hepatology. 2012;56(2):422–33.
21. Ioannou GN. Hepatitis B virus in the United States: infection, exposure, and immunity rates in a nationally representative survey. Ann Intern Med. 2011; 154(5):319–28. Epub 2011/03/02
22. Ezzikouri S, Pineau P, Benjelloun S. Hepatitis B virus in the Maghreb region: from epidemiology to prospective research. Liver Int. 2013;33(6):811–9.
23. O'Flanagan D, Cotter S, Mereckiene J. Hepatitis B vaccination in Europe. The Health Protection Surveillance Centre European Centre for disease Control VENICE II project. 2009; Available from: http://venice.cineca.org/Report_Hepatitis_B_Vaccination.pdf
24. Rechel B, Mladovsky P, Ingleby D, Mackenbach JP, McKee M. Migration and health in an increasingly diverse Europe. Lancet. 2013;381(9873):1235–45. Epub 2013/04/02
25. Rossi C, Schwartzman K, Oxlade O, Klein MB, Greenaway C. Hepatitis B screening and vaccination strategies for newly arrived adult Canadian immigrants and refugees: a cost-effectiveness analysis. PLoS One. 2013;8(10):e78548.
26. Evlampidou I, Hickman M, Irish C, Young N, Oliver I, Gillett S, Cochrane A. Low hepatitis B testing among migrants: a cross-sectional study in a UK city. Br J Gen Pract. 2016;66(647):e382–91.
27. Lutgehetmann M, Meyer F, Volz T, Lohse AW, Fischer C, Dandri M, Petersen J. Knowledge about HBV, prevention behaviour and treatment adherence of patients with chronic hepatitis B in a large referral centre in Germany. Z Gastroenterol. 2010;48(9):1126–32.
28. The HEPscreen Project. 2015; Available from: www.hepscreen.eu
29. Clandestino – Database on irregular migration. http://irregular-migration.net/
30. Richter C, Ter Beest G, Gisolf EH, Van Bentum P, Waegemaekers C, Swanink C, et al. Screening for chronic hepatitis B and C in migrants from Afghanistan, Iran, Iraq, the former soviet republics, and Vietnam in the Arnhem region, the Netherlands. Epidemiol Infect. 2014;142(10):2140–6.
31. Milionis C. Serological markers of hepatitis B and C among juvenile immigrants from Albania settled in Greece. Eur J Gen Pract. 2010;16(4):236–40.
32. Uddin G, Shoeb D, Solaiman S, Marley R, Gore C, Ramsay M, et al. Prevalence of chronic viral hepatitis in people of south Asian ethnicity living in England: the prevalence cannot necessarily be predicted from the prevalence in the country of origin. J Viral Hepatitis. 2010;17(5):327–35.
33. McPherson S, Valappil M, Moses SE, Eltringham G, Miller C, Baxter K, et al. Targeted case finding for hepatitis B using dry blood spot testing in the British-Chinese and south Asian populations of the north-east of England. J Viral Hepatitis. 2013;20(9):638–44.
34. Veldhuijzen IK, Wolter R, Rijckborst V, Mostert M, Voeten HA, Cheung Y, et al. Identification and treatment of chronic hepatitis B in Chinese migrants: results of a project offering on-site testing in Rotterdam, the Netherlands. J Hepatol. 2012;57(6):1171–6.
35. Veldhuijzen IK, van Driel HF, Vos D, de Zwart O, van Doornum GJJ, de Man RA, et al. Viral hepatitis in a multi-ethnic neighborhood in the Netherlands: results of a community-based study in a low prevalence country. Int J Infect Dis. 2009;13(1):e9–e13.
36. Zuure FR, Bouman J, Martens M, Vanhommerig JW, Urbanus AT, Davidovich U, et al. Screening for hepatitis B and C in first-generation Egyptian migrants living in the Netherlands. Liver Int. 2013;33(5):727–38.
37. Zacharakis G, Kotsiou S, Papoutselis M, Vafiadis N, Tzara F, Pouliou E, et al. Changes in the epidemiology of hepatitis B virus infection following the implementation of immunisation programmes in northeastern Greece. Euro Surveill. 2009;14(32):1–6.
38. O'Leary MC, Sarwar M, Hutchinson SJ, Weir A, Schofield J, McLeod A, et al. The prevalence of hepatitis C virus among people of south Asian origin in Glasgow - results from a community based survey and laboratory surveillance. Travel Med Infect Dis. 2013;11(5):301–9.
39. Baaten GG, Sonder GJ, Dukers NH, Coutinho RA, Van den Hoek JA. Population-based study on the seroprevalence of hepatitis a, B, and C virus infection in Amsterdam, 2004. J Med Virol. 2007;79(12):1802–10. Epub 2007/10/16
40. Bjerke SEY, Holter E, Vangen S, Stray-Pedersen B. Sexually transmitted infections among Pakistani pregnant women and their husbands in Norway. Int J Womens Health. 2010;2:303–9.

16

Hepatitis a virus genotypes and strains from an endemic area of Europe, Bulgaria 2012–2014

Roberto Bruni[1*], Stefania Taffon[1], Michele Equestre[2], Eleonora Cella[3], Alessandra Lo Presti[3], Angela Costantino[1], Paola Chionne[1], Elisabetta Madonna[1], Elitsa Golkocheva-Markova[4], Diljana Bankova[4], Massimo Ciccozzi[3], Pavel Teoharov[4] and Anna Rita Ciccaglione[1]

Abstract

Background: Hepatitis A virus (HAV) infection is endemic in Eastern European and Balkan region countries. In 2012, Bulgaria showed the highest rate (67.13 cases per 100,000) in Europe. Nevertheless, HAV genotypes and strains circulating in this country have never been described. The present study reports the molecular characterization of HAV from 105 patients from Bulgaria.

Methods: Anti-HAV IgM positive serum samples collected in 2012–2014 from different towns and villages in Bulgaria were analysed by nested RT-PCR, sequencing of the VP1/2A region and phylogenetic analysis; the results were analysed together with patient and geographical data.

Results: Phylogenetic analysis revealed two main sequence groups corresponding to the IA (78/105, 74%) and IB (27/105, 26%) sub-genotypes.

In the IA group, a major and a minor cluster were observed (62 and 16 sequences, respectively). Most sequences from the major cluster (44/62, 71%) belonged to either of two strains, termed "strain 1" and "strain 2", differing only for a single specific nucleotide; the remaining sequences (18/62, 29%) showed few (1 to 4) nucleotide variations respect to strain 1 and 2. Strain 2 is identical to the strain previously responsible for an outbreak in the Czech Republic in 2008 and a large multi-country European outbreak caused by contaminated mixed frozen berries in 2013.

Most sequences of the IA minor cluster and the IB group were detected in large/medium centers (LMCs). Overall, sequences from the IA major cluster were more frequent in small centers (SCs), but strain 1 and strain 2 showed an opposite relative frequency in SCs and LMCs (strain 1 more frequent in SCs, strain 2 in LMCs).

Conclusions: Genotype IA predominated in Bulgaria in 2012–2014 and phylogenetic analysis identified a major cluster of highly related or identical IA sequences, representing 59% of the analysed cases; these isolates were mostly detected in SCs, in which HAV shows higher endemicity than in LMCs. The distribution of viral sequences suggests the existence of some differences between the transmission routes in SCs and LMCs.

Molecular characterization of an increased number of isolates from Bulgaria, regularly collected over time, will be useful to explore specific transmission routes and plan appropriate preventing measures.

Keywords: Hepatitis a virus, HAV, Hepatitis, Phylogenetic analysis, Sequencing, Bulgaria

* Correspondence: roberto.bruni@iss.it
[1]National Reference Laboratory for HAV, Viral Hepatitis Unit, Department of Infectious Diseases, Istituto Superiore di Sanità, Rome, Italy
Full list of author information is available at the end of the article

Background

Hepatitis A virus (HAV) is one of the major causes of acute hepatitis throughout the world and causes substantial morbidity in both developed and developing countries [1, 2]. On the basis of genome sequence divergence, all viruses infecting humans have been classified in three genotypes (I, II, III), further divided into two sub-genotypes (A and B). Genotypes and subtypes tend to show different geographic distribution [3].

HAV is mainly transmitted by the faecal-oral route. HAV can survive for long in water and numerous waterborne epidemics have been observed following consumption of contaminated drinking water [4], food produce [5, 6], or shellfish [7].

The infection is usually asymptomatic or mild in children under five years, while in adults more frequently occurs with symptoms and jaundice. Clearance of infection confers lifelong immunity. In high endemicity countries, HAV infection is acquired in early childhood and most adult population is positive for anti-HAV IgG and protected from re-infection. In contrast, in low endemicity countries most adult population is susceptible: as a result, infections are more likely to occur in adults, in which are frequently symptomatic [8].

In Europe, the epidemiology of the HAV infection is characterized by countries with variable endemicity. In 2012, the European Centre for Disease Prevention and Control (ECDC) reported a mean rate of infection in Europe of 2.6 cases per 100,000 inhabitants (13,156 total confirmed cases). The majority of them were from an endemic area which included Eastern European and Balkan region countries [9]. Among them, Bulgaria is a country with intermediate hepatitis A endemicity, with annual incidence between 25 and 94 cases per 100,000 population (data since 2000). In 2011 and 2012 the cases increased to 75.88/100,000 (5588 cases) and 67.13/100,000 (4919 cases), respectively, then decreased to 25.05/100,000 in 2013 (1825 cases) [10].

In 2011–2013, the most affected population group was children aged 5–9 years, followed by the 10–14 years and 1–4 years age groups, which are the main risk groups for the disease in Bulgaria in general. During this time, 28 outbreaks of hepatitis A were detected in different Bulgarian districts, affecting dominantly minority Roma neighbourhoods [9, 10]. The prevalence of anti-HAV antibodies in general population in Bulgaria is poorly known. The only available data were from a small study carried out in Plovdiv, the second largest town in Bulgaria, in which two quarters with very different hygienic and sanitary conditions were sampled [11]. The mean seroprevalence was 68.3%, but it reached 90.2% in the quarter with poor hygienic and sanitary conditions and 44.8% in the other with normal conditions [11]. Vaccination in Bulgaria is recommended for people at risk [12]; however, targeted immunization campaigns are launched in response to outbreaks, such as in 2006 [13].

Molecular analysis of HAV isolates has proved to be crucial for understanding the demographic, social and environmental factors that have given rise to the current epidemiological patterns in Europe. Several studies described circulation of different HAV genotypes from both autochthonous and travel-related cases [14–21]. Nevertheless, HAV strains from Bulgaria and other European endemic countries have never been described. This gap delays the comprehension of the local transmission routes and the implementation of control measures in areas that urgently need them.

In the present study, serum samples from 105 patients with acute hepatitis A, collected in different towns and villages in Bulgaria during 2012–2014, were analysed by nested RT-PCR and sequencing to characterize HAV isolates. Phylogenetic analysis of sequences was performed to describe, for the first time, HAV genotypes and strains circulating in Bulgaria.

Methods

Patients

The Department of Virology of the National Center of Infectious and Parasitic Diseases in Bulgaria receives serum samples from patients with acute hepatitis (according to the clinical definition by World Health Organization (WHO) [22]) from all over the country for laboratory testing. One hundred and five anti-HAV IgM positive sera from cases occurred during 2012–2014 in several towns/villages, mostly in West Bulgaria, had been randomly stored and were available for the present study. Anti-HAV IgM antibodies had been detected by the HAV IgM ELISA kit (Dia.Pro, Diagnostic BioProbes s.r.l., Italy). All the 105 cases were classified as confirmed HAV infections on the basis of specific IgM antibody detection according to the recommended case definition by WHO [22]. Among them, 91.4% were Bulgarian, 51.4% were males, the mean age of the patients was 21 years, ranging from 2 to 78. HAV characterization by nested RT-PCR and sequencing was carried out in Italy at the National Reference Laboratory for Hepatitis Viruses - Istituto Superiore di Sanità (NRL-ISS) (see next paragraph). Informed consent for participation in the study had been obtained before patient discharge. The study was approved by the Ethics Committee at the National Center of Infectious and Parasitic Diseases, Sofia, Bulgaria.

Nested RT-PCR and sequencing

Viral RNA was extracted from 140 μL serum by using the QIAmp viral RNA extraction kit (Qiagen, Hilden, Germany). One sixth extracted RNA (10 μL) was reverse transcribed by the SuperScript III First-Strand Synthesis System for RT-PCR (Invitrogen) with random hexamers.

Nested PCR was carried out as previously reported [14, 15]. To control for possible PCR contamination, negative control sera were included in each run: they were extracted, reverse transcribed and amplified by nested PCR along with the sera under study. Double strand sequencing of purified PCR products obtained from human sera was carried out by using the GenomeLab Dye Terminator Cycle Sequencing (DTCS) Quick Start Kit and an automated DNA sequencer (both kit and instrument by Beckman Coulter, Inc., Fullerton, CA). The sequencing reaction was carried out according to the manufacturer instructions. In brief, 20–40 ng purified DNA was used as template with 3.2 pmoles of primer and DTCS Quick Start Master Mix, in a 20 μL final volume. The reaction was subjected to 30 cycles of: 96 °C, 20 s; 50 °C, 20 s; 60 °C, 4 min.

The sequenced region encompassed the VP1/2A region of HAV genome (460 nt, positions 2915 to 3374 in the HM-175 reference sequence Acc.No. NC_001489).

Sequence analysis

Genotype was assigned by phylogenetic analysis of a dataset containing 105 HAV sequences from Bulgaria [GenBank:KX858970 to KX859074] plus 13 HAV reference sequences representative of genotypes and sub-genotypes (sub-genotype IA [GenBank:EF406357; KC182590; X75215; X83302], sub-genotype IB [GenBank:AF314208; M20273; NC001489; AF268396], sub-genotype IIA [GenBank:AY644676], sub-genotype IIB [GenBank:AY644670], sub-genotype IIIA [GenBank:AJ299464; KF706410], sub-genotype IIIB [GenBank:AB258387]).

Phylogenetic relationships were analysed by constructing a Neighbor-Joining phylogenetic tree by MEGA 6.0 [23]. The best substitution model (T92 + G) was selected by analysis of sequences with the Models tool in MEGA. Tree reliability was assessed by setting bootstrap replicates to 1000. Bootstrap values >70 were considered significant.

Mean intra-group identity level was calculated from the output identity matrix obtained by the Sequence Identity Matrix function in BioEdit 7.2.5 [24].

Results

Distribution of patients according to age and size of urban centers

According to official data of 2011 census, urban centers were classified in large to medium centers (LMCs) (>30,000 inhabitants, range 44,000–1,203,000) and small centers (SCs) (<30,000 inhabitants, range 132–27,000). One hundred and five patients with acute HAV infection were evaluated in the study. Among them, 46 (43.8%) were from large to medium centers (LMCs) and 50 47.6%) from small centers (SCs). Nine subjects (8.6%), of unknown nationality, were from a refugee camp in Bulgaria. The age was known for 102 patients and their classification into three age categories (Children: 0–12; Teens: >12 to 19; Adults: >19) indicated that 48 (47.1%) were children, 13 (12.7%) teens and 41 (40.2%) adults.

Distribution of hepatitis A cases according to the size of urban centers revealed an opposite age distribution pattern in LMCs and SCs (Fig. 1). The percentages of children and adults were 33.3% and 53.3%, respectively, in patients from LMCs, while they were 54.0% and 32.0% in patients from SCs ($p < 0.05$, Fisher's exact test). The percentage of teens was similar in the two groups.

Genotyping of HAV strains

Phylogenetic analysis of the 105 HAV isolates from Bulgaria and reference sequences with known genotype revealed two main groups corresponding to the IA ($n = 78$) and IB ($n = 27$) sub-genotypes (Fig. 2). No genotype II or III isolates were observed.

In the IA group two main statistically supported clusters can be observed (Fig. 2, labelled as "MAJOR cluster" and "minor cluster"). The major cluster included sequences ($n = 62$, 79.5% of IA isolates) showing a very high intra-cluster identity level (mean value 99.6%, range 98%–100%).

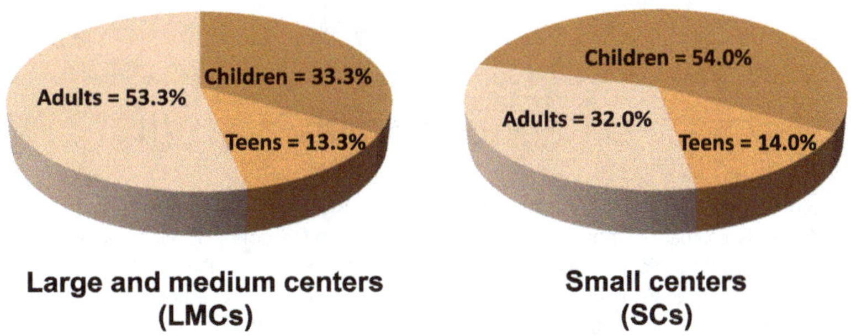

Fig. 1 Distribution of molecularly characterized hepatitis A cases according to age categories and size of urban centers. The distribution in three age groups (Children: 0–12 years; Teens: >12 to 19 years; Adults: > 19 years) according to the size of urban centers (Large and medium centers: >30,000 inhabitants, range 44,000–1,203,000; Small centers: <30,000 inhabitants, range 132–27,000) is reported

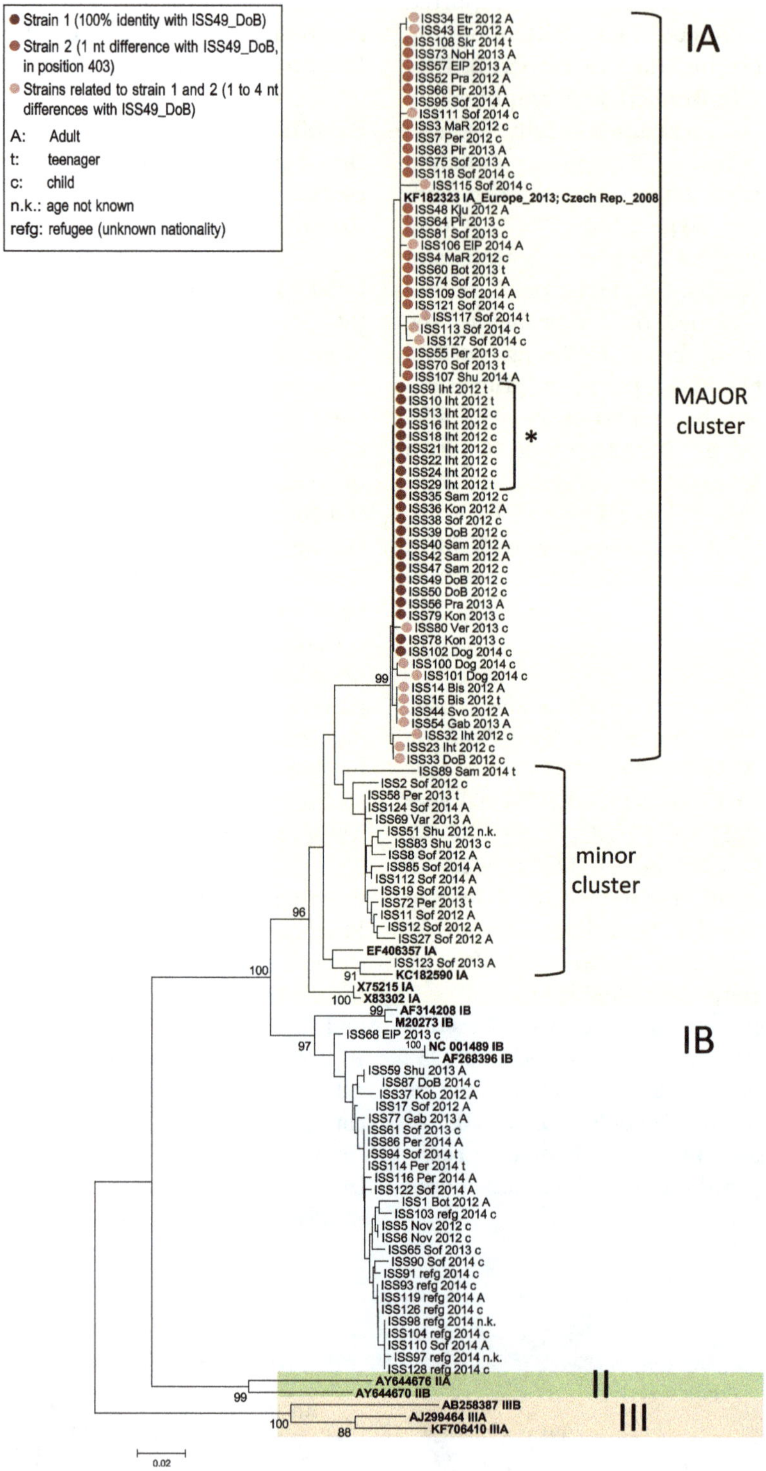

Fig. 2 Neighbour-Joining phylogenetic tree (Substitution model: T92 + G) of the 105 HAV isolates from Bulgaria. For each sequence, the town/village (Bis: Bistritsa; Bot: Botevgrad; DoB: Dolna Banja; Dog: Doganovo; ElP: Elin Pelin; Etr: Etropole; Gab: Gabrovo; Iht: Ihtiman; Kju: Kjustendil; Kob: Kostinbrod; Kon: Kostenets; MaR: Manaselska Reka; NoH: Novi Han; Nov: Novachene; Per: Pernik; Pir: Pirdop; Pra: Pravetz; Sam: Samokov; Shu: Shumen; Skr: Skravena; Sof: Sofia; Svo: Svoge; Var: Varna; Ver: Verinsko; refg: refugee, village information not available), the isolation year (2012, 2013, 2014) and the age group of the patient (A: Adult; t: teenager; c: child; n.k.: not known) are reported after the sequence ID. Reference strains with known genotype (IA, IB, IIA, IIB, IIIA, IIIB) were included in the analysis and are reported (in bold) by Accession number followed by the sub-genotype they belong to. Significant bootstrap values are reported. The asterisk shows a small outbreak of 9 cases from Ihtiman occurred between 25 June and 8 August 2012 and involving 6 children and 3 teenagers: the complete nucleotide identity of the isolates confirms a local small outbreak caused by the same strain

The minor cluster contained IA sequences (n = 16, 20.5% of IA isolates) characterized by a lower intra-cluster identity level (mean value 98.1%, range 93.7%–100%).

In the IB group, the 27 sequences showed a high identity level (mean value 99.1%, range 98%–100%). Among the IB isolates from 9 patients living in a refugee camp in Bulgaria, 2 small clusters (each containing 3 isolates) of identical sequences were observed. Although the sequences from refugees showed a tendency to cluster separately from the other IB isolates, bootstrap values were not significant: sequences from refugees showed high identity (1 to 4 nt differences) with several sequences from Bulgarian patients circulating in the same (2014) and in the previous years (2012 and 2013) suggesting that refugees got infected with local strains.

To include in the phylogenetic analysis also the proposed sub-genotype IC [17], a separate analysis limited to a shorter region (261 nt) had to be carried out; in fact the available reference IC sequences only partially overlapped with the region sequenced in the present study. IC isolates formed a separate cluster, intermediate between IA and IB; however, none of the Bulgarian isolates grouped with them (data not shown).

Nucleotide variations in strains from the IA major cluster

To better compare HAV isolates from the IA major cluster, one of them, the ISS49_DoB, was chosen as reference sequence. Based on this, the 62 isolates from the major cluster were classified into three groups as follows (see also Fig. 2): (1) "strain 1" group, including 22 (35.5%) sequences (21 sequences showing 100% identity with ISS49_DoB plus the reference sequence itself); (2) "strain 2" group, including 22 (35.5%) sequences presenting only 1 nucleotide (nt) difference with ISS49_DoB, with all isolates showing the same nt difference in the same position (nt 403, C → T, numeration of [GenBank:KF182323]); strain 2 is identical to a strain (reference sequence [GenBank:KF182323] in Fig. 2) previously reported to be responsible for both an outbreak in the Czech Republic in 2008 and a large European outbreak caused by mixed frozen berries in 2013 [15]; (3) "strains related to strain 1 and 2" group, including 18 (29%) sequences showing 1 to 4 nucleotide differences versus ISS49_DoB (individual nucleotide variations were scattered in different positions) (Fig. 2, see the box). Overall, strain 1 and strain 2 represent 44/62 (71%) isolates of the major cluster; 12 distinct variants could be recognised in the remaining 18/62 (29%) isolates of this cluster.

By linking epidemiological and sequence data, a small outbreak of 9 cases could be clearly identified in the major cluster. All cases were from Ihtiman village and occurred between 25 June and 8 August 2012, involving 6 children and 3 teenagers: the complete identity of the isolates confirms a local small outbreak caused by the strain 1 during a period of two months (Fig. 2, MAJOR cluster, labelled by the asterisk).

Distribution of HAV genotypes and strains in urban centers of different size

Distribution of HAV genotypes according to the size of the town/village of patients showed that the percentages of isolates belonging to IA major cluster, IA minor cluster and IB group were 42.2%, 31.1% and 26.7%, respectively, in patients from LMCs and 86.0%, 2.0% and 12.0% in patients from SCs (Fig. 3a). Most isolates from the IA major cluster (43/62, 69.4%) were identified in patients from SCs. In contrast, all but one strains from the IA minor cluster were observed in patients from LMCs, suggesting that different transmission routes, linked to urbanization, operate in these cases. Among the IB subgenotype, isolates were identified in both LMCs and SCs, however the frequency was higher in patients from LMCs (26.7% in LMCs vs 12% in SCs) (Fig. 3a). Analysis of the 62 isolates from the IA major cluster revealed a different frequency of strain 1 and strain 2 in LMCs and SCs (Fig. 3b): strain 1 largely prevailed in SCs (5.3% in LMCs vs. 48.8% in SCs), strain 2 prevailed in LMCs (63.1% in LMCs vs. 23.3% in SCs) (p < 0.001, Fisher's exact test); in contrast, the strains related to strain 1 and 2 showed similar frequency (31.6% vs. 27.9%).

Analysis of the geographical localization of the strains in Bulgaria map showed that strain 1 was preferentially detected in a restricted area south-east of Sofia, strain 2 and strains related to strain 1 and 2 showed a more scattered distribution, whereas most strains from the IA minor cluster and IB strains were observed in large towns such as Sofia, Pernik, Shumen, Gabrovo and Varna (Fig. 4).

Discussion

The ECDC surveillance report of food- and waterborne diseases, published in 2014, defined Bulgaria as the European country that reported the highest number of hepatitis A cases in 2011 (5587 cases) and 2012 (4919 cases). Investigation of a large outbreak in Bulgaria, occurred in 2012 in the Iskra village in the Plovdiv region, indicated that unregulated and/or frequently failing water supply and sewage system are associated with virus spread in this area [9]. Despite the level of endemicity, molecular epidemiology of HAV in Bulgaria has never been described. Thus, the studied samples represent an extremely rare resource, if not unique, to obtain information on HAV strains that have circulated and might still be circulating in an Eastern Europe country. The results of the present study represent the first analysis of the HAV genotypes and strains circulating in Bulgaria.

Analysis of the age distribution showed that patients were younger in SCs than in LMCs, suggesting different endemicity among these areas. In SCs, high HAV

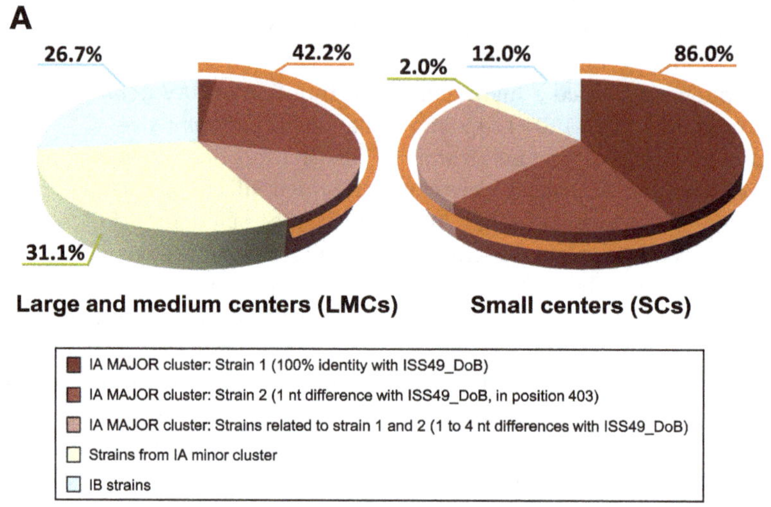

B

	LMCs		SCs	
	cases	%	cases	%
Strain 1 (n = 22 cases)	1	5.3%	21	48.8%
Strain 2 (n = 22 cases)	12	63.1%	10	23.3%
Strains related to Strain 1 and 2 (n = 18 cases)	6	31.6%	12	27.9%

Fig. 3 Distribution of strains according to the size of urban centers. **a** Distribution of the strains from the IA Major cluster, IA minor cluster and IB cluster according to the size of urban centers (see the legend of Fig. 1). The percent values are shown. **b** Detail of the number of cases and relative frequency of the strains from the IA Major cluster (strain 1, strain 2 and strains related to strain 1 and 2) in LMCs and SCs

endemicity results in a large proportion of adults protected by antibodies developed in childhood and, thus, HAV circulation mainly in children. High endemicity in SCs is likely related to poor hygienic conditions and health education of the population, as suggested by a study investigating an outbreak occurred in 2012 in a SC (Iskra village) [25].

Molecular characterization of HAV from 105 acute hepatitis A cases, collected between 2012 and 2014, indicated that both IA and IB sub-genotypes circulate in Bulgaria; however, about 74% of the isolates were assigned to sub-genotype IA that, thus, seems to be dominant.

Interestingly, IA strains grouped in two distinct phylogenetic clusters. The major cluster, that included 79.5% of the IA cases and 59% of the total cases, contained highly related viruses. Sequence analysis indicated that isolates were either identical (at least over the analysed genomic region), as observed in strain 1 or strain 2 groups, or showed very few (1 to 4) nucleotide variations. Strain 1 and strain 2 groups differed each other for a single specific nucleotide, that was T in strain 1 and C in strain 2. The very low level of variability observed in the IA major cluster might be the result of a common origin of the two main strains and of their spread in the local population, with random generation of new variants, highly related to the main strains, in the course of endemic and epidemic circulation.

The distribution of strains according to urban size (Fig. 3b) and the geographical localization of the involved urban centers (Fig. 4) indicate that strain 1 preferentially circulated in small urban centers and villages south-east of Sofia, where transmission was likely maintained by poor water supply and lack of infrastructures. Although the relative frequency of strain 2 was higher in LMCs than in SCs (Fig. 3b), strain 2 showed wider geographical distribution than strain 1 (Fig. 4) and it was detected both in large urban centers, such as Sofia, Pernik and Shumen, and in small villages.

A completely different pattern of circulation was observed for isolates from the IA minor cluster and from the IB cluster. In fact, all but one patients infected with strains from the IA minor cluster and two thirds of cases infected with IB strains were from LMCs (Fig. 3a), suggesting that different transmission routes, linked to urbanization, might operate in these cases (e.g. consumption of shellfish or other food, contaminated in the same or other countries).

Assuming the distribution of HAV genotypes and strains reported in the present study roughly represents isolates circulating in Bulgaria in 2012–2014, it is conceivable that the IA strains from the IA major cluster, accounting for 59% of sequenced cases, were responsible for the epidemic peak observed in Bulgaria in 2011 and

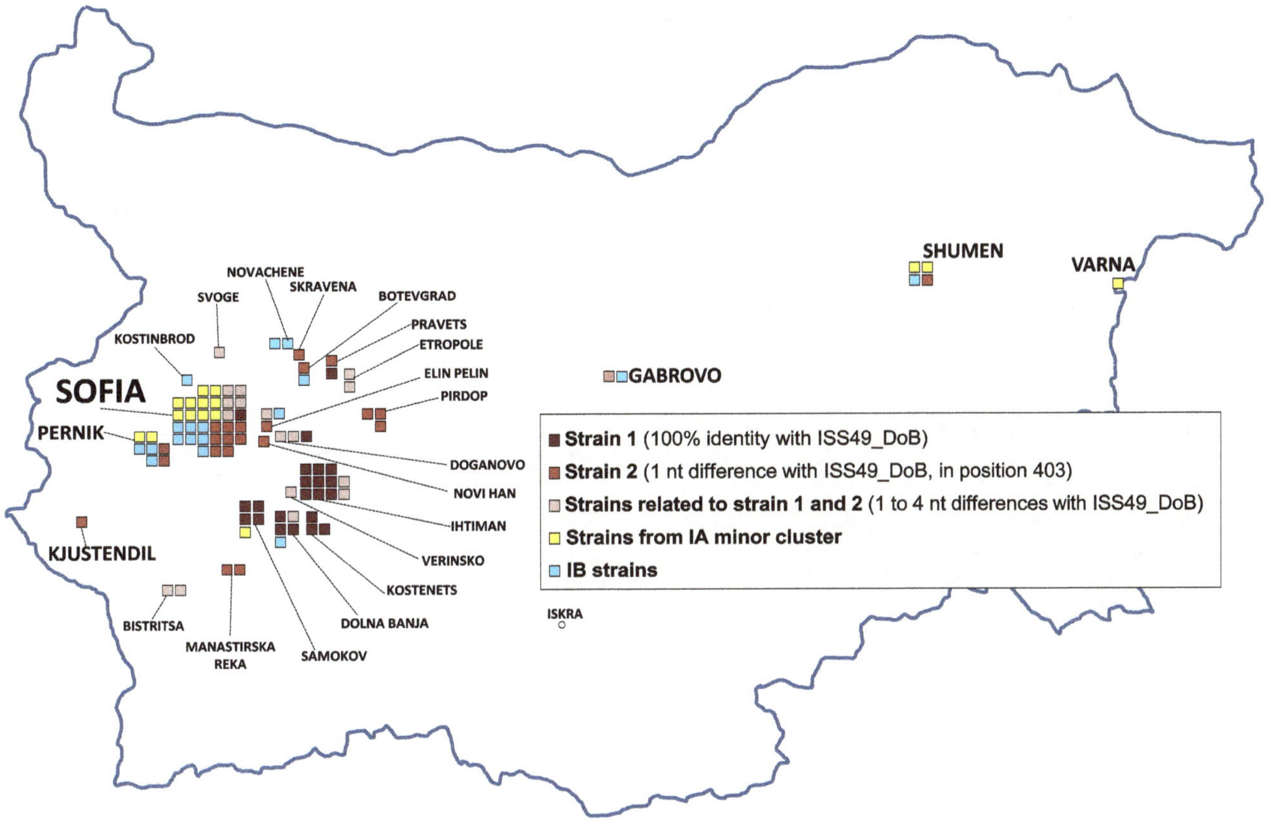

Fig. 4 Geographical localization of the characterized strains in Bulgarian towns/villages. The name of centers >30,000 inhabitants is reported in larger font size than the name of centers <30,000 inhabitants

2012 and, most likely, for the multiple outbreaks detected in different Bulgarian districts during those years [9, 10].

Conclusions

This is the first study describing the HAV genotypes and strains circulating in Bulgaria, one of the European countries with intermediate endemicity. Genotype IA predominates, with several highly related strains. Further studies need to be carried out to increase the number of molecularly characterised isolates from Bulgaria and from other countries of Eastern Europe that, by a phylogenetic approach, can be useful to investigate the factors underlying the spread of HAV infections and to implement appropriate preventing measures, at both national and European level.

Abbreviations

HAV: Hepatitis A Virus; LMCs: Large/Medium Centers; RT-PCR: Reverse Transcription and Polymerase Chain Reaction; SCs: Small Centers

Acknowledgements

The authors are very grateful to the many physicians and employees of Bulgarian health system for their silent but valuable work that allowed the present study.

Authors' contribution

ARC, RB, PT and MC conceived the study and participated in its design and coordination; ST, ME, AC, PC and EM conceived the experimental design of PCR and sequencing, carried out the experiments and elaborated raw data; ST, EC and ALP performed editing, alignment and quality control of sequences; RB and ARC performed phylogenetic and statistical analysis, prepared visualization of data and drafted the manuscript; RB, EG, DB, PT and ARC critically reviewed and edited the draft. All authors critically revised the intellectual content of the paper and approved the final manuscript.

Funding

The study received no specific funding.

Consent for publication

Not applicable (no individual person's data).

Competing interests

The authors declare that they have no competing interests.

Author details

[1]National Reference Laboratory for HAV, Viral Hepatitis Unit, Department of Infectious Diseases, Istituto Superiore di Sanità, Rome, Italy. [2]Department of Neurosciences, Istituto Superiore di Sanità, Rome, Italy. [3]Epidemiology Unit, Department of Infectious Diseases, Istituto Superiore di Sanità, Rome, Italy. [4]Department of Virology, National Center of Infectious and Parasitic Diseases, Sofia, Bulgaria.

References

1. Franco E, Meleleo C, Serino L, Sorbara D, Zaratti L. Hepatitis A: Epidemiology and prevention in developing countries. World J Hepatol. 2012;4:68–73.
2. Koff RS, Hepatitis A. Lancet. 1998;351:1643–9.
3. Vaughan G, Goncalves Rossi LM, Forbi JC, de Paula VS, Purdy MA, Xia G, Khudyakov YE. Hepatitis a virus: host interactions, molecular epidemiology and evolution. Infect Genet Evol. 2014;21:227–43. doi:10.1016/j.meegid.2013.10.023. Review
4. Bosch A, Guix S, Sano D, Pintò RM. New tools for the study and surveillance of viral pathogens in water. Curr Opin Biotechnol. 2008;19:295–301.
5. Dentinger CM, Bower WA, Nainan OV, Cotter SM, Myers G, Dubusky LM, Fowler S, Salehi ED, Bell BP. An outbreak of hepatitis a associated with green onions. J Infect Dis. 2001;183:1273–6.
6. Fiore AE. Hepatitis a transmitted by food. Clin Infec Dis. 2004;38:705–15.
7. Legeay O, Caudrelier Y, Cordevant C, Rigottier-Gois L, Lange M. Simplified procedure for detection of enteric pathogenic viruses in shellfish by RT-PCR. J Virol Methods. 2000;90:1–14.
8. Jacobsen KH, Wiersma ST. Hepatitis A virus seroprevalence by age and world region, 1990 and 2005. Vaccine. 2010; 28:6653–6657. doi:10.1016/j.vaccine.2010.08.037.
9. European Centre for Disease Prevention and Control. Annual epidemiological report 2014 – food- and waterborne diseases and zoonoses. Stockholm: ECDC; 2014. Available from: http://ecdc.europa.eu/en/publications/Publications/food-waterborne-diseases-annual-epidemiological-report-2014.pdf . Accessed 10 July 2017.
10. European Food Safety Authority, 2014. Tracing of food items in connection to the multinational hepatitis a virus outbreak in Europe. EFSA journal. 2014; 12(9):3821, 186 pp. doi:10.2903/j.efsa.2014.3821. Available from: http://onlinelibrary.wiley.com/doi/10.2903/j.efsa.2014.3821/epdf. Accessed 10 July 2017.
11. Vatev NT, Atanasova MV, Stoilova YD, Chervenyakova TP, Troyancheva MG. Seroprevalence of hepatitis a viral infection in Plovdiv, Bulgaria. Folia Med (Plovdiv). 2009;51(1):70–3.
12. Haverkate M, D'Ancona F, Giambi C, Johansen K, Lopalco PL, Cozza V, Appelgren E. on behalf of the VENICE project gatekeepers and contact points. Mandatory and recommended vaccination in the EU, Iceland and Norway: results of the VENICE 2010 survey on the ways of implementing national vaccination programmes. Euro Surveill. 2012;17(22):-20183.
13. Kojouharova M; Editorial team. Current outbreak of hepatitis A in Bulgaria 2006. Euro Surveill. 2006; 11(10):E061005.1.
14. Petrignani M, Verhoef L, Vennema H, van Hunen R, Baas D, van Steenbergen JE, Koopmans MP. Underdiagnosis of foodborne hepatitis a, The Netherlands, 2008-2010. Emerg Infect Dis. 2014;20(4):596–602. doi:10.3201/eid2004.130753.
15. Bruni R, Taffon S, Equestre M, Chionne P, Madonna E, Rizzo C, Tosti ME, Alfonsi V, Ricotta L, De Medici D, Di Pasquale S, Scavia G, Pavoni E, Losio MN, Romanò L, Zanetti AR, Morea A, Pacenti M, Palù G, Capobianchi MR, Chironna M, Pompa MG, Ciccaglione AR; Italian National Task Force on Hepatitis A. Key Role of Sequencing to Trace Hepatitis A Viruses Circulating in Italy During a Large Multi-Country European Foodborne Outbreak in 2013 PLoS One 2016;11(2):e0149642. doi:10.1371/journal.pone.0149642.
16. Pérez-Sautu U, Costafreda MI, Lite J, Sala R, Barrabeig I, Bosch A, Pintó RM. Molecular epidemiology of hepatitis a virus infections in Catalonia, Spain, 2005-2009: circulation of newly emerging strainsJ Clin Virol. 2011;52(2): 98–102. doi:10.1016/j.jcv.2011.06.011. Epub 2011 Jul 27
17. MacDonald E, Steens A, Stene-Johansen K, Gillesberg Lassen S, Midgley S, Lawrence J, Crofts J, Ngui SL, Balogun K, Frank C, Faber M, Gertler M, Verhoef L, Koopmans M, Sane J, van Pelt W, Sundqvist L, Vold L. Increase in hepatitis A in tourists from Denmark, England, Germany, the Netherlands, Norway and Sweden returning from Egypt, November 2012 to March 2013. Euro Surveill. 2013; 18(17):20468. No abstract available. Erratum in: Euro Surveill. 2013;18(18). pii: 20473.
18. Desbois D, Couturier E, Mackiewicz V, Graube A, Letort MJ, Dussaix E, Roque-Afonso AM. Epidemiology and genetic characterization of hepatitis a virus genotype IIA. J Clin Microbiol. 2010;48(9):3306–15. doi:10.1128/JCM.00667-10. Epub 2010 Jun 30
19. Ngui SL, Granerod J, Jewes LA, Crowcroft NS. Teo CG; 2002 hepatitis a outbreaks investigation network. Outbreaks of hepatitis a in England and Wales associated with two co-circulating hepatitis a virus strains. J Med Virol. 2008;80(7):1181–8. doi:10.1002/jmv.21207.
20. Guzman-Herrador BR, Panning M, Stene-Johansen K, Borgen K, Einöder-Moreno M, Huzly D, Jensvoll L, Lange H, Maassen S, Myking S, Myrmel M, Neumann-Haefelin C, Nygård K, Wenzel JJ, Øye AK, Vold L. Importance of molecular typing in confirmation of the source of a national hepatitis a virus outbreak in Norway and the detection of a related cluster in Germany. Arch Virol. 2015;160(11):2823–6. doi:10.1007/s00705-015-2531-y. Epub 2015 Aug 7
21. Faber MS, Stark K, Behnke SC, Schreier E, Frank C. Epidemiology of hepatitis a virus infections, Germany, 2007-2008. Emerg Infect Dis. 2009;15(11):1760–8. doi:10.3201/eid1511.090214.
22. WHO–recommended standards for surveillance of selected vaccine-preventable diseases, 2003; revised: July 2008. Available at: http://www.who.int/immunization/monitoring_surveillance/burden/vpd/surveillance_type/passive/hepatitis_standards/en/. Accessed 10 July 2017.
23. Tamura K, Stecher G, Peterson D, Filipski A, Kumar S. MEGA6: molecular evolutionary genetics analysis version 6.0. Mol Biol Evol. 2013;30:2725–9.
24. Hall TA. BioEdit: a user-friendly biological sequence alignment editor and analysis program for windows 95/98/NT. Nucl Acids Symp Ser. 1999;41:95–8.
25. Vatev N, Petrov A, Troyancheva M, Stoycheva M, Georgieva V. Clinical, epidemiological and laboratory characteristics of hepatitis a outbreak in the village of Iskra (Plovdiv region - Bulgaria), January - march 2012. International Journal of Pharmaceutical Science Invention. 2013;2(1):8–11.

Characterization of hepatitis B and delta coinfection in Israel

Rachel Shirazi[1], Daniela Ram[1], Aviya Rakovsky[1], Efrat Bucris[1], Yael Gozlan[1], Yaniv Lustig[1], Pninit Shaked-Mishan[2], Orit Picard[3], Yonat Shemer-Avni[4], Haim Ben-Zvi[5], Ora Halutz[6], Yoav Lurie[7], Ella Veizman[8], Matthias Carlebach[9], Marius Braun[10], Michal Cohen-Naftaly[10], Amir Shlomai[10,11], Rifaat Safadi[12], Ella Mendelson[1,13], Ella H. Sklan[11], Ziv Ben-Ari[11,14] and Orna Mor[1,13]*

Abstract

Background: Characteristics of hepatitis B (HBV) and delta (HDV) coinfection in various geographical regions, including Israel, remain unclear. Here we studied HDV seroprevalence in Israel, assessed HDV/HBV viral loads, circulating genotypes and hepatitis delta antigen (HDAg) conservation.

Methods: Serological anti HDV IgG results from 8969 HBsAg positive individuals tested in 2010-2015 were retrospectively analyzed to determine HDV seroprevalence. In a cohort of HBV/HDV coinfected (n=58) and HBV monoinfected (n=27) patients, quantitative real-time PCR (qRT-PCR) and sequencing were performed to determine viral loads, genotypes and hepatitis delta antigen (HDAg) protein sequence.

Results: 6.5% (587/8969) of the HBsAg positive patients were positive for anti HDV antibodies. HDV viral load was >2 log copies/ml higher than HBV viral load in most of the coinfected patients with detectable HDV RNA (86%, 50/58). HDV genotype 1 was identified in all patients, most of whom did not express HBV. While 66.6% (4/6) of the HBV/HDV co-expressing patients carried HBV-D2 only 18.5% (5/27) of the HBV monoinfections had HBV-D2 (p=0.03). Higher genetic variability in the HDAg protein sequence was associated with higher HDV viral load.

Conclusions: The overall significant prevalence of HDV (6.5%) mandates HDV RNA testing for all coinfected patients. Patients positive for HDV RNA (characterized by low HBV DNA blood levels) carried HDV genotype 1. Taken together, the significant HDV seroprevalence and the lack of effective anti-HDV therapy, necessitates strict clinical surveillance especially in patients with higher HDV viral loads and increased viral evolution.

Keywords: Hepatitis delta (HDV), HDV genotype, Seroprevalence, Hepatitis B (HBV), HBV genotype, HBV/HDV viral load

Background

More than 350 million people worldwide are chronically infected with hepatitis B virus (HBV). Fifteen to twenty millions of these individuals are considered to be coinfected with hepatitis delta virus (HDV) [1]. While HBV is a DNA virus coding for several proteins, HDV is a circular single-strand negative-sense ribonucleic acid (RNA) virus that codes for a single protein, the HDV antigen (HDAg) [2] and requires HBV surface antigen (HBsAg) for infection, thus can only be detected in HBV positive individuals. Infection with HBV and HDV leads to the most severe form of chronic viral hepatitis, causing liver cirrhosis and hepatocellular carcinoma [3]. Patients with HBV and HDV chronic infection have a twofold higher risk to develop cirrhosis, a threefold higher risk to develop hepatocellular carcinoma and a twofold increased mortality rate compared with HBV monoinfected individuals [4, 5]. The severity of the liver disease caused by HBV/HDV is thought to be associated with the HDV genotype and viral loads [6, 7]. HBV genome is divided into 10 genotypes (A-J). The most common HBV genotype in Europe is genotype D. There are eight reported genotypes of HDV with unexplained

* Correspondence: orna.mor@sheba.health.gov.il
[1]Central Virology Laboratory, Ministry of Health, Chaim Sheba Medical Center, Tel - Hashomer, 52621 Ramat Gan, Israel
[13]School of Public Health, Sackler School of Medicine, Tel Aviv University, Tel Aviv, Israel
Full list of author information is available at the end of the article

variations in their geographical distribution and pathogenicity [8]. The most common, worldwide distributed HDV genotype is genotype 1, found mainly in Europe and North America. While drugs for HBV are available and several anti-HDV drugs are now in clinical development [9, 10] there is still no specific therapy approved for HDV.

In Israel, the incidence of HBV has declined dramatically since the introduction of the vaccination program in 1992, and was estimated to be 0.5/100,000 in 2015 [11]. The prevalence of HBV was lately estimated to be 0.96% [12] suggesting that approximately 72,000 individuals in Israel are HBV carriers. On the other hand, the frequency of HBV/HDV infection has not been reported and information on the local genotypes which may be relevant when anti-HDV therapy will be available, is lacking.

Here, the seroprevalence of HDV was determined in a large sample of HBsAg positive patients. HBV and HDV viral loads and genotypes were assessed in a separate sample of patients positive for HDV RNA (n=58) and in 27 HBV monoinfected patients. In addition, the full HDAg coding region was determined and compared between HDV/HBV patients.

Methods

Patients and samples

Seroprevalence of HDV in Israel was determined by a retrospective analysis of anti HDV immunoglobulin G (IgG) antibody results obtained from all HBsAg positive patients (n=8969) tested for anti HDV between 2010 and 2015. The medical reason for requesting HDV serology by the physicians was not recorded.. The data was not obtained from a specific group of individuals (e.g. routine blood donors). The data was collected anonymously from approximately a quarter of the clinical virology laboratories engaged in HBV and HDV testing in Israel. These laboratories are located in five medical centers (Carmel, Soroka, Sheba, Rabin and Sorasky) from different regions in Israel. HDV IgG positivity was determined using an ELISA assay (ETI-AB-DELTAK-2, DiaSorin, Italy). All serological tests were performed following the manufacturer's instructions. Whenever possible, information on sex and age was also collected. To reduce redundancy as much as possible, if multiple results from a single individual were identified, they were removed prior to data analysis. The presence of HDV-RNA, which was assessed by a qualitative assay [13] in HDV IgG positive samples identified in the clinical virology laboratory of Soroka, was also recorded. The study was approved by the Ethical Committee of the Sheba Medical Center (approval number SMC 2890-15) and informed consent was deemed unnecessary.

Molecular analysis (quantification of HDV and HBV viral load, genotyping and in HBV/HDV samples-comparison of HDAg predicted protein sequences) was performed on samples from 58 patients positive for HDV RNA and 27 HBV monoinfected patients (who failed anti HBV therapy and for whom HBV resistance analysis was requested). Blood samples (5 ml) collected from these patients between January 2013 and December 2016 were transferred to the national HIV and viral hepatitis reference center where plasma was separated and stored at -20^{0}C until used.

HDV and HBV viral load

Nucleic acids were extracted from 0.5 ml plasma using the NucliSENS Easy MAG total nucleic acid extraction system (Biomerieux, Marcy l'Etoile, France), according to the manufacturer's protocol. HDV viral load was determined with Primerdesign HDV genesig assay (Primerdesign Ltd, United Kingdom) which is characterized by high priming efficiencies of >95% and can detect less than 100 copies of target template and was validated with an external control program (QCMD HDV14, QCMD, Glasgow, Scotland). HBV viral load was determined as previously described [14]. This assay, with an estimated 20 IU/ml detection limit, was validated using an external control program (HBVDNA2017, QCMD, Glasgow, Scotland).

HDV and HBV genotyping

Genotypes were determined in samples with viral load >1000 copies/ml (HBV or HDV). HDV genotype was determined following PCR amplification of the whole HDAg region with ORF891F 5'- ATGCCGACCCGAAGAGGA-3' and ORF1680R 5'- GTCCAGCRGTCTCCTCTTTA-3' by single step RT-PCR using 7 µl HDV RNA and sequencing with previously published primers [13, 15]. Genotyping of HBV was performed following PCR amplification of a fragment from the polymerase region with 2F-5-'GCGGGCCGGCTACTCTTCTTTC and 6r 5'-GTGGGGGTTGCGTCAGCAAA-3' with 5µl HBV DNA. Direct sequencing of all PCR products was performed using an automatic sequencer (ABI PRISM 3100 genetic analyzer DNA Sequencer, Applied Biosystems, Foster City, CA, USA) and BigDye Terminator v1.1 Cycle Sequencing kit (Applied Biosystems, Foster City, CA, USA).

Phylogenetic analyses

HDV and HBV nucleotide sequences were aligned using the Open-gene system (Siemens, Malvern PA, United States). Reference sequences were GeneBank accession X04451 for HDV and the references sequences from Open-gene system module for HBV. Representative nucleotide sequences for HDV genotypes 1-8 from GenBank (Genotype 1a: U81989-Etiopia, U81988-Somalia; Genotype 1b: JX888099-Nigeria Genotype 1c: KJ744240-Iran; M58829-Nauru; Genotype1d:

AM779588_tk34_Turkey; LT594475_Romania; KJ744214_Iran; KJ744218_Iran KR363258_1054_China; genotype2_AF104264; genotype3_L22063; genotype 4_AF018077; genotype5_AM183326; genotype6_AM 183332; genotype7_AM183333; genotype8_AM183327) and of HBV (D1_ AB674425,M32138, D2_EU594433, JF754621, D3_X85254, AB674437, A1_AF09084, FM19 9974, A2_GQ477460, X51970, C1_X04615,AB014381, C2_AB117758 , B3_AB033554, B1_D00329,B2_AF1003 09) were aligned using Sequencher 5.0, and clustered with the Clustal X algorithm (bootstrap value of 1000). Phylogenetic trees (375 nucleotides, 1200-1573 in HDV X04451 and 442 nucleotides, 458-897 in HBV AB6 74436) were constructed by neighbor joining method and produced by Mega 6.0.

Comparison of HDAg protein sequences

Full length HDAg sequences were translated via online Expasy translation tool [16]. To investigate the mutational pattern of functional domains within the HDAg protein, the amino acid sequences of the different isolates were compared with each other using LOGO [17]. Shannon entropy was used to assess the degree of amino acid conservation [18]. Conserved residues are those with zero Shannon entropy.

Statistical analysis

The association between HDV seropositivity, age and sex was assessed using the $\chi2$ test for categorical variables and t-test for numeric variables. Univariate logistic regression model, Odds ratios (OR) and 95% confidence intervals were calculated. Fisher exact test was used to assess the association between HDV and HBV genotypes and between HDAg amino acid conservation in low (<5 log copies/ml) and high (>5 log copies/ml) HDV viral load patients. P-value <0.05 was considered statistically significant. Data were analyzed using the SAS software (version 9.1.3).

Results

HDV seroprevalence

Retrospective study of anti HDV IgG results obtained for samples from 8969 HBsAg positives was conducted, 587 (6.5%) were found positive (Table 1). Patients positive for anti IgG HDV were, on average, slightly older than HDV seronegative HBsAg positive patients (47.5 ±13.8 versus 45.2±16 years, $p<0.01$). No significant difference in HDV prevalence was found between males and females (6.2% versus 6.9%, respectively). The presence of HDV RNA was assessed in the Soroka virology laboratory for a limited number of samples found to be anti HDV positive (n=196). 23% (45/196) were HDV-RNA positive.

HDV and HBV viral load and genotypes

The mean and median HDV and HBV viral loads, assessed in a separate cohort of HBV/HDV patients (n=58) positive for HDV RNA, were 5.78±1.42 and 5.79 (IQR 2.3); 1.34±1.39 and 1.51 (IQR 1.58) log copies/ml, respectively, p<0.05. In most of these coinfection cases (86%, 50/58) HDV viral load was at least 2 log higher than HBV viral load. In samples from HBV monoinfected patients who failed anti HBV therapy (n=27), the mean and median HBV viral load was 4.8±1.66 and 4.6 (IQR 2.0) log copies/ml, respectively.

HDV genotype was successfully determined for 95% (55/58) of the HDV/HBV patients, all with >1000 copies/ml HDV viral load (Fig. 1). All were infected with HDV genotype 1. Le Gal et al., recently suggested classification of HDV-1 into four subtypes [19]. Accordingly, the majority (n=48) of the patients carried subtype HDV-1d and a small group (n=5) carried HDV-1c or HDV-1a (n=2). Of 55 samples in which HDV genotypes were determined, 41 had known birth place. While those from Eastern Europe (35/41, former Soviet Union, Ukraine, Romania) and Israel (2/41) carried HDV-1d or HDV-1c (2/41, Russia), both of the two patients born in Ethiopia carried HDV-1a which corresponds mainly to Africa [19, 20].

HBV genotype could be determined in samples from 33 patients: 6 HBV/HDV patients (those with plasma viral load >1000 copies/ml, enabling sequencing of both viruses) and in 27 HBV monoinfected patients.

Of 6 HBV/HDV patients, the distribution of HBV genotypes and subgenotypes was as below: 4 (66.7%), 1 (16.7%), and 1 (16.7%) were D2, D1 and D3 respectively.

Table 1 Prevalence of HDV infection in Israel

	Samples tested, N	HDV negative samples	HDV seropositive samples	% seropositive (95% CI)	Odds Ratio (95% CI)	*p*-value
Total	8969	8382	587	6.5 (6.1-7.1)		
Age (mean± SD)	8452[a]	45.2± 16 (n=7919)	47.5± 13.8 (n=533)		1.0 (1.0-1.1)	<0.01
Gender (n=8744)[a]						
Male	5046	4734	312	6.2 (5.6-6.9)	Reference	0.18
Female	3698	3443	255	6.9 (61.-7.8)	1.1 (0.9-1.3)	

[a]The number of samples for which this information was available

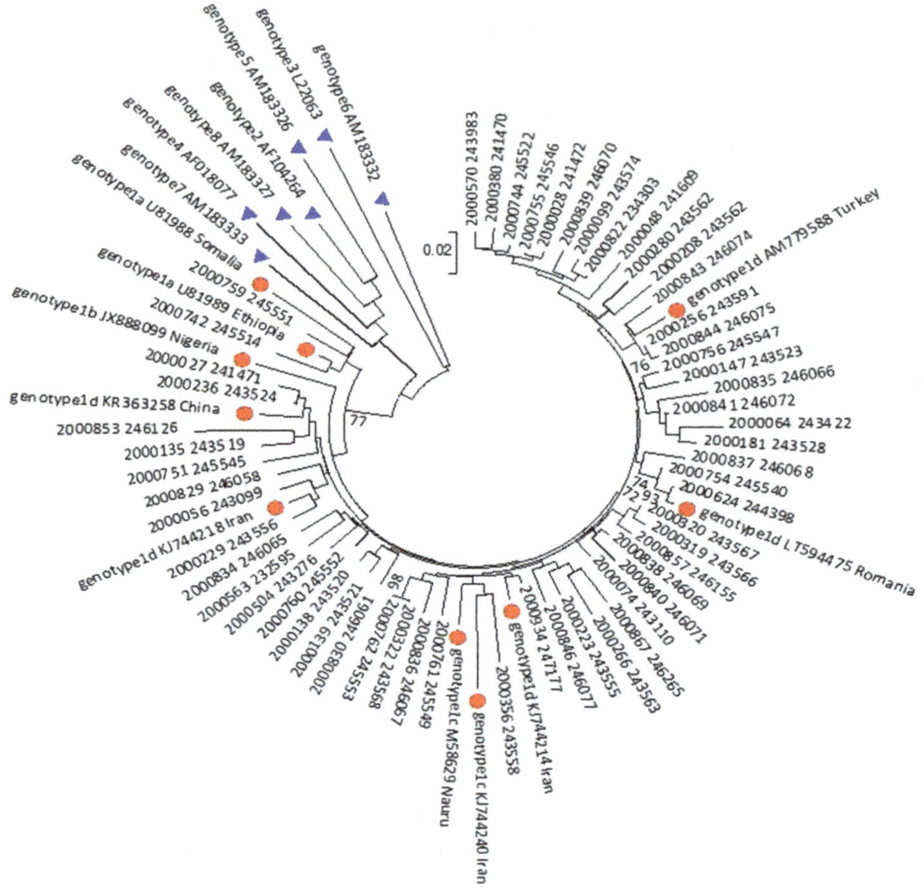

Fig. 1 Phylogenetic Analysis of HDV nucleotide sequences. Phylogenetic tree of 55 HDV nucleic acid (n.a) patient sequences, 1 HDV-RNA sequence derived from HK293 cells transfected with HDV plasmid (2000504), and 17 prototype sequences obtained from GeneBank (dots, HDV genotype 1; triangle, HDV genotype 2-8) was constructed by Clustal W pairwise alignment with the 375 n.a. from HDVAg. The prototype sequences are identified by the HDV genotype and subtype [19], GeneBank accession number and the name of the country of origin (if known). The Israeli-identified sequences are defined by their patient and sample numbers. Bootstrap values are indicated for the major nodes as data obtained from 1000 replicates.

In contrast, of 27 HBV mono-infected patients, the distribution was as follow: D1 (59.3%), D2 (18.5%) D3 (11.1%) and A1, A2 and C2 (3.7% each). The prevalence of genotype HBV-D2 was significantly different between mono-infected and co-infected groups (4 (66.7%) vs 5 (18.5%), p=0.03).

HDAg analysis

Full HDAg sequence (214 amino acids) was successfully determined in 48 of the 55 HBV/HDV patients with HDV sequences. It is possible that the considerable heterogeneity and strong internal base pairing of HDV did not allow analysis of the complete HDAg region in seven of the sampled [21]. Multiple sequence alignment of the full HDAg sequences revealed that although major regulatory sites [2, 22–28] were conserved in all patients, high amino-acid diversity was observed between the sequences. To better assess this phenomenon, the amino acid variability (as measured by Shannon Entropy) between 12 patients with low HDV viremia (<5log copies/ml, mean viral load 4.2±0.63 log copies/ml) and 36 with high HDV viremia (=>5 log copies/ml, mean viral load 6.6±1.42 log copies/ml) was compared. For this comparison, the same reference sequence was used (CAQ16911.1 large Hepatitis delta antigen dTk5 Turkey). In the 12 patients with low HDV viremia, the HDAg predicted protein sequence was more conserved (69.2%, 148/214 conserved residues) compared to the amino acid sequence of HDAg in the high viremic patients (56.1%, 120/214 conserved residues, p<0.05) versus. Substitutions in amino acids K26R, E29D, L34I/S/V, N58H/Y and Q100R/E located in the coiled coil and RNA binding domains were observed in high viremic patients only (Fig. 2).

Discussion

HDV infection in patients with chronic HBV infection, which continues to be a public health concern

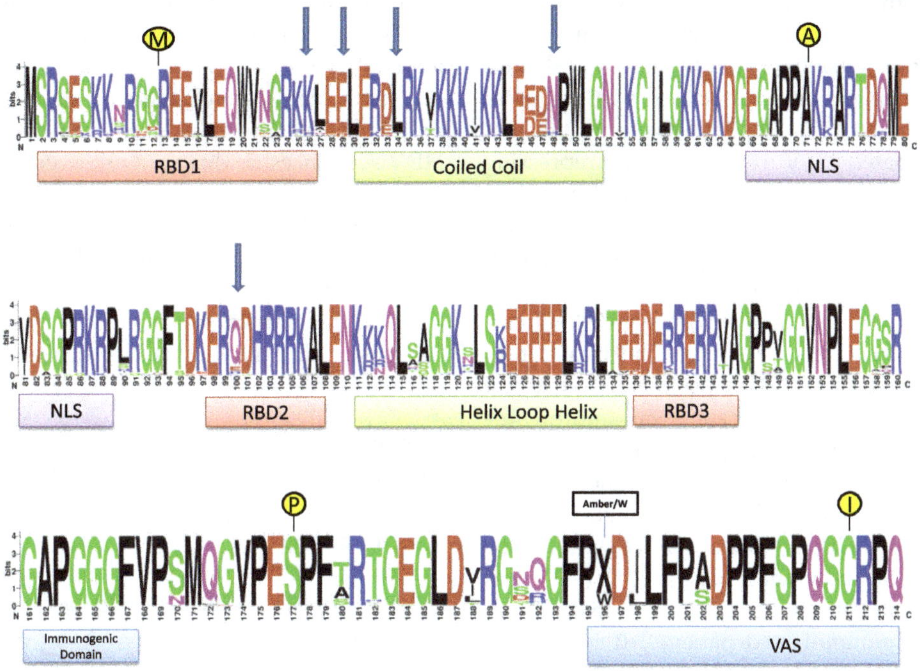

Fig. 2: HDAg sequence alignment logo. Amino-acid logo of full HDAg sequences obtained from 48 HDV- RNA positive patients. Functional domains (presented by boxes) and post-transcriptional modification sites (illustrated as circles) are indicated. Arrows indicate residues in regulatory regions found to be less conserved in high viremic patients.

worldwide, results in the most severe form of viral hepatitis. However, testing for hepatitis delta is limited and the rate of HDV infection in many countries is unknown [29]. To the best of our knowledge the rate of HDV seropositivity in Israel has not yet been reported nor have the circulating genotypes been assessed. Moreover, molecular detection of HDV by real-time PCR is rarely performed and HDV viral load is not monitored.

Here, 6.5% of HBsAg positive patients in Israel were found to be HDV seropositive, a higher rate than the estimated 5% worldwide prevalence [30]. Reported HDV prevalence varies in different European countries between very low (0.23%) in Slovenia to high (35.3%) prevalence in Greece [31]. In Lebanon HDV prevalence reported in 258 HBV positive individuals was only 1.2% [32]. A higher seroprevalence, 8.3%, was reported in Egypt among 121 HBV carriers [33]. As both studies assessed HDV seroprevalence in a small number of HBV seropositive individuals, the results may not fully represent the overall HDV infection rate in these countries. In a previous study performed in Israel on 400 injecting drug users, 22 were found HBsAg positive and 18% of them (4/22) were also anti HDV positive [34]. This high prevalence may be misleading as the study was performed on a small number of a specific group of individuals, before the initiation of HBV vaccination program and thus may not fully represent the current serological and demographic status of the population in Israel. The 6.5% rate for anti HDV antibodies found here amongst nearly 9000 HBsAg positives (>10% of the individuals considered to be HBV positive, [12]), may better present the current status of HDV infection in Israel. HDV RNA was detected in 24% of the samples tested for the presence of virus. These results, which may underestimate HDV RNA positivity due to low sensitivity of the assay and which were obtained in only a limited number of HDV seropositive patients, call for molecular analysis of HDV in all seropositive cases.

Genotyping revealed that HDV patients, most of whom were born in Eastern Europe, carried HDV-1 sequences which clustered with HDV isolates from Europe (Italy, Romania) and Asia (Iran, Turkey). The only two patients with HDV born in Ethiopia clustered with strains identified in Africa. Predominance of HDV-1 has been described worldwide [28, 35]. HDV-1 was also the only genotype identified in other Mediterranean countries like Turkey [36] and Tunisia [37].

Almost all (>90%) of HBV positive cases were infected with genotype D, the most prevalent genotype worldwide. However, while D1 was the most frequent subtype in HBV monoinfected patients (59.3%, 16/27) and D2 was identified in only 18.5% of these monoinfected patients, HBV/HDV patients were mainly (66.7%) infected with HBV-D2. HBV genotypes other than genotype D were not observed. This analysis was performed in a limited number of patients only, as most HBV/HDV coinfections had low or undetectable HBV viral load. Low viral loads of HBV in samples positive for plasma HDV RNA were previously reported by others [38], suggesting that HDV replication is associated with suppression of HBV replication [39]. Evidence has indicated that HDAg down regulates HBV replication by repressing activity of the two HBV enhancer regions, and by transactivating the interferon-inducible MxA gene, which inhibits HBV replication by reducing the export of viral mRNA from the nucleus [40]. In a study conducted in Spain which assessed viral loads of HDV in HBV-D carriers [7], higher HDV levels were significantly and persistently found compared to HBV. Specifically, this effect was HBV genotype dependent and was more pronounced in HBV-A than HBV-D genotypes (median of 4.48 and 3.49 log copies/ml for HBV-A and HBV-D, respectively). The authors concluded that higher inhibitory effect of HDV on HBV replication is HBV genotype specific. Our results show that subtype HBV-D2 was more frequently found in HBV/HDV coinfected individuals than in HBV monoinfected patients. It is possible that HBV-D2 overcomes the repression conferred by HDV-1 better than other HBV genotypes. The correlation between HDV and HBV genotypes and reciprocal repression has practical consequences. It may cause misdiagnoses of the viral load of HDV or HBV in coinfection and underrepresentation of slow replicating genotypes. Future studies are needed to better establish the association between HBV/HDV genotypes and co-replication interference.

HDAg protein is considered to display more amino acid changes compared to structural proteins of other RNA viruses [39]. Analysis of HDAg predicted amino acid sequences of 48 patients showed increased variability in high compared to low viremic patients in protein domains involved in viral replication. The functional and clinical relevance of the specific amino acid changes observed herein (including the changes in amino acid 202 observed in several patients not connected to viral load status) requires further studies especially as no direct acting HDV antiviral is yet available. Indeed, a major obstacle in developing treatment of HDV infection is lack of self-replicative function to be directly targeted by antivirals. Peg-Interferon remains the mainstay of treatment however interferon therapy is associated with frequent side effects and low response rate. Clinical studies exploring prenylation inhibitors, viral entry inhibitors and nucleic acid polymers to block particle release demonstrate progress towards cure of HDV infection [41].

One of the limitations of this study is that HDV-RNA measurements are not done routinely in all HDV seropositive cases, therefore, the rate of RNA positivity could be defined in only a limited number of cases. Also, HDV viral load was not routinely assessed. In addition, another limitation of this study is that data on disease status (e.g. cirrhosis), HBsAg levels, a known risk factor for HDV viremia [42] or risk factors for HDV infection (e.g. birth place, use of injection drugs) for the 586 seropositive HDV individuals was lacking. Although most HDV sequences in this study derived from patients born in Eastern European countries and a few in Ethiopia, countries with a high prevalence of HBV infection [43], this information was not available for all HDV seropositive individuals. The ethnic group of the HBV/HDV coninfected individuals, which may also be a risk factor for HBV positivity [42, 44] was also unknown.

Conclusions

This study identified a 6.5% rate of HDV seroprevalence in HBsAg positive patients. This high rate suggests that screening for HDV in HBV positive patients in Israel is mandatory and should be continued. Furthermore, the presence of HDV-RNA should be assessed in all HDV IgG positive cases. In HDV-RNA positive cases, HDV viral load measurements could be beneficial. Patients with high HDV viral load and higher degree of viral diversity should be more closely monitored. Whenever possible, analysis of HBV/HDV genotypes will also be beneficial especially as the most common HDV genotype observed in this study, HDV-1, is considered to worsen the liver disease more than other HDV genotypes. Moreover, as the clinical efficacy of future anti-HDV therapy may also be influenced by HBV/HDV genotypes and subtypes, deciphering the local HBV/HDV status will be advantageous.

Abbreviations

HBV: Hepatitis B; HDV: Hepatitis delta; HDAg: Hepatitis delta antigen; IgG: Immunoglobulin G; HIV: Human immunodeficiency virus; ml: Microliters; PCR: Polymerase chain reaction; RT-PCR: reverse transcription PCR; qRT-PCR: Quantitative real-time PCR

Acknowledgments

The authors would like to acknowledge Ravit Bassal for her assistance in statistical analysis, Zehava Yossefi for her excellent administrative services and Keren Tsaraf, Yael Harif and Rimma Kramsky for their ongoing technical assistance. This work was presented at the meeting of the European association of the study of the liver (EASL) 2017.

Funding

None

Authors' contributions

RS, DR, AR, EB and YG preformed all the experiments. YL, YS, EHS, EM and ZBA were major contributors in writing the manuscript. PSM, OP, HBZ, OH, and YS analyzed and interpreted the patient serological data. YL, EV, MB, MC, MCN, AS, RS, ZBA saw the patients and provided clinical information. OM was in charge of the whole project and wrote the manuscript. All authors read and approved the final manuscript.

Consent for publication
Not applicable

Competing interests
The authors declare that they have no competing interests.

Author details
[1]Central Virology Laboratory, Ministry of Health, Chaim Sheba Medical Center, Tel - Hashomer, 52621 Ramat Gan, Israel. [2]Microbiology Laboratory, Carmel Medical Center, Haifa, Israel. [3]Gastroenterology Laboratory, Sheba Medical Center, Ramat Gan, Israel. [4]Laboratory of Clinical Virology, Soroka University Medical Center, Beer Sheva, Israel. [5]Microbiology Laboratory, Rabin Medical Center, Petach Tikva, Israel. [6]Microbiology Laboratory, Sorasky Medical Center, Tel Aviv, Israel. [7]Liver Unit, Shaare Zedek Medical Center, Jerusalem, Israel. [8]Liver Unit, Rambam Medical Center, Haifa, Israel. [9]Liver Unit, Bnai Zion Medical Center, Haifa, Israel. [10]Liver Institute, Rabin Medical Center, Petah-Tikva, Israel. [11]The Sackler School of Medicine, Tel Aviv University, Tel Aviv, Israel. [12]Liver Unit, Hadassah Hebrew University Hospital, Jerusalem, Israel. [13]School of Public Health, Sackler School of Medicine, Tel Aviv University, Tel Aviv, Israel. [14]Liver Disease Center, Sheba Medical Center, Ramat Gan, Israel.

References

1. Wedemeyer H, Manns MP. Epidemiology, pathogenesis and management of hepatitis D: update and challenges ahead. Nat Rev Gastroenterol Hepatol. 2010;7(1):31–40.
2. Wang KS, Choo QL, Weiner AJ, Ou JH, Najarian RC, Thayer RM, Mullenbach GT, Denniston KJ, Gerin JL, Houghton M. Structure, sequence and expression of the hepatitis delta (delta) viral genome. Nature. 1986; 323(6088):508–14.
3. Lempp FA, Ni Y, Urban S. Hepatitis delta virus: insights into a peculiar pathogen and novel treatment options. Nat Rev Gastroenterol Hepatol. 2016;13(10):580–9.
4. Fattovich G, Bortolotti F, Donato F. Natural history of chronic hepatitis B: special emphasis on disease progression and prognostic factors. J Hepatol. 2008;48(2):335–52.
5. Fattovich G, Giustina G, Christensen E, Pantalena M, Zagni I, Realdi G, Schalm SW. Influence of hepatitis delta virus infection on morbidity and mortality in compensated cirrhosis type B. The European Concerted Action on Viral Hepatitis (Eurohep). Gut. 2000;46(3):420–6.
6. Braga WS, de Oliveira CM, de Araujo JR, Castilho Mda C, Rocha JM, Gimaque JB, Silva ML, Vasconcelos HL, Ramasawmy R, Parana R. Chronic HDV/HBV co-infection: predictors of disease stage—a case series of HDV-3 patients. J Hepatol. 2014;61(6):1205–11.
7. Madejon A, Romero M, Hernandez A, Garcia-Sanchez A, Sanchez-Carrillo M, Olveira A, Garcia-Samaniego J. Hepatitis B and D viruses replication interference: Influence of hepatitis B genotype. World J Gastroenterol. 2016; 22(11):3165–74.
8. Le Gal F, Gault E, Ripault MP, Serpaggi J, Trinchet JC, Gordien E, Deny P. Eighth major clade for hepatitis delta virus. Emerg Infect Dis. 2006;12(9): 1447–50.
9. Koh C, Canini L, Dahari H, Zhao X, Uprichard SL, Haynes-Williams V, Winters MA, Subramanya G, Cooper SL, Pinto P, Wolff EF, Bishop R, Ai Thanda Han M, Cotler SJ, Kleiner DE, Keskin O, Idilman R, Yurdaydin C, Glenn JS, Heller T. Oral prenylation inhibition with lonafarnib in chronic hepatitis D infection: a proof-of-concept randomised, double-blind, placebo-controlled phase 2A trial. Lancet Infect Dis. 2015;15(10):1167–74.
10. Bogomolov P, Alexandrov A, Voronkova N, Macievich M, Kokina K, Petrachenkova M, Lehr T, Lempp FA, Wedemeyer H, Haag M, Schwab M, Haefeli WE, Blank A, Urban S. Treatment of chronic hepatitis D with the entry inhibitor myrcludex B: First results of a phase Ib/IIa study. J Hepatol. 2016;65(3):490–8.
11. Farias A, Re V, Mengarelli S, Kremer L, Pisano MB, Allende L, Nicolas J, Elbarcha O, Contigiani M. Detection of hepatitis C virus (HCV) in body fluids from HCV monoinfected and HCV/HIV coinfected patients. Hepatogastroenterology. 2010;57(98):300–4.
12. Schweitzer A, Horn J, Mikolajczyk RT, Krause G, Ott JJ. Estimations of worldwide prevalence of chronic hepatitis B virus infection: a systematic review of data published between 1965 and 2013. Lancet. 2015;386 (10003):1546–55.
13. Mederacke I, Bremer B, Heidrich B, Kirschner J, Deterding K, Bock T, Wursthorn K, Manns MP, Wedemeyer H. Establishment of a novel quantitative hepatitis D virus (HDV) RNA assay using the Cobas TaqMan platform to study HDV RNA kinetics. J Clin Microbiol. 2010;48(6):2022–9.
14. Mixson-Hayden T, Lee D, Ganova-Raeva L, Drobeniuc J, Stauffer WM, Teshale E, Kamili S. Hepatitis B virus and hepatitis C virus infections in United States-bound refugees from Asia and Africa. Am J Trop Med Hyg. 2014;90(6):1014–20.
15. Celik I, Karatayli E, Cevik E, Kabakci SG, Karatayli SC, Dinc B, Cinar K, Yalcin K, Idilman R, Yurdaydin C, Bozdayi AM. Complete genome sequences and phylogenetic analysis of hepatitis delta viruses isolated from nine Turkish patients. Arch Virol. 2011;156(12):2215–20.
16. Artimo P, Jonnalagedda M, Arnold K, Baratin D, Csardi G, de Castro E, Duvaud S, Flegel V, Fortier A, Gasteiger E, Grosdidier A, Hernandez C, Ioannidis V, Kuznetsov D, Liechti R, Moretti S, Mostaguir K, Redaschi N, Rossier G, Xenarios I, Stockinger H. ExPASy: SIB bioinformatics resource portal. Nucleic Acids Res. 2012;40(Web Server issue):W597–603.
17. Crooks GE, Hon G, Chandonia JM, Brenner SE. WebLogo: a sequence logo generator. Genome Res. 2004;14(6):1188–90.
18. Yusim K, Richardson R, Tao N, Dalwani A, Agrawal A, Szinger J, Funkhouser R, Korber B, Kuiken C. Los alamos hepatitis C immunology database. Appl Bioinformatics. 2005;4(4):217–25.
19. Le Gal F, Brichler S, Drugan T, Alloui C, Roulot D, Pawlotsky JM, Deny P, Gordien E. Genetic diversity and worldwide distribution of the deltavirus genus: A study of 2,152 clinical strains. Hepatology. 2017;66(6):1826–41.
20. Zhang YY, Tsega E, Hansson BG. Phylogenetic analysis of hepatitis D viruses indicating a new genotype I subgroup among African isolates. J Clin Microbiol. 1996;34(12):3023–30.
21. Homs M, Giersch K, Blasi M, Lutgehetmann M, Buti M, Esteban R, Dandri M, Rodriguez-Frias F. Relevance of a full-length genomic RNA standard and a thermal-shock step for optimal hepatitis delta virus quantification. J Clin Microbiol. 2014;52(9):3334–8.
22. Alves C, Freitas N, Cunha C. Characterization of the nuclear localization signal of the hepatitis delta virus antigen. Virology. 2008;370(1):12–21.
23. Poisson F, Roingeard P, Baillou A, Dubois F, Bonelli F, Calogero RA, Goudeau A. Characterization of RNA-binding domains of hepatitis delta antigen. J Gen Virol. 1993;74(Pt 11):2473–8.
24. Alves C, Branco C, Cunha C. Hepatitis delta virus: a peculiar virus. Adv Virol. 2013;2013:560105.
25. Mu JJ, Chen DS, Chen PJ. The conserved serine 177 in the delta antigen of hepatitis delta virus is one putative phosphorylation site and is required for efficient viral RNA replication. J Virol. 2001;75(19): 9087–95.
26. Glenn JS, Watson JA, Havel CM, White JM. Identification of a prenylation site in delta virus large antigen. Science. 1992;256(5061):1331–3.
27. Shih HH, Shih C, Wang HW, Su CW, Sheen IJ, Wu JC. Pro-205 of large hepatitis delta antigen and Pro-62 of major hepatitis B surface antigen influence the assembly of different genotypes of hepatitis D virus. J Gen Virol. 2010;91(Pt 4):1004–12.
28. Perveen S, Nasir MI, Shahid SM, Azhar A, Khan OY. Phylogenetic analysis of HDV isolates from HBsAg positive patients in Karachi, Pakistan. Virol J. 2012;9:162.
29. Eduardo B. Martins JG (2017) Sa1486 – Prevalence of Hepatitis Delta Virus (HDV) Infection in the United States: Results from an ICD-10 Review. Gastroenterology Volume 152, Issue 5, Supplement 1, April 2017, Pages S1085
30. Meng XJ. Recent advances in Hepatitis E virus. J Viral Hepat. 2010; 17(3):153–61.
31. Jelen MM, Hosnjak L, Stunf S, Zagozen A, Fujs Komlos K, Markocic P, Poljak M, Seme K. Hepatitis D virus infection in Slovenian patients with chronic hepatitis B virus infection: a national prevalence study and literature review. Acta Dermatovenerol Alp Pannonica Adriat. 2016;25 (3):49–53.
32. Ramia S, El-Zaatari M, Sharara AI, Ramlawi F, Farhat B. Current prevalence of hepatitis delta virus (HDV) infection and the range of HDV genotypes in Lebanon. Epidemiol Infect. 2007;135(6):959–62.

33. Fouad R, Abdo M, Eldeen HG, Sabry D, Atef M, Ahmed R, Zayed N. Influence of delta virus infection on the virologic status in Egyptian patients with chronic hepatitis B virus genotype D. J Med Virol. 2016;88(5):837–42.
34. Dan M, Rock M, Lilos P, Shany SB. Seroepidemiology of hepatitis B and D virus infection among intravenous drug addicts in Israel. Int J Epidemiol. 1993;22(1):140–3.
35. El Bouzidi K, Elamin W, Kranzer K, Irish DN, Ferns B, Kennedy P, Rosenberg W, Dusheiko G, Sabin CA, Smith BC, Nastouli E. Hepatitis delta virus testing, epidemiology and management: a multicentre cross-sectional study of patients in London. J Clin Virol. 2015;66:33–7.
36. Altuglu I, Ozacar T, Sertoz RY, Erensoy S. Hepatitis delta virus (HDV) genotypes in patients with chronic hepatitis: molecular epidemiology of HDV in Turkey. Int J Infect Dis. 2007;11(1):58–62.
37. Yacoubi L, Brichler S, Mansour W, Le Gal F, Hammami W, Sadraoui A, Ben Mami N, Msaddek A, Cheikh I, Triki H, Gordien E. Molecular epidemiology of hepatitis B and Delta virus strains that spread in the Mediterranean North East Coast of Tunisia. J Clin Virol. 2015;72:126–32.
38. Gish RG, Yi DH, Kane S, Clark M, Mangahas M, Baqai S, Winters MA, Proudfoot J, Glenn JS. Coinfection with hepatitis B and D: epidemiology, prevalence and disease in patients in Northern California. J Gastroenterol Hepatol. 2013;28(9):1521–5.
39. Shirvani-Dastgerdi E, Tacke F. Molecular interactions between hepatitis B virus and delta virus. World J Virol. 2015;4(2):36–41.
40. Alfaiate D, Lucifora J, Abeywickrama-Samarakoon N, Michelet M, Testoni B, Cortay JC, Sureau C, Zoulim F, Deny P, Durantel D. HDV RNA replication is associated with HBV repression and interferon-stimulated genes induction in super-infected hepatocytes. Antiviral Res. 2016;136:19–31.
41. Wranke A, Wedemeyer H. Antiviral therapy of hepatitis delta virus infection - progress and challenges towards cure. Curr Opin Virol. 2016;20:112–8.
42. Lin HH, Lee SS, Yu ML, Chang TT, Su CW, Hu BS, Chen YS, Huang CK, Lai CH, Lin JN, Wu JC. Changing hepatitis D virus epidemiology in a hepatitis B virus endemic area with a national vaccination program. Hepatology. 2015; 61(6):1870–9.
43. Loebstein R, Mahagna R, Maor Y, Kurnik D, Elbaz E, Halkin H, Olchovsky D, Ezra D, Almog S. Hepatitis C, B, and human immunodeficiency virus infections in illicit drug users in Israel: prevalence and risk factors. Isr Med Assoc J. 2008;10(11):775–8.
44. Sandler SG, Nath N, Biger Y. Seroepidemiology of hepatitis B virus in Israel. Results of a pilot study in Jerusalem. Am J Epidemiol. 1977;106(1):76–82.

18

Seroprevalence of hepatitis B virus infection and associated factors among healthcare workers in northern Tanzania

Elichilia R. Shao[1,2,4,5*], Innocent B. Mboya[2], Daniel W. Gunda[3], Flora G. Ruhangisa[1,2], Elizabeth M. Temu[1], Mercy L. Nkwama[1], Jeremia J. Pyuza[1,2], Kajiru G. Kilonzo[1,2], Furaha S. Lyamuya[1,2] and Venance P. Maro[2]

Abstract

Background: Hepatitis B virus infection is a global health problem with the highest prevalence in East Asia and Sub-Saharan Africa. The majority of infected people, including healthcare workers are unaware of their status. This study is aimed to determining seroprevalence of hepatitis B virus infection and associated factors among healthcare workers in northern Tanzania.

Methods: This cross-sectional study included 442 healthcare workers (HCWs) from a tertiary and teaching hospital in Tanzania before the nationwide hepatitis B vaccination campaign in 2004. Questionnaire- based interviews were used to obtain detailed histories of the following: demographic characteristics; occupation risks such splash and needle stick injuries or other invasive procedure such as intravenous, intramuscular or subcutaneous injections; history of blood transfusion and surgeries, as well as HCWs'knowledge of HBV. Serological markers of HBV were done using Laborex HBsAg rapid test. Serology was done at zero months and repeated after six months (bioscienceinternational.co.ke/rapid-test-laborex.html HBsAg Piazzale-milano-2, Italy [Accessed on November 2017]). Chi-square (χ^2) tests were used to compare proportion of HBV infection by different HCWs characteristics. Multivariable logistic regression was used to determine factors associated with HBV infection.

Results: A total of 450 surveys were sent out, with a 98.2% response rate. Among the 442 HCWs who answered the questionnaire, the prevalence of chronic hepatitis B virus infection was 5.7% (25/442). Only 50 (11.3%) of HCWs were aware of the HBV status. During the second HBsAg testing which was done after six months one participant sero-converted hence was excluded. Adjusted for other factors, history of blood transfusion significantly increased the odds of HBV infection (OR = 21.44, 95%CI 6.05, 76.01, $p < 0.001$) while HBV vaccine uptake was protective against HBV infection (OR = 0.06, 95%CI 0.02, 0.26, $p < 0.001$). The majority of HCWs with chronic HBV infection had poor to fare knowledge about HBV infection but this was not statistically significant when controlled for confounding.

Conclusions: Prevalence of HBV among health care workers was 5.7% which is similar to national prevalence. Although the response rate to take part in the study was good but knowledge on HBV infection among HCWs was unsatisfactory. History of blood transfusion increased risks while vaccine uptake decreased the risk of HBV infection. This study recommends continues vaccinating HCWs together with continues medical education all over the country. We also recommend documentation of vaccination evidence should be asked before employment of HCWs in order to sensitize more uptakes of vaccinations. Although we didn't assess the use of personal protective equipment but we encourage HCWs to abide strictly on universal protections against nosocomial infections.

Keywords: Hepatitis B virus, Risk factors, Healthcare workers, Tanzania

* Correspondence: elichilia2004@yahoo.co.uk
[1]Internal Medicine Department, Kilimanjaro Christian Medical Center, P.O.Box3010, Moshi, United Republic of Tanzania
[2]Institute of Public Health, Community Health Department, Kilimanjaro Christian Medical University College, P.O.Box2240, Moshi, Tanzania
Full list of author information is available at the end of the article

Background

About 240 million people are living with chronic hepatitis B virus (HBV) infection worldwide, majority of them from low-and middle income countries. HBV is a major causative agent of chronic hepatitis and can cause liver cirrhosis and hepatocellular carcinoma [1, 2]. Most people including health care workers (HCWs) are unaware of their HBV serological statues. Antiretroviral drugs like Entecavir and tenofovir reduces aggressiveness of the disease and reduces mortality [3–5]. However, due to unawareness of HBV status in most of developing countries, implementation of treatment strategies has not been well established. HCWs have an increased risk of hepatitis B infection about four times as compared to general population because of their direct contact with infectious material such as blood, needle stick injuries and other contaminated body fluids [6]. Prevalence of hepatitis B infection among general population in Tanzania is 6%; HCWs are at increased risk to infection because of their working environment [7–10].About 3 million HCWs globally, experience percutaneous exposure to blood pathogens each year. Those who perform invasive procedures such as surgeons, emergency medicine expertise, laboratory personnel and pathologists shown to have higher prevalence as compared to others specialities. The different in prevalence can be explained by the different degree of exposures to the risks [11].Other factors which might increase the risks to contract HBV includes medical procedures such as surgeries, blood and blood products transfusions, endoscopic procedures and dialysis. Sexual behaviour such as unprotected sex with multiple partners in endemic area is among important an aspect which is associated with increased risks to HBV infection [12].

Risk factors to contract HBV have been studied by different authors basing on the questions such as HBV is presents in high concentration in blood fluids. Hepatitis B virus infection is more infectious than HIV, can cause liver cancer; can stay alive out of blood for seven days [13]. Factors such as unprotected sexual intercourse, blood transfusion, needle stick injuries, splash, intravenous and/or intramuscular injections, and unvaccinated population has been associated with increased risks toward hepatitis B infections [14, 15]. Knowledge about HBV infection has a big impact on a person's decision toward preventive measures hence can influence sero-positivity. There is growing body of literature in Tanzania on HBV infection but there limited information on associated risk factors among HCWs. This article contributes information on the sero-prevalence and associated risk factors towards HBV infection among HCWs.

Methods

Setting and study population

This study was conducted among HCWs from January 2015 to December 2016 at Kilimanjaro Christian Medical Centre (KCMC) in Moshi, Tanzania. KCMC is a referral and teaching hospital which serve over 15 million people in Northern Tanzania. It is a huge complex facility with 800 inpatients, 1852 students and 1300 employees [16]. Study design, sampling and participant's recruitmentA total of 442 HCWs aged 18 years and above participated in this study; making a response rate of 98.2%.Enrolled was done in two categories, those from surgical and none surgical departments. Our research team had one group dealing with workers at night shift and the other group with day shift. Category A: Surgical departments (that included Obstetrics and Gynaecology, General surgery, Orthopaedic surgery, Eye Nose and Throat, Urology and Eye department). Category B: None-surgical department (that included medical, paediatrics, dermatology, emergency/OPD, Orthopaedic workshop, as well as laboratory and administration). After consent, HCWs participated in this study were voluntary enrolled consecutively until desired number was met. Consenting participants were asked to fill a self-administered questionnaire after they had provided a blood sample. Unique identification number was used to link participant's laboratory results and the questionnaire. The standardized questionnaire was used to collect information like demographic data, years at work, medical history, education level and professional. The questionnaire had four sections: demographic and academic characteristics, knowledge of the risk factors for HBV infection and vaccine and history of accidental exposure to blood and its products. A detailed history was obtained from the HCW on hepatitis B vaccination and infection history, any occupation risks such (splash and needle stick injuries). Other invasive procedure such as Intravenous (IV), Intramuscular (IM), subcutaneous (SC) injections, blood transfusion history, surgery and all these findings were all recorded. Other risk behaviours like multiple sexual partners without using protection were also asked from the participants. Knowledge measurements were done by adopting an approach used by Abdul-Hakeem et al. 2016. In this study, each correct response "answered Yes") to the 16 questions on knowledge on HBV infection and vaccination was scored one mark while none or don't know was scored zero. The total scores were converted to percentage and grouped as poor (< 50%), fair (50–74%) and good (≥75%) [17].

Ethical issues

Ethically this study was approved by KCMUCo Research and Ethics Review Committee with permission number 916. All participants signed an informed consent. Counselling and blood collection were done at the private room and no names was used instead identification numbers was used. All questionnaires were stored in the secure room at KCMC while data for this study were secured in a password protected laptop. Those who tested positive for HBsAg were counselled and channelled to the physician for further evaluation. Benefit for the study participantTo date no antiviral treatment is licensed for treating chronic HBV infection in Tanzania. But knowing your hepatitis status is a step towards monitoring and treatment. We invited family members and sexual partners of infected participants for testing and further assessment.

Serological analysis for HBV

Under aseptic technique about (4 mL) of blood was obtained through venipuncture from all subjects using sterilized disposable 5 ml syringes and 20 gauge needles by laboratory technologist who is experienced phlebotomist at KCMC.All collected blood samples were tested using Laborex HBsAg rapid test [18], Milan Italy for positive hepatitis B surface antigen. The test strip was removed from the foil pouch and dipped into the specimen for at least 10 s until thoroughly wet. Then the strip was removed from the specimen and placed in the dry flat surfaces to wait for the red lines to appear. Interpretation of the results: Positive; when two distinct red lines appears, one line in the control region (C) and another one in the test region (T).Negative: One red line appears in the control (C). No apparent red or pink line appears in the test region (T). Invalid: Control line fails to appear. Quality control: appearance of red line in the control region (C) was the internal procedural control. It confirms sufficient specimen volume and correct procedure technique. For those which turned to be positive participants were counselled and informed to come and repeat the test after six months. Those who still turned positive after six months were termed chronic hepatitis B infected HCWs. All the methods used were proved by laboratory standard in Tanzania.

Statistical analysis

Data were entered in Microsoft excel and analysis was performed using STATA version 13.1. Descriptive analysis was performed whereby numeric variables were summarized using measures of central tendency and the corresponding measures of dispersion. Categorical variables were summarized using frequency and percentages. Chi-square ($\chi 2$) test was used to compare the prevalence of hepatitis B infection by participant characteristics. Multivariable logistic regression (Odds ratio and the corresponding 95% confidence interval) was used to determine factors associated with hepatitis B infection among health care workers at KCMC. A cut-off point of 10% ($p > 0.1$) was used to select variables to be included in further analysis. After controlling for potential confounders, variables with $p < 0.05$ was considered statistically associated with hepatitis B infection.

Results

Patient characteristics

A total of 442 health workers was included in this study. The median age of participants was 37 years and interquartile range (IQR) of 31–46 years. About 189 (43%) were aged above 40 years while 165 (37.3%) were aged between 30 and 39 years. Over 270 (60%) of all participants were females and above three quarter 344 (78.5%) had tertiary education level. Also 275 (62%) of all participants were married or cohabiting 378 (85.7%) The majority of the participants were from none-surgical 248(56.1%) departments (Table 1). Majority of HCWs who were seropositive for HBsAg were mainly medical doctors 6(24%), nurses 5(20%) followed by laboratory personnel 4(16%) and ward attendants 4(16%).

Exposure to the risk of HBV infection

Among all participants in this study, 145 (32.8%) had history of surgery, 121 (27.4%) had history of blood splash to the eyes or mouth, 367 (83.0%) every had intravenous injections, 387 (87.6%) had intramuscular injections, 167 (37.9%) had a history of needle stick injury, less than 10% had history of invasive procedure such as endoscopy and about 8% ever had blood transfusion. Prevalence of HBV vaccine uptake in this study was 67.4% (Table 2).

Prevalence of HBV

Prevalence of chronic HBV infection (HBsAg) was reported to be 5.7% (25/442). During the second testing which was done after six months one participant sero-converted hence was excluded. There was no significant difference in contracting HBV between males and females ($\chi 2 = 0.432$; $p = 0.51$). Majority of seropositive HCWs were > =30 yrs. but the difference was not significant ($p = 0.93$). Years of practices were not associated with seropositivity ($p = 0.13$), Table 3.

Sixty percent of chronic HBV infection was found among none-surgical HCWs with no statistical significance difference between these groups ($p = 0.47$). We found that history of blood transfusion and surgery were associated with seropositivity (p-value = 0.001 and 0.003) respectively. Likewise, history of vaccine uptake was also associated with HBV infection ($p < 0.001$), Table 4. Among HCWs who were positive for HBV, 6(20%) were medical doctors; two from none-surgical department and the rest were from surgical department (Tables 4).

Knowledge on HBV infection

The median knowledge score was 62.5% and interquartile range of 50–75%. Nearly a quarter (25.4%) of all

Table 1 Demographic characteristics of HCWs at KCMC Moshi Tanzania 2016/17 ($N = 442$)

Variable	Frequency (n)	Percentage (%)
Age (years)		
Median (IQR)	37	(31, 46)
20–29	88	19.9
30–39	165	37.3
40+	189	42.8
Sex		
Male	166	37.6
Female	276	62.4
Education level		
Primary	27	6.2
Secondary	67	15.3
Tertiary	344	78.5
Marital status		
Single	140	31.7
Married/Cohabiting	275	62.2
Widow/Divorced	27	6.1
Religion*		
Christian	378	85.7
Muslim	63	14.3
Area of residence		
Rural	187	42.3
Urban	255	57.7
Department		
Surgical	194	43.9
Non-surgical	129	29.2
Outpatient/Emergency	21	4.8
Administrative/Supportive	42	9.5
Laboratory/Pathology	56	12.7
Specialty		
Doctor	130	29.4
Nurse	137	31.0
Laboratory	37	8.4
Other health professions	56	12.7
Administrative/ Supportive staff	82	18.6
Work in clinical area		
Yes	350	79.2
No	92	20.8
Years of practice*		
< 5	91	21.0
≥5	342	79.0

*Frequency do not tally to the total due to missing information on religion

Table 2 Exposure to the risk of HBV infection among healthcare workers at KCMC Moshi Tanzania 2016/17

Variable	n	%
History of surgery		
Yes	145	32.8
No	297	67.2
History of blood splash to the eyes or mouth		
Yes	121	27.4
No	319	72.2
Don't know	2	0.5
Ever had intravenous injections		
Yes	367	83.0
No	75	17.0
Ever had intramuscular injections		
Yes	387	87.6
No	55	12.4
History of needle stick injury*		
Yes	167	37.9
No	274	62.1
History of invasive procedure such as endoscopy*		
Yes	40	9.1
No	399	90.5
Don't know	2	0.5
Ever had blood transfusion		
Yes	34	7.9
No	399	92.2
HBV Vaccine uptake*		
Yes	295	67.4
No	143	32.6

*Frequency do not tally to the total due to missing values

participants had good knowledge and about half (49.6%) had fair knowledge about HBV infection (Table 5). Only 17.9% of participants were aware, that unprotected sex with multiple partners was the risks for HBV infection. Most of the participants (85.9%) correctly identified that HBV is more contagious than HIV, while (91.3%) knew that there is effective and safe hepatitis B vaccine. About (23.4%) of HCWs wrongly understood that you can get HBV infection from DNA-recombinant vaccine.

Factors associated with HBV

Several factors showed significant association with HBV seropositivity in the crude analysis. This includes history of surgery (OR = 3.31, 95%CI 1.44, 7.58), history of blood transfusion (OR = 19.24, 95%CI 7.64, 48.47) and having good knowledge on HBV infection (OR = 0.18, 95%CI 0.04, 0.82) compared to those with poor knowledge (Table 6). The final model was adjusted for religion, history of surgery, history of blood transfusion, HBV

Table 3 Demographic characteristics associated with Hepatitis B virus infection among HCWs at KCMC Moshi, Tanzania 2016/17

Variable	Total	Serology n (%)		χ^{2*}	p-value
		Negative	Positive		
Age (years)				0.278	0.93**
20–29	88	84 (95.4)	4 (4.6)		
30–39	164	154 (93.9)	10 (6.1)		
40+	187	176 (94.1)	11 (5.9)		
Sex				0.432	0.51
Male	166	155 (93.4)	11 (6.6)		
Female	273	259 (94.9)	14 (5.1)		
Education level				1.835	0.30**
Primary	26	24 (92.3)	2 (7.7)		
Secondary	67	61 (91.0)	6 (9.0)		
Tertiary	342	325 (95.0)	17 (5.0)		
Marital status				4.212	0.14**
Single	140	128 (91.4)	12 (8.6)		
Married/Cohabiting	272	259 (95.2)	13 (4.8)		
Widow/Divorced	27	27 (100)	0 (0)		
Religion				3.992	0.05
Christian	375	357 (95.2)	18 (4.8)		
Muslim	63	56 (88.9)	7 (11.1)		
Area of residence				1.001	0.32
Rural	186	173 (93.0)	13 (7.0)		
Urban	253	241 (95.3)	12 (4.7)		
Department				2.653	0.47**
Surgical	193	183 (94.8)	10 (5.2)		
Non-surgical	129	122 (96.1)	5 (3.9)		
Outpatient/Emergency	21	19 (90.5)	2 (9.5)		
Administrative/Supportive	42	39 (92.9)	3 (7.1)		
Laboratory/Pathology	56	51 (91.1)	5 (8.9)		
Specialty				3.076	0.48**
Doctor	130	123 (94.6)	7 (5.4)		
Nurse	135	130 (96.3)	5 (3.7)		
Laboratory	37	33 (89.2)	4 (10.8)		
Other health professions	56	52 (92.9)	5 (7.1)		
Administrative/ Supportive staff	81	76 (93.8)	5 (6.2)		
Work in clinical area				1.229	0.32**
Yes	348	326 (93.7)	22 (6.3)		
No	91	88 (96.7)	3 (3.3)		
Years of practice				2.756	0.13**
< 5	91	89 (97.8)	2 (2.2)		
≥5	339	316 (93.2)	23 (6.8)		

*Chi-square; **p-value by Fisher's exact estimation

vaccine uptake and HBV knowledge. History of blood transfusion and HBV vaccine uptake were the only factors associated with HBV infection (Table 6). HCWs with history of blood transfusion had over 21 times the higher odds of HBV infection compared to those without transfusion (OR = 21.44, 95%CI 6.05, 76.01) while

Table 4 HBV infection by past exposure to potential risk factors among HCWs at KCMC Moshi Tanzania 2016/17

Variable	Total	Serology n (%)		χ^{2*}	p-value
		Negative	Positive		
History of surgery*				8.897	0.003**
Yes	144	129 (89.6)	15 (10.4)		
No	295	285 (96.6)	10 (3.4)		
History of blood splash to the eyes or mouth*				2.137	2.26**
Yes	121	111 (91.7)	10 (8.3)		
No	316	301 (95.3)	15 (4.7)		
Don't know	2	2 (100)	0 (0)		
Ever had intravenous injections*				0.446	0.78**
Yes	365	343 (94.0)	22 (6.0)		
No	74	71 (96.0)	3 (4.0)		
Ever had intramuscular injections*				0.414	0.75**
Yes	386	363 (94.0)	23 (6.0)		
No	53	51 (96.2)	2 (3.8)		
History of needle stick injury*				0.452	0.50
Yes	165	154 (93.3)	11 (6.8)		
No	273	259 (94.9)	14 (5.1)		
History of invasive procedure such as endoscopy*				0.151	1.00**
Yes	39	37 (94.9)	2 (5.1)		
No	397	374 (94.2)	23 (5.8)		
Don't know	2	2 (100)	0 (0)		
Ever had blood transfusion*				65.946	< 0.001
Yes	34	22 (64.7)	12 (35.3)		
No	399	388 (97.2)	11 (2.8)		
HBV Vaccine uptake*				23.420	< 0.001**
Yes	293	289 (98.6)	4 (1.4)		
No	142	125 (88.0)	17 (12.0)		
Knowledge on HBV infection				5.886	0.04**
Poor	108	98 (90.7)	10 (9.3)		
Fair	217	204 (94.0)	13 (6.0)		
Good	114	112 (98.2)	2 (1.8)		

*Frequencies do not tally to the total due to missing values either in the outcome variable (serology status) or the independent variables, this also causes variations from numbers in Table 4; **p-value by Fisher's exact estimation

those with history of vaccine uptake were protected against HBV infection (OR = 0.06, 95%CI 0.02, 0.26).

Discussion

This study was carried out to determine seroprevalence of chronic HBV infection and risk factors associated with seropositivity among HCWs in a Tanzanian tertiary and teaching hospital. Serological testing revealed that 5.7% of HCWs were chronic carriers while 94.3% were susceptible to HBV infection. These workers were infected with hepatitis B virus were counselled and given feedbacks to do a further workout and channelled to the respective clinics. The response rate of 98.2% out of 450 study participants was achieved because of the good relationship between participants and research team. There were two groups of research team, night team dealing with those workers at night shift and day team for day shift. These HCWs might transmit HBV infection to the patients as well as their family members. We counselled them to bring their sexual partners and children to be tested for HBV infection. A similar study conducted in Mwanza among HCWs showed the prevalence of 7%, but was almost twice the prevalence among pregnant women, and less than pregnant women who were HIV positive and blood donors. The slight different in this study as compared to the previous study by

Table 5 Knowledge on HBV infection and vaccination among healthcare workers at KCMC* Moshi Tanzania 2016/17 (N = 442)

Statement	n	%
1. HBV can be transmitted through sexual intercourse	354	80.6
2. HBV can be transmitted through unprotected sex with multiple sexual partner	79	17.9
3. HBV is the most contagious blood-borne pathogen through accidental exposure to blood and its products	379	85.9
4. Injury with needle contaminated with infected blood is the risk factor of HBV infection	391	89.1
5. Contact with broken skin with infected body fluid is a risk factor of HBV infection	365	83.0
6. Contact to mucous membrane in the eyes or mouth with infected blood is a risk factor of HBV infection	321	72.8
7. Contact of healthy skin with infected blood or products is a risk factor of HBV infection	144	32.7
8. HBV infection can be transmitted through oral-fecal route	134	30.4
9. HBV could be transmitted from a mother to her fetus	290	65.9
10. Immunoglobulin against HBV can prevent infection after exposure	233	53.0
11. There is a vaccine which is available against HBV	398	91.3
12. If Hepatitis B vaccination is taken properly as per protocol, it is more than 95% protective against HBV infection	340	77.3
13. The minimum numbers of doses for a complete primary HBV vaccination is three doses	278	63.0
14. An immune response test should be done after HBV vaccination	199	46.5
15. Antibody titer above 10 IU is the recommended amount which is protective	138	31.3
16. You can get HBV infection from recombinant HBV vaccination	103	23.4
Knowledge level		
Median (IQR)	62.5	(50, 75)
Poor	109	24.7
Fair	219	49.6
Good	114	25.8

*Frequency and percentage distributions of only those who answered correctly in these statements

Table 6 Univariate and multivariate logistic regression for factors associated with HBV infection among HCWs at KCMC Moshi, Tanzania 2016/17

Variable	Total	+Ve serology n (%)	cOR* (95%CI)	*p*-value	aOR** (95%CI)	*p*-value
Religion						
Muslim	63	7 (11.1)	Reference		Reference	
Christian	375	18 (4.8)	0.40 (0.16, 1.01)	0.05	1.05 (0.26, 4.18)	0.94
History of surgery						
No	295	10 (3.4)	Reference		Reference	
Yes	144	15 (10.4)	3.31 (1.44, 7.58)	0.005	2.31 (0.77, 6.90)	0.13
Ever had blood transfusion						
No	399	11 (2.8)	Reference		Reference	
Yes	34	12 (35.3)	19.24 (7.64, 48.47)	< 0.001	21.44 (6.05, 76.01)	< 0.001
HBV Vaccine uptake*						
No	142	17 (12.0)	Reference		Reference	
Yes	293	4 (1.4)	0.10 (0.03, 0.31)	< 0.001	0.06 (0.02, 0.26)	< 0.001
Knowledge on HBV infection						
Poor	108	10 (9.3)	Reference		Reference	
Fair	217	13 (6.0)	0.62 (0.26, 1.47)	0.28	0.48 (0.14, 1.65)	0.25
Good	114	2 (1.8)	0.18 (0.04, 0.82)	0.03	0.38 (0.07, 2.09)	0.25

*Crude odds ratio; **Adjusted odds ratio

Mueller et al. might be explained by the methodological components. The recent mini review article by Kilonzo et al., presented the national prevalence of HBsAg among general population to be 6% which is similar to our study [7, 15–17, 19–22]. In this study we only did HBsAg and not anti-HBc + which might tell us the HCWs who cleared the infection [9].

In a similar study in the neighbouring country, Uganda showed the prevalence of 8.1%. Other studies of HBsAg among HCWs reported the prevalence ranging from 1.5–8.1% in Nigeria, Rwanda and Uganda. Nigeria is among the countries with high prevalence in the general population when compared to Tanzania. Furthermore in the study which was done by Abiola et al., the prevalence of HBsAg was as low as 1.5% which might be explained by the low sample size of participants as compared to our study [23–26]. Majority of seropositive HCWs in this study were medical doctors, nurses followed by laboratory personel. This was different from Uganda study by Ziraba et al., who showed that nursing assistant was leading followed by laboratory technicians [6]. The difference might be explained by the different levels of risk of exposure to potential risks environment. Out of six medical doctors who were seropositive for HBV, 66.7% were from none surgical-department as compared to the rest who were from the surgical departments. Different level of potential risks exposure might affect the prevalence of the particular nosocomial infection. However, we asked about the sexual history, but it was prone to bias because the researchers were from the same institutions. But we believe it was controlled in one way or another because no names were used instead identification number was used. Other factors such as ethnicity, region of origin, years of practices and religion might influence the chance of HCWs to be infected or not. In the current study we could not compare the seroprevalence among different religious groups because of unequal distribution of this group [27].

In this study we found greater than 19-fold higher risk for HCWs to acquire HBV infection if they ever had the blood transfusion (odds ratio 19.24, $p < =0.001$). This might be explained by the methodology used for screening as well as the incubation period of the disease. Furthermore the occult HBV infection can explain this because for the donated blood is always screened by doing HBsAg and hepatitis core-antibody but studies have revealed an HBV DNA positivity rate of 0–15% when HBV nucleic acid testing (NAT) was employed [20].Therefore in order to reduce transfusion transmissible infection we might opt for HBV nucleic acid instead of our traditional methods which has some challenges due to the pathogenesis of HBV. The study found higher rate of HBV infection in older workers as compared to younger ones. This could be explained by more exposure during life time to among older HCWs or less exposure among younger HCWs.Also, we learned that majority about 92% of seropositive HCWs have more than five years working experience which support the assumption of more exposure. Our findings are similar to the study by Mueller et al., in Lake Zone Mwanza Tanzania [8]. Many years in practice means increased occupational exposure in clinical services which increases the chances of acquiring HBV infection, this in similar in other studies [6, 26].

This study was conducted before nationwide vaccination campaign against all HCWs which was started January 2015. Therefore, the vaccination coverage was 19.6% which was similar with the one reported in Mwanza study among HCWs. We could not get complete information about the number of doses and if they did screening before vaccination. These vaccinations were done among HCWs who were involved in different research projects runned by KCMC in collaboration with international agents. This proportion seems to be higher as compared to other studies in SSA [8, 26, 27]. There was association between vaccination uptake and seropositive of HBV infection. After adjustment for the confounding effect, HBV vaccine uptake remained to be statistically significant. Although the vaccination coverage in this study was very low when compared to developed countries in Europe [28, 29].In resource limited settings like Tanzania, most HBV infection take place during childhood due to high endemicity nature of hepatitis B virus infection. This has been supported by our study which didn't show any association between age and years of practices, which means many HCWs, has been infected during childhood rather adulthood as occupational hazards. HCWs can be infected via occupational exposure to infected clients or vice versa. Therefore, vaccination is still the main soul for the control of new infections in this region.

The percentage of good knowledge was very low as compared to the studies in Nigeria which was 69% [19]. About half of the participants didn't know that antibody titer should be done after finishing the third dose. This was similar to other studies in Cameroon where about one-fourth of the HCWs had good knowledge about hepatitis B infection and vaccination [15]. Good level of knowledge was protective towards hepatitis B infection, therefore those with poor knowledge has more chances of been infected. After adjusting for other confounders there was no statistical significant between knowledge level and seropositivity for HBV. We had about 20% of HCWs who responded that hepatitis B cannot be transmitted through unprotected sexual intercourse. About quarter of the participants responded that HBV cannot be transmitted through contact with mucous membrane in the eyes and mouth. Furthermore 30 % of participants wrongly perceived that hepatitis B can be transmitted through feaco-oral route. It seems that many HCWs are not knowledgeable about many aspects of HBV from its pathogenesis, transmission as well as preventive measures. The percentage of poor knowledge is this study was higher than the study in Northwest Ethiopia [11]. One third of the workers didn't understand that HBV can be transmitted from mother to child; surprisingly 10% of the HCWs had no information about the availability of effective and safe hepatitis B vaccine. More than 50 % of HCWs didn't understand that they needed to do antibody titters after finishing three doses of hepatitis B vaccination. Quarter of the workers responded that you could get hepatitis B infection from the DNA recombinant Hepatitis B vaccine. This is less than the finding from South Korea where about 56% of family medicine residence declined to take hepatitis B infection because of the fear that they might develop infection from the given recombinant vaccine [5, 25]. Continues medical education is very crucial for HCWs, but vaccination against HBV infection remain the most effective and safe method toward elimination of hepatitis B infection.

Limitations of the study

We only did HBsAg therefore we cannot conclude about the number of HCWs exposed to hepatitis B virus which can be done by HBsAb. Since we were dealing with our colleagues, some questions might be too personal, hence respond, will have bias. Also, most of the information given by HCWs was prone to recall bias due to time interval between the event and the time we asked questions. Questions like unprotected sex with multiple sexual partners faced some challenges where some HCWs didn't respond.

Conclusions

The prevalence of hepatitis B virus infection among healthcare workers was high. Majority of HCWs were exposed to potential risks of infection but only small percentages were vaccinated against HBV. These findings highlight the need for continues improving the working environment of HCWS by provision of hepatitis B vaccination. Continuous medical education to HCWs should be reinforced to improve their knowledge in order to protect them. Vaccination program to HCWs should continue to be implemented either mandatory or optional framework. It is the right time to expand this study to involve other health facilities in order to be able to formulate evidenced national data for action. Although we didn't assess the use of personal protective equipment but we encourage strictly abide on universal protections against nosocomial infections.

Abbreviations

AIDS: Acquired Immune Deficiency Syndrome; ALT: Alanine aminotrasnferase; Ant-HBC: Antibody to Hepatitis B core protein; Ant-HBe: Antibody to Hepatitis B e antigen; Anti HBC IgM: Hepatitis B core protein antibody immunoglobulin mu; Anti-HBs: Antibody Hepatitis B surface; APRI score: Aspartate and platelets ratio index score; AST: Aspartate aminotrasnferase; CBC: Complete Blood Count; cccDNA: covalently closed circular DNA; CDC: Centre for Disease Control; CHB: Chronic hepatitis B; CI: Confidence interval; CMV: Cytomegalovirus; DNA: Deoxyribonucleic acid; HbcAg: Hepatitis B core antigen; HbeAg: Hepatitis B e antigen; HBIG: Hepatitis B immune globulin; HbsAb: Hepatitis B surface antibody; HBsAg: Hepatitis B surface antigen; HBV: Hepatitis B Virus; HbxAg: Hepatitis B Virus X antigen; HCC: Hepatocellular Carcinoma; HCV: Hepatitis C Virus; HCW's: Health Care Workers.

Acknowledgments

We thank all nurses at KCMC Obstetrics Gynaecology outpatients for their great job of performing phlebotomy for all the participants. We thank all healthcare workers of KCMC (including post-graduate students) of KCMUCo for taking part in this study.

Consent to publication

Not Applicable.

Funding

Not Applicable.

Author's contributions

ES and VM conceptualized the study and FL, FR and KK participated in its design and coordination.ES, DG and VM drafted the manuscript. ES, JP, ET and MN collected the data and carried out serological assays. IM, ET, MN and ES contributed to the analysis and interpretation of data. IM wrote the statistical analysis and results sections. All authors have read and approved the final manuscript.

Competing interests

The authors declare that they have no competing interests.

Author details

[1]Internal Medicine Department, Kilimanjaro Christian Medical Center, P.O.Box3010, Moshi, United Republic of Tanzania. [2]Institute of Public Health, Community Health Department, Kilimanjaro Christian Medical University College, P.O.Box2240, Moshi, Tanzania. [3]CUHAS, P.O.Box 1370, Mwanza, Tanzania. [4]Better Human Health Foundation, P.O.Box1348, Moshi, Tanzania. [5]Imagedoctors International, P.O.Box16341, Arusha, Tanzania.

References

1. Bian T, Yan H, Shen L, Wang F, Zhang S, Cao Y, Zhang S, Zhang Y and Bi S (2013) Change in Hepatitis B Virus Large Surface Antigen Variant Prevalence 13 Years after Implementation of a Universal Vaccination Program in. 87(22): 12196–12206.
2. WHO (2016). Global health sector strategy on viral hepatitis 2016–2021. Toward ending viral hepatitis. www.who.int/hepatitis/strategy2016-2021/ghss-hep/en/. [Accessed on November 2017].
3. Ashraf H, Alam NH, Rothermundt C, Brooks A, Bardhan P, Hossain L, Salam MA, Hassan MS, Beglinger C, Gyr N. Prevalence and risk factors of hepatitis B and C virus infections in an impoverished urban community in Dhaka. Bangladesh. 2010:1–8.
4. La Torre G, Scalingi S, Garruto V, Siclari M, Chiarini M, Knowledge MA. Attitude and Behaviours towards recommended vaccinations among healthcare workers. Multidisciplinary digital publishing institute. In Healthcare. 2017;5(1):13.

5. Ko K, Kim S, Kim SH, Son KY, Lee J, Lee DR. Knowledge, current status, and barriers toward healthcare worker vaccination among family medicine resident participants in a web-based survey in Korea. Korean journal of family medicine 2017 1;38(1):21–27.
6. Ziraba AK, Bwogi J, Namale A, Wainaina CW, Mayanja-Kizza H. Sero-prevalence and risk factors for hepatitis B virus infection among health care workers in a tertiary hospital in Uganda. BMC Infect Dis. 2010;10:191.
7. Kilonzo SB, Gunda DW, Mpondo BC, Bakshi FA, Jaka H. Hepatitis B virus infection in Tanzania: current status and challenges. Journal of tropical medicine. 2018;2018.
8. Sabria R, Kilewo C, Said A. Seroprevalence of hepatitis B virus infection among antenatal clinic attendees at a tertiary hospital in Dar Es Salaam, Tanzania. Tanzania Journal of health research. 2014;16(1).
9. Mueller A, Stoetter L, Kalluvya S, Stich A, Majinge C, Weissbrich B, Kasang C. Prevalence of hepatitis B virus infection among health care workers in a tertiary hospital in Tanzania. BMC Infect Dis 2015 :23;15:386.
10. Debes JD, Kayandabila J, Pogemiller H. Knowledge of hepatitis B transmission risks among health Workers in Tanzania. Am J Trop Med Hyg 2016 ; 4;94(5):1100–1102.
11. Abeje G, Azage M. Hepatitis B vaccine knowledge and vaccination status among health care workers of Bahir Dar City Administration, Northwest Ethiopia: a cross sectional study. BMC Infect Dis. 2015;15:30.
12. Malewezi B, Omer SB, Mwagomba B, Araru T. Protecting health workers from nosocomial hepatitis B infections: a review of strategies and challenges for implementation of hepatitis B vaccination among health workers in sub-Saharan Africa. Journal of epidemiology and global health. 2016;6(4):229–41.
13. Schillie S, Murphy TV, Sawyer M, Ly K, Hughes E, Jiles R, de Perio MA, Reilly M, Byrd K, Ward JW, Centers for disease control and prevention (CDC). CDC guidance for evaluating health-care personnel for hepatitis B virus protection and for administering postexposure management. MMWR Recomm Rep 2013 Dec 20;62(10):1–9.
14. Hassan M, Awosan KJ, Tinau NS, Burodo K, Yakubu A, Oche MO. Knowledge, risk perception and hepatitis B vaccination status of healthcare workers in Usmanu Danfodiyo University teaching hospital, Sokoto Nigeria. J Public Health Epidemiol. 2016;8(4):53–9.
15. Tatsilong HO, Noubiap JJ, Nansseu JR, Aminde LN, Bigna JJ, Ndze VN, Moyou RS. Hepatitis B infection awareness, vaccine perceptions and uptake, and serological profile of a group of health care workers in Yaoundé, Cameroon. BMC Public Health. 2016;15:706.
16. https://www.kcmc.ac.tz [Accessed on November 2017].
17. Al-Hazmi AH. Knowledge, attitudes and practice of dentists concerning the occupational risks of hepatitis B virus in Al Jouf Province, Saudi Arabia. Nigerian journal of clinical practices. 2015;18(3).
18. bioscienceinternational.co.ke/rapid-test-laborex.html HBsAg Piazzale-milano-2, Italy [Accessed on November 2017].
19. Abiola AH, Oke OA, Balogun MR, Olatona FA, Adegbesan-Omilabu MA. Knowledge, attitude, and practice of abortion among female students of two public senior secondary schools in Lagos mainland local government area, Lagos state. Journal of Clinical Sciences. 2016;13(2):82.
20. WHO (2015).HepatitisB [https://www.who.int/medicentre/factsheets/fs204/en]. Accessed on November2017.
21. Matee MI, Magesa PM, Lyamuya EF. Seroprevalence of human immunodeficiency virus, hepatitis B and C viruses and syphilis infections among blood donors at the Muhimbili National Hospital in Dar Es Salaam, Tanzania. BMC Public Health 2006 30; 6(1):21.
22. Manyahi J, Msigwa Y, Mhimbira F, Majigo M. High sero-prevalence of hepatitis B virus and human immunodeficiency virus infections among pregnant women attending antenatal clinic at Temeke municipal health facilities, Dar Es Salaam, Tanzania: a cross sectional study. BMC pregnancy and childbirth. 2017;17(1):109.
23. Bwogi J, Braka F, Makumbi I, Mishra V, Bakamutumaho B, Nanyunja M, Opio A, Downing R, Biryahwaho B, Lewis RF. Hepatitis B infection is highly endemic in Uganda: findings from a national serosurvey. African health sciences. 2009;9(2).
24. Nouetchognou JS, Ateudjieu J, Jemea B, Mbanya D. Accidental exposures to blood and body fluids among health care workers in a referral Hospital of Cameroon. BMC research notes. 2016;9(1):94.
25. WHO (2015). Guidelines for the prevention, care and treatments of persons with chronic hepatitis B infection. March 2015. [Accessed on November 2017].
26. Braka F, Nanyunja M, Makumbi I, Mbabazi W, Kasasa S, Lewis RF. Hepatitis B infection among health workers in Uganda: evidence of the need for health worker protection. Vaccine. 2006;24(47):6930–7.
27. Meschi S, Schepisi MS, Nicastri E, Bevilacqua N, Castilletti C, Sciarrone MR, Paglia MG, Fumakule R, Mohamed J, Kitwa A, Mangi S. The prevalence of antibodies to human herpesvirus 8 and hepatitis B virus in patients in two hospitals in Tanzania. J Med Virol. 2010;82(9):1569–75.
28. Rachiotis G, Goritsas C, Alikakou V, Ferti A, Roumeliotou ANASTASIA. Vaccination against hepatitis B virus in workers of a general hospital in Athens. La Medicina del lavoro. 2005;96(1):80–6.
29. Maltezou HC, Poland GA. Vaccination policies for healthcare workers in Europe. Vaccine. 2014;32(38):4876–80.

19

Risk factors for hepatitis E virus seropositivity in Dutch blood donors

Sofie H. Mooij[1], Boris M. Hogema[2], Anna D. Tulen[1*], Wilfrid van Pelt[1], Eelco Franz[1], Hans L. Zaaijer[2], Michel Molier[2] and Agnetha Hofhuis[1]

Abstract

Background: A marked increase of hepatitis E cases has recently been observed in the Netherlands. Causes of the (re-)emergence of hepatitis E virus (HEV) and exact sources and routes of transmission of HEV infection are currently unknown. We aimed to identify risk factors for HEV seropositivity.

Methods: Using the Wantai EIA, 2100 plasma samples of blood donors from all over the Netherlands aged 18-70 years were tested for anti-HEV IgG antibodies. A questionnaire on socio-demographic characteristics, health, and potential risk factors for HEV exposure was sent to these participants.

Results: The overall IgG-seroprevalence was 31% (648/2100) and increased with age. Several food products were independently associated with IgG-seropositivity in a multivariate analysis adjusting for age and gender among 1562 participants who completed the questionnaire: traditional Dutch dry raw sausages called "cervelaat", "fijnkost", "salami" and "salametti" which are generally made from raw pork and beef (aOR 1.5; 95%CI 1.2-1.9), frequent consumption of bovine steak (aOR 1.3; 95%CI 1.0-1.7), and frequent consumption of smoked beef (aOR 1.3 95%CI 1.0-1.7). Although not frequently reported, contact with contaminated water was also a risk factor for seropositivity (aOR 2.5; 95%CI 1.5-4.4). Lower seroprevalence was associated with eating raspberries, going out for dinner, and contact with wild animals and dogs.

Conclusion: Several pork food products, mainly dry raw sausages, and contact with contaminated water were associated with past HEV infection in the Netherlands. Further investigation is needed into the prevalence and infectivity of HEV in these risk factor food products, as well as investigation of the production methods and possible origin of HEV-contamination within these sausages, e.g. very small amounts of pork liver, pig-derived blood products as food additive, or the pork muscle tissue.

Keywords: Hepatitis E, Risk factors, Zoonoses, Blood donors, Netherlands

Background

Hepatitis E has long been considered a disease mainly affecting developing countries and returning travelers [1]. However, over the last decade it became clear that autochthonous infection with hepatitis E virus (HEV) is common in some industrialized countries, and that in Europe the incidence has increased by ten times [2–4]. The vast majority of HEV-infections in Western Europe are caused by genotype 3, which is known to be a zoonosis with domestic swine, wild boar and deer as the main reservoir [3, 5]. Autochthonous cases may be caused by transmission via food (e.g., consumption of contaminated undercooked meat from pigs, pig-derived blood products used in the food industry, or wild animals) or the environment (e.g., contaminated water or direct contact with infected animals and their feces) [5, 6], but the exact sources and routes of transmission are unknown. Recently Slot et al. demonstrated that the incidence of HEV infection is significantly lower among donors not eating meat compared with meat-eating donors [7]. Moreover, reasons for the current increase of HEV infections in the Netherlands and surrounding countries [4], as observed among young Dutch blood

* Correspondence: lola.tulen@rivm.nl
[1]Epidemiology and surveillance unit, Centre for Infectious Disease Control Netherlands, National Institute for Public Health and the Environment (RIVM), Antonie van Leeuwenhoeklaan 9, 3721 MA Bilthoven, the Netherlands
Full list of author information is available at the end of the article

donors [8] and in our national sentinel laboratory surveillance system [9], are currently unclear.

The Netherlands is densely populated by both humans and livestock, including 5.8 million fattening pigs, 1.2 million breeding sows and 5.6 million piglets in 2015 [10]. HEV genotype 3 RNA has been detected in 53% of pig farms, 4% of wild boar feces, and 17% of surface water samples in the Netherlands from 2004 to 2006 [6]. A recent study (2017) showed that residential proximity to pig farms was not associated with increased presence of antibodies against HEV in humans who live in a pig livestock-dense area in the South of the Netherlands [11], which might indicate a primarily food-borne transmission of HEV. Recently in the Netherlands HEV-RNA genotype 3 was detected in a large majority of "liver sausages" (43/55) and "pork liver pâté samples" (12/15) [12], and in 33/36 nonheated liquid pig derived blood products and 7/24 spray dried powder products from pig blood [13]. Other developed countries also reported a broad distribution of HEV-RNA genotype 3 in pork products, among others in liver sausages and dry raw sausages [14–19]. It is currently unclear whether these pork products contained viable and infectious virus, however the level of HEV-RNA-positive samples among common food products is alarmingly high.

Most human infections by HEV genotype 3 are asymptomatic, or present with mild self-limiting symptoms of hepatitis including jaundice, fever, abdominal pain and fatigue. Most symptomatic cases occur among middle-aged and elderly men [1]. In immunocompromised patients there is a risk of chronic infection which can quickly progress to liver cirrhosis, with substantial morbidity and mortality [1]. Therefore, prevention of HEV infection is especially urgent in these high-risk groups. Increased insight in the epidemiology, risk factors and transmission routes of HEV are essential to be able to formulate and implement food regulatory and public health measures for prevention of hepatitis E infection. In this study, we aimed to identify risk factors for HEV seropositivity.

Methods

Data collection

This study was performed among blood donors aged 18-70 years who donate plasma at the Dutch blood bank Sanquin. A random selection of 2100 plasma samples collected between March and May 2016 from unique blood donors from all over the Netherlands was tested using an anti-HEV IgG assay (Wantai Biological Pharmacy Enterprise Co., Ltd) according to the manufacturer's instructions. Borderline reactive samples were considered negative. A detailed, self-administered questionnaire regarding socio-demographic characteristics, health, and potential risk factors for HEV-infection e.g., comprehensive food consumption habits with a focus on meat, contact with (contaminated) water and animals, travel history and outdoor activities was sent to these tested blood donors by post. The recall period used to assess risk factors in the questionnaire was set to 2 months, assuming that food consumption and other habits are relatively constant throughout large periods in life.

Written informed consent was obtained from each participant included in the study. The link between laboratory results, personal identifiers (including postal address) and study number was exclusively retained at Sanquin. Anonymized data were processed and analyzed by the researchers at the National Institute for Public Health and the Environment (RIVM). The ethics committee of Sanquin approved this study, titled "HEV-ID" (acronym for Hepatitis E Virus In Donors).

Statistical analyses

Associations between determinants and anti-HEV IgG seropositivity (as dichotomous outcome, i.e., yes or no) were assessed using Chi-square tests and univariate logistic regression analyses. Variables associated with seropositivity with a P-value < 0.15 in univariate logistic regression analyses were entered into a multivariate logistic regression model. Gender and categories of age were forced into each model, because these were significant confounders of seropositivity being related to many variables that were associated with seropositivity. Subsequently, variables were removed by backward selection to yield a model with the most relevant independent risk factors. With the variables that were included in the multivariate model, additional multivariate logistic regression analyses were performed to assess whether there could be a dose-response effect for food products, by assessing the risk of participants who reported consumption of food products more frequently. Frequency of food consumption was categorized as "often" (several times per week), "regularly" (once per week), "occasionally" (several times per month) and "sometimes" (less than once per month). P-values were 2-sided and considered significant at $P < 0.05$. All analyses were performed using Stata software package version 14.

Results

Characteristics of the study population and anti-HEV IgG seroprevalence

The overall seroprevalence of anti-HEV IgG was 31% (648 out of 2100 donors) and increased with age. In total, 1562/2100 (74%) donors who were invited into the study completed the questionnaire and could be included in the current analyses. The 538 donors who did not respond to the questionnaire were significantly relatively more often male and significantly younger than the 1562 included participants. Out of 1562 participants who responded to the questionnaire, 1234 (79%) were male and the median age was 58 years (interquartile range 51-64 years); 488 (31%) were anti-HEV IgG-seropositive, and the seroprevalence was highest in males above 60 years of age (39%). There were no significant differences in seropositivity between men and women (32% and 28%, respectively). Seropositivity was similar to results from a previous study by Sanquin among Dutch blood donors [8], in which donations collected in 2011/2012 were analyzed for anti-HEV IgG antibodies using the same assay as in the current study. Nearly all participants reported to be born in the Netherlands (98%) and around half of them reported a high level of education (college or university). In general, the study population consisted of healthy individuals with relatively few health complaints or underlying diseases (Table 1).

Risk factors for hepatitis E seropositivity

Factors related to food, contact with water, animals and lifestyle

In the univariate analyses, age, level of education, lifestyle-related factors like alcohol consumption and going out for dinner, multiple food products including pork products containing pork liver and pork products without pork liver, and factors related to contact with contaminated water or animals, showed a significant association with anti-HEV IgG-seropositivity (Table 2).

In multivariate analyses, gender and categories of age were forced into each model, because these were significant confounders of seropositivity being related to many variables that were associated with seropositivity. Seropositivity significantly increased with age, with an adjusted odds ratio (aOR) of 2.4 (95% confidence interval (CI) 0.8-7.2) for age category > 60 years compared to < 30 years. Consumption of traditional Dutch dry sausages generally made from raw pork and beef (called "cervelaat", "fijnkost", "salami" and "salametti") was also significantly associated with seropositivity with an aOR of 1.5 ($n = 889$, 95% CI 1.2-1.9). These traditional Dutch dry raw sausages do not contain pork liver. However, consumption of traditional Dutch dry raw sausages was significantly correlated with consumption of pork liver pâté and liver sausages ($P < 0.001$).

Also, consumption of "other dry sausages" showed an aOR of 1.6 (95% CI 1.1-2.4). This was an open question and included very diverse both national and international (local) meat products (fuet ($n = 12$, 10.3%), saucisson d'Ardenne ($n = 10$, 8.6%), French dry sausage ($n = 9$, 7.8%), grilled sausage ($n = 8$, 6.9%) and smoked bacon called "katenspek" ($n = 6$, 5.2%) were most reported). Bovine steak and smoked beef were also significantly associated ($n = 891$; aOR 1.3 95% CI 1.0-1.7) and ($n = 455$; aOR 1.3 95% CI 1.0-1.7), respectively. Furthermore, among 65 persons (4.3% of our subjects) who reported to have had contact with contaminated water (i.e., removed water from a stable, worked with a septic tank or had contact with sewage) we observed increased OR's (aOR 2.5; 95% CI 1.5-4.4). Interestingly, consumption of raspberries and going out for dinner more than once per month showed a negative association on seropositivity, as well as having had contact with dogs or wild animals in the last 2 months. Consumption of seafood (e.g., mussels, oysters) showed no significant association with anti-HEV IgG seropositivity.

We assessed whether there could be a dose-response effect for food products, using the same variables as included in the previous multivariate model. Within the group of participants who reported consumption of traditional Dutch dry raw sausages, risk significantly increased for participants who reported consumption most frequently as compared to those reported least frequently ($n = 233$; aOR 2.5 95% CI 1.8-3.6) and ($n = 192$; aOR 1.1 95% CI 0.8-1.7), respectively.

Health-related factors

None of the health-related factors assessed were significantly associated with anti-HEV IgG-seropositivity in univariate or multivariate analyses adjusting for gender and age and mostly cases per factor were low. In a multivariate model assessing health complaints in the last 2 months only reporting diarrhea less than 3 times per day was borderline significantly associated ($n = 125$; aOR 1.6; 95% CI 1.0-2.5; $P = 0.052$), reporting diarrhea more than 3 times per day was not significantly associated to seropositivity. There were no significant associations between underlying diseases in the last 6 months reported by > 50 participants and seropositivity.

Discussion

With this study we identified risk factors for past hepatitis E infection that were primarily related to consumption of (pork) food products and contact with contaminated water. The pork food products "traditional Dutch dry raw sausages (called "cervelaat", "fijnkost", "salami" and "salametti")" and "other dry sausages" were independent risk factors for hepatitis E seropositivity. These dry raw sausages are generally eaten unheated, as they are meant to be consumed sliced on bread. While it is currently unknown whether these products, generally made from raw pork and beef, indeed contain (infectious) HEV, transmission of HEV via raw [20] and processed [21] pork products has been suggested before and is biologically plausible. To completely inactivate HEV it is necessary to heat food to an internal temperature of 70° Celsius for at least 20 min [22]. Production and consumption of raw dry sausages like the Dutch "cervelaat",

Table 1 Demographic characteristics of 1562 study participants: blood donors from all over the Netherlands 2016

	Overall (*n* = 1562)		Anti-HEV IgG-negative (*n* = 1074)		Anti-HEV IgG-positive (*n* = 488)	
	N	%	N	%	N	%
Total	1562	100	1074	68.8	488	31.2
A. Socio-demographic characteristics						
Gender						
Men	1234	79.0	837	77.9	397	81.4
Women	328	21.0	237	22.1	91	18.7
Median age in years (IQR)	58.1	(50.7-63.9)	56.9	(49.6-63.1)	60.2	(54.5-65.4)
Age groups						
< 30 years of age	24	1.5	20	1.9	4	0.8
30-40 years of age	75	4.8	68	6.3	7	1.4
40-50 years of age	255	16.3	194	18.1	61	12.5
50-60 years of age	561	35.9	392	36.5	169	34.6
> 60 years of age	647	41.4	400	37.2	247	50.6
Country of birth[a]						
The Netherlands	1519	97.8	1041	97.6	478	98.2
Any other country	35	2.3	26	2.4	9	1.8
Level of education[b]						
Low/intermediate	780	50.3	508	47.7	272	56.1
High	770	49.7	557	52.3	213	43.9
B. Health-related characteristics						
Previous HEV-test for medical reasons[c]						
No	1368	88.4	927	87.2	441	90.9
Yes	8	0.5	6	0.6	2	0.4
Unknown	172	11.1	130	12.2	42	8.7
Health complaints last 2 months[f]						
Fever	56	3.7	39	3.7	17	3.6
Nausea	54	3.5	41	3.9	13	2.7
Diarrhea < 3 times/day	125	8.2	83	7.9	42	8.8
Stomach ache	91	6.0	67	6.4	24	5.0
Headache	282	18.4	216	20.5	66	13.8
Tiredness	306	20.1	228	21.7	78	16.4
Dark urine	73	4.8	52	5.9	21	4.4
Itching	163	10.6	116	11.0	47	9.8
Neurological symptoms	75	4.9	51	4.9	24	5.0
Underlying diseases last 6 months[f]						
High blood pressure	214	13.7	143	13.3	71	14.5
Diabetes	51	3.3	30	2.8	21	4.3
High cholesterol	126	8.1	82	7.6	44	9.0
Alcohol consumption[d]						
< =6 drinks per week	938	62.5	661	64.2	277	58.7
> 7 drinks per week	564	37.6	369	35.8	195	41.3
Smoking[e]						
No, never	710	46.8	503	48.4	207	43.4
Past smoker	665	43.8	445	42.8	220	46.1

Table 1 Demographic characteristics of 1562 study participants: blood donors from all over the Netherlands 2016 *(Continued)*

	Overall (*n* = 1562)		Anti-HEV IgG-negative (*n* = 1074)		Anti-HEV IgG-positive (*n* = 488)	
	N	%	N	%	N	%
Current smoker	142	9.4	92	8.9	50	10.5
Traveling history (lifetime)						
Asia	687	44.0	479	44.6	208	42.6
Africa	528	33.8	362	33.7	166	34.0
North-America	585	37.5	410	38.2	175	35.9
Central/South-America	417	26.7	306	28.5	111	22.8
C. Consumption of meat[g]						
No, never	5	0.3	5	0.5	0	0
No, only in the past	24	1.6	20	1.9	4	0.8
Yes	1518	98.1	1036	97.6	482	99.2

[a]8 missing values
[b]12 missing values
[c]14 missing values
[d]60 missing values
[e]45 missing values
[f]shown if reported by > = 50 participants
[g]15 missing values

"fijnkost", "salami" and "salametti" mainly takes place in Europe. The sausages can vary slightly between different regions and countries. In general, this type of sausages is produced from uncooked, cured pork belly meat mixed with beef. Regularly, the mix of raw meat is fermented, filled in a porous synthetic casing and is hung out to dry until it is solid enough to cut. Remarkably, the pork food products that we found to be risk factors for anti-HEV IgG seropositivity do not contain pork liver tissue. In our study, pork food products that do contain liver ("liver sausages" and "pork liver pâté") were only independent risk factors in the univariate model, and were no longer significant risk factors in the multivariate model. However, a correlation between the consumption of pork food products that do contain liver and consumption of traditional Dutch dry raw sausages was found. Usually diaphragm tissue is added to Dutch dry raw sausages, which could lead to the presence of very small amounts of liver in the sausages [23].

Besides the liver, HEV is present as well in blood and muscle tissue of pigs during infection with the virus [24, 25]. Pig meat might contain HEV due to the presence of residual blood (1-2%), however the viral dose is probably low due to the small amount of blood. In addition, pig-derived blood products (e.g. spray-dried plasma, red blood cells, globin and collagen) might be used as additives to enhance color and texture of the sausages [26]. Unfortunately, we could not measure the consumption of pig-derived blood products directly, as it is not possible to query about blood products in the questionnaire. Whether HEV transmission might occur following consumption of products containing pig-derived blood products is still unclear. Recently, HEV RNA was detected in 33/36 porcine blood product samples, which are produced for application in the food industry. According to Boxman et al. the liquid blood products are not heat-treated during production, leaving the HEV detected most likely infectious [13]. A study of Szabo et al. detected HEV RNA in 20% of raw sausages that did not contain liver [19]. Furthermore, it might be possible that traditional Dutch dry raw sausages contain residual infectious virus as they do not have a long period of curing, while pork liver sausages are often briefly cooked during processing. It might be possible that although pork products containing liver contain a high amount of HEV RNA, this is associated with heat-inactivated virus particles that are unable to cause infection. Possibly, the level of HEV RNA in the traditional Dutch dry raw sausages is much lower, but associated with viable virus particles.

We found that eating bovine steak and smoked beef were positively associated with seropositivity. However, participants who reported consumption of bovine steak were more likely to report consumption of traditional Dutch dry raw sausages (61.8% versus 50.4%; OR 1.6 95% CI 1.3-2.0), and consumption of "other dry sausages" (10.2% versus 5.2%; OR 2.1 95% CI 1.4-3.1). Also, participants who reported consumption of smoked beef were more likely to report consumption of traditional Dutch dry raw sausages (65.7% versus 53.3%; OR 1.7 95% CI 1.3-2.1).

Participants who reported to have had contact with contaminated water (i.e., removed water from a stable, worked with a septic tank or had contact with sewage) showed relatively high seroprevalence (46%). This is not an unexpected finding, as it is known that in sewage water,

Table 2 Univariate and multivariate analyses of risk factors associated with anti-HEV IgG-seropositivity among 1562 blood donors. Only variables with $P < 0.05$ in uni- and/or multivariate analyses are shown. The multivariate logistic regression model, adjusted for age and gender, was based on backward selection of variables with $P < 0.15$ in univariate analyses

	Univariate analyses			Multivariate analyses	
	Seropositivity n/N (%)	OR (95% CI)	*P*-value	aOR (95% CI)	*P*-value
A. General factors					
Gender			0.121		0.692
Men	397/1234 (32.2%)	1.0		1.0	
Women	91/328 (27.7%)	0.8 (0.6-1.1)		0.9 (0.7-1.3)	
Age groups in years			< 0.001		< 0.001
< 30	4/24 (16.7)	1.0		1.0	
30-40	7/75 (9.3)	0.5 (0.1-1.9)		0.4 (0.1-1.5)	
40-50	61/255 (23.9)	1.6 (0.5-4.8)		1.2 (0.4-3.8)	
50-60	169/561 (30.1)	2.2 (0.7-6.4)		1.7 (0.5-5.1)	
> 60	247/647 (38.2)	3.1 (1.0-9.1)		2.4 (0.8-7.2)	
Level of education			0.002		
Low/intermediate	272/780 (34.9%)	1.0			
High	213/770 (27.7%)	0.7 (0.6-0.9)			
Alcohol consumption			0.042		
< =6 drinks per week	277/938 (29.5%)	1.0			
> 7	195/564 (34.6%)	1.3 (1.0-1.6)			
Traveling history to South America			0.016		
No	377/1145 (32.9%)	1.0			
Yes	111/416 (26.6%)	0.7 (0.6-0.9)			
B. Food consumption last 2 months					
Pork food products					
Pork tenderloin			0.009		
No	247/867 (28.5%)	1.0			
Yes	241/695 (34.7%)	1.3 (1.1-1.7)			
Pork chop			0.001		
No	311/1083 (28.7%)	1.0			
Yes	177/479 (37.0%)	1.5 (1.2-1.8)			
Pork belly			0.037		
No	267/915 (29.2%)	1.0			
Yes	221/647 (34.2%)	1.3 (1.0-1.6)			
Smoked sausage			0.044		
No	201/702 (28.6%)	1.0			
Yes	287/860 (33.4%)	1.2 (1.0-1.6)			
Raw or dry sausages					
Farmer sausage			0.006		
No	340/1159 (29.3%)	1.0			
Yes	148/403 (36.7%)	1.4 (1.1-1.8)			
Traditional Dutch dry raw sausages[a] ("salami" "salametti" "cervelaat" "fijnkost")			< 0.001		< 0.001
No	176/673 (26.2%)	1.5		1.0	
Yes	312/889 (35.1%)	1.3 (1.2-1.9)		1.5 (1.2-1.9)	
Liver cheese/ Leberkäse			0.001		

Table 2 Univariate and multivariate analyses of risk factors associated with anti-HEV IgG-seropositivity among 1562 blood donors. Only variables with $P < 0.05$ in uni- and/or multivariate analyses are shown. The multivariate logistic regression model, adjusted for age and gender, was based on backward selection of variables with $P < 0.15$ in univariate analyses *(Continued)*

	Univariate analyses			Multivariate analyses	
	Seropositivity n/N (%)	OR (95% CI)	*P*-value	aOR (95% CI)	*P*-value
No	371/1267 (29.3%)	1.0			
Yes	117/295 (39.7%)	1.6 (1.2-2.1)			
Pork liver slices			0.001		
No	408/1370 (29.8%)	1.0			
Yes	80/192 (41.7%)	1.7 (1.2-2.3)			
Other dry sausages[e]			0.033		0.022
No	438/1436 (30.5%)	1.0		1.0	
Yes	50/126 (39.7%)	1.5 (1.0-2.2)		1.6 (1.1-2.4)	
Spreadable pork					
Regional raw pork sausage "Brabantse metworst"			0.036		
No	471/1526 (30.9%)	1.0			
Yes	17/36 (47.2%)	2.0 (1.0-3.9)			
Tea sausage			0.017		
No	467/1518 (30.8%)	1.0			
Yes	21/44 (47.7%)	2.1 (1.1-3.7)			
Pâté / liver sausage[b]			0.011		
No	197/704 (27.9%)	1.0			
Yes	291/858 (33.9%)	1.3 (1.1-1.6)			
Beef					
Steak			0.023		0.022
No	189/671 (28.2%)	1.0		1.0	
Yes	299/891 (33.6%)	1.3 (1.0-1.6)		1.3 (1.0-1.7)	
Smoked beef					0.020
No	318/1107 (28.7%)	1.0	0.001	1.0	
Yes	170/455 (37.4%)	1.5 (1.2-1.9)		1.3 (1.0-1.7)	
Ox sausage			0.021		
No	375/1254 (29.9%)	1.0			
Yes	113/308 (36.7%)	1.4 (1.0-1.8)			
Fruits and vegetables					
Raspberries			0.031		0.039
No	429/1328 (32.3%)	1.0		1.0	
Yes	59/234 (25.2%)	0.7 (0.5-1.0)		0.7 (0.5-1.0)	
C. Food outside the home					
Restaurant visit			0.003		0.009
< 1 time per month	234/667 (35.1%)	1.0		1.0	
> 1 time per month	234/868 (28.0%)	0.7 (0.6-0.9)		0.7 (0.6-0.9)	
D. Contact with water or animals in the last 2 months					
Contact with contaminated water[c]			0.008		0.001
No	458/1497 (30.6%)	1.0		1.0	
Yes	30/65 (46.2%)	1.9 (1.2-3.2)		2.5 (1.5-4.4)	
Contact with dogs			0.066		0.013

Table 2 Univariate and multivariate analyses of risk factors associated with anti-HEV IgG-seropositivity among 1562 blood donors. Only variables with $P < 0.05$ in uni- and/or multivariate analyses are shown. The multivariate logistic regression model, adjusted for age and gender, was based on backward selection of variables with $P < 0.15$ in univariate analyses *(Continued)*

	Univariate analyses			Multivariate analyses	
	Seropositivity n/N (%)	OR (95% CI)	*P*-value	aOR (95% CI)	*P*-value
No	214/632 (33.9%)	1.0		1.0	
Yes	274/930 (29.5%)	0.8 (0.7-1.0)		0.7 (0.6-0.9)	
Contact with wild animals[d]			0.072		0.025
No	470/1481 (31.7%)	1.0		1.0	
Yes	18/81 (22.2%)	0.6 (0.4-1.0)		0.5 (0.3-0.9)	

aOR: Odds ratio adjusted for age and gender
95% CI: 95%-confidence interval
[a]Combined variable, created based on "salami", "salametti", "cervelaat" and "fijnkost"
[b]Combined variable, created based on several (open) questions
[c]Combined variable, created based on "removed water from a stable", "worked with a septic tank" and "contact with sewage"
[d]Combined variable based on contact with deer ($n = 7$), roe ($n = 4$), wild boar ($n = 0$), hare ($n = 7$), rat ($n = 9$), mice ($n = 54$), and/or other wild animals ($n = 21$)
[e]Variable based on an open question, including very diverse both national and international (local) meat products, five most reported: fuet ($n = 12$, 10.3%), saucisson d'Ardenne ($n = 10$, 8.6%), French dry sausage ($n = 9$, 7.8%), grilled sausage ($n = 8$, 6.9%), smoked bacon called "katenspek" ($n = 6$, 5.2%)

surface water and waste water, HEV RNA sequences can be detected that cluster with sequences found in autochthonous cases, swine and wildlife from the same geographical area [5]. Surprisingly, however, we found an independent negative association between anti-HEV IgG-seropositivity and contact with wild animals and dogs, which is in contrast with previous studies [27]. Participants that reported to go out for dinner more than once per month, or to have eaten raspberries in the last 2 months, were less likely to have had past hepatitis E infection, even after adjusting for age and gender. The level of education was significantly higher among participants who reported raspberry consumption and going out for dinner more than monthly, which were negatively associated with anti-HEV IgG-seropositivity. These negative associations with anti-HEV IgG-seropositivity may possibly be due to a higher level of education of these participants and may indicate a healthy lifestyle in general with less exposure to HEV due to for example less meat consumption and less occupations that involve contact with contaminated water. Indeed, a lower level of education was observed among participants who reported contact with contaminated water, which we identified as a risk factor for anti-HEV IgG-seropositivity.

As most infections go unnoticed, serology studies can provide valuable information on prevalence and incidence of HEV infection over different geographical regions and periods in time. In a recent review among European countries the prevalence of anti-HEV IgG antibodies in blood donors ranged from 1.3% (DIAPRO assay, Italy) to 52% (Wantai assay, France) [3]. Among Dutch blood donors seroprevalence was 27% among donations collected in 2011/2012 (Wantai assay) [28]. Our results of the anti-HEV IgG-seropositivity among blood donors in the Netherlands were very similar to those observed 5 years ago [8], i.e. high (31%), unrelated to gender and increasing with age. In this study, we tried to identify risk factors for anti-HEV IgG seropositivity instead of risk factors for acute infection, to identify risk factors associated with past infection and (eating) habits. Moreover, only 0.076% of 59,474 blood donations collected in 2013/2014 in the Netherlands was PCR positive for HEV-RNA [29]. However, in a group of PCR positive donors we would expect recent consumption of a food product with a particularly high risk for HEV, besides the regular (pork) eating habits. For example, in England and Wales consumption of pork pie and consumption of ham and sausages purchased from a major UK supermarket chain was found to be associated with indigenous infection [21].

Strengths of this study include the relatively large number of participants and the use of a detailed questionnaire specifically designed to assess risk factors for hepatitis E infection. A limitation is the discrepancy in timing between the moment of infection and recall period of the questionnaire. The recall period used to assess risk factors in the questionnaire was set on 2 months, thereby assuming that food consumption and other habits are relatively constant throughout large periods in life. The persistence of anti-HEV IgG antibodies after infection still needs further elucidation, as wide population variation in the extent and timing of anti-HEV IgG antibody decay is reported in literature, in which variation between antibody assays probably plays a large role [30]. In addition, the study population consisted of healthy individuals with relatively few health complaints or underlying diseases, and might therefore be not completely representative for the entire population.

Conclusions

In conclusion, this study identified specific raw pork food products and contact with contaminated water as independent risk factors for past hepatitis E infection. This confirms the general working hypothesis that consumption of pork products is the primary route of transmission in the Netherlands. Raw pork food products that do not contain liver might contain a low amount of infectious HEV, while pork food products that do contain liver might contain high levels of inactivated HEV. There could be some additional transmission of HEV via the environment but our study could show this only in case of intense exposure. Contact with animals seems not to be an important transmission route of HEV for the general population. Further studies are needed to elucidate the role of pig-derived blood products used as additives in food in HEV transmission and it should be determined whether the food products we found as a risk factor indeed contain infectious viral particles. As long as the reasons for the current increase in autochthonous hepatitis E cases in the Netherlands are not understood, it is important for people at risk of chronic hepatitis E infection (e.g., immunocompromised and transplant patients) to avoid eating raw or processed pork products and products that might contain pig-derived blood products.

Acknowledgements

The authors would like to thank the analysts of Sanquin for plasma sample testing; Willem Miellet for data entry; above all, we gratefully acknowledge all study participants for their co-operation.

Funding

This study was financed by, and conducted on behalf of Sanquin and the ministry of Health, Welfare and Sport of the Netherlands.

Authors' contributions

The study concept and design was developed by WvP, AH, BH and HZ. Acquisition of data was performed by BH, HZ, SM and AH. SM, AH and AT analyzed and interpreted the data. Statistical analysis was performed by SM, AT and AH. Drafting of the manuscript was performed by SM and AT. WvP and HZ obtained funding. BH and MM performed antibody testing. The study was supervised by AH, WvP and EF. All authors were involved in critical revision of the manuscript and all authors read and approved the final manuscript.

Competing interests

The authors declare that they have no competing interests.

Author details

[1]Epidemiology and surveillance unit, Centre for Infectious Disease Control Netherlands, National Institute for Public Health and the Environment (RIVM), Antonie van Leeuwenhoeklaan 9, 3721 MA Bilthoven, the Netherlands. [2]Sanquin Research, Department of Blood-borne Infections, Amsterdam, the Netherlands.

References

1. Kamar N, Bendall R, Legrand-Abravanel F, Xia NS, Ijaz S, Izopet J, et al. Hepatitis E. Lancet. 2012;379:2477–88.
2. European Centre for Disease Prevention and Control. Hepatitis E in the EU/EEA, 2005-2015. Stockholm: ECDC; 2017.
3. Lapa D, Capobianchi MR, Garbuglia AR. Epidemiology of hepatitis E virus in European countries. Int J Mol Sci. 2015;16:25711–43.
4. Adlhoch C, Avellon A, Baylis SA, Ciccaglione AR, Couturier E, de Sousa R, et al. Hepatitis E virus: assessment of the epidemiological situation in humans in Europe, 2014/15. J Clin Virol. 2016;82:9–16.
5. Van der Poel WH. Food and environmental routes of hepatitis E virus transmission. Curr Opin Virol. 2014;4:91–6.
6. Rutjes SA, Lodder WJ, Lodder-Verschoor F, Van den Berg HH, Vennema H, Duizer E, et al. Sources of hepatitis E virus genotype 3 in the Netherlands. Emerg Infect Dis. 2009;15:381–7.
7. Slot E, Zaaijer HL, Molier M, van den Hurk K, Prinsze F, Hogema BM. Meat consumption is a major risk factor for hepatitis E virus infection. PLoS One. 2017;12:e0176414.
8. Hogema BM, Molier M, Slot E, Zaaijer HL. Past and present of hepatitis E in the Netherlands. Transfusion. 2014;54:3092–6.
9. Dutch Working Group for Clinical Virology. Reports of Weekly Sentinel Surveillance System. Bilthoven: RIVM; 2016.
10. National Institute for Public Health and the Environment. Zoonotic Diseases Report. Bilthoven: RIVM; 2015.
11. van Gageldonk-Lafeber AB, van der Hoek W, Borlée F, Heederik DJ, Mooij SH, Maassen CB, et al. Hepatitis E virus seroprevalence among the general population in a livestock-dense area in the Netherlands. BMC Infect Dis. 2017;17:21.
12. National Institute for Public Health and the Environment. Hepatitis E Virus RNA in diverse pork liver products. Weekly overview of Infectious Disease Signals 25. Bilthoven: RIVM; 2016.
13. Boxman IL, Jansen CC, Hägele G, Zwartkruis-Nahuis A, Cremer J, Vennema H, et al. Porcine blood used as ingedrient in meat productions may serve as a vehicle for hepatitis E virus transmission. Int J Food Microbiol. 2017;257:225–31.
14. Heldt FH, et al. Hepatitis E virus in surface water, sediments, and pork products marketed in southern Brazil. Food Environ Virol. 2016;8(3):200–5.
15. Di Bartolo I, Angeloni G, Ponterio E, Ostanello F, Ruggeri FM. Detection of hepatitis E virus in pork liver sausages. Int J Food Microbiol. 2015;193:29–33.
16. Wilhelm B, Leblanc D, Houde A, Brassard J, Gagné MJ, Plante D, et al. Survey of Canadian retail pork chops and pork livers for detection of hepatitis E virus, norovirus, and rotavirus using real time RT-PCR. Int J Food Microbiol. 2014;185:33–40.
17. Berto A, Grierson S. Hakze- van der Honing R, Martelli F, Johne R, Reetz J, et al. Hepatitis E virus in pork liver sausage, France. Emerg Infect Dis. 2013;19:264–6.
18. Mykytczuk O, Harlow J, Bidawid S, Corneau N, Nasheri N. Prevalence and molecular characterization of the hepatitis E virus in retail pork products marketed in Canada. Food Environ Virol. 2017;9:208–18.
19. Szabo K, Trojnar E, Anheyer-Behmenburg H, Binder A, Schotte U, Ellenbroek L, et al. Detection of hepatitis E virus RNA in raw sausages and liver sausages from retail in Germany using an optimized method. Int J Food Microbiol. 2015;215:149–56.
20. Colson P, Borentain P, Queyriaux B, Kaba M, Moal V, Gallian P, et al. Pig liver sausage as a source of hepatitis E virus transmission to humans. J Infect Dis. 2010;202:825–34.
21. Said B, Ijaz S, Chand MA, Kafatos G, Tedder R, Morgan D. Hepatitis E virus in England and Wales: indigenous infection is associated with the consumption of processed pork products. Epidemiol Infect. 2014;142:1467–75.
22. Barnaud E, Rogée S, Garry P, Rose N, Pavio N. Thermal inactivation of infectious hepatitis E virus in experimentally contaminated food. Appl Environ Microbiol. 2012;78:5153–9.
23. Puolanne E. Cooked sausages. Handbook of meat and processing. Wiley: New York; 2010. p. 313–77.
24. Bouwknegt M, Rutjes SA, Reusken CB, Stockhofe-Zurwieden N, Frankena K, de Jong MC, et al. The course of hepatitis E virus infection in pigs after contact-infection and intravenous inoculation. BMC Vet Res. 2009;5:7.

25. Williams TPE, Kasorndorkbua C, Halbur PG, Haqshenas G, Guenette DK, Toth TE, et al. Evidence of extrahepatic sites of replication of the hepatitis E virus in a swine model. J Clin Microbiol. 2001;39:3040–6.
26. Ofori JA, Hsieh YHP. The Use of Blood and Derived Products as Food Additives. In: El-Samragy Y editor. Food additive. InTech; 2012. https://doi.org/10.5772/32374.
27. Hartl J, Otto B, Madden RG, Webb G, Woolson KL, Kriston L, et al. Hepatitis E Seroprevalence in Europe: a meta-analysis. Viruses. 2016;8:211.
28. Slot E, Hogema BM, Riezebos-Brilman A, Kok TM, Molier M, Zaaijer HL. Silent hepatitis E virus infection in Dutch blood donors, 2011 to 2012. Euro Surveill. 2013;18:20550.
29. Hogema BM, Molier M, Sjerps M, de Waal M, van Swieten P, van de Laar T, et al. Incidence and duration of hepatitis E virus infection in Dutch blood donors. Transfusion. 2016;56:722–728.30.
30. Krain LJ, Nelson KE, Labrique AB. Host immune status and response to hepatitis E virus infection. Clin Microbiol Rev. 2014;27:139–65.

20

Seroprevalence and risk factors of recent infection with hepatitis E virus during an acute outbreak in an urban setting in Chad, 2017

Larissa Vernier[1,2†], Annick Lenglet[2*†], Boris M. Hogema[3], Ali M. Moussa[4], Cono Ariti[5], Simone Vollmer[1], Andrea Irwin[1], Prince Alfani[1], Sibylle Sang[2] and Charity Kamau[2]

Abstract

Background: From September 2016–April 2017, Am Timan, Chad, experienced a large HEV outbreak in an urban setting with a limited impact in terms of morbidity and mortality. To better understand HEV epidemiology in this context, we estimated the seroprevalence of anti-HEV antibodies (IgM and IgG) and assessed the risk factors for recent HEV infections (positive anti-HEV IgM) during this outbreak.

Methods: A serological survey using simple random sampling was implemented in Am Timan at the tail-end of the outbreak (sample size aim = 384 household). Household members provided us with blood samples and household heads answered questions around water, sanitation and hygiene practices and animal ownership. Blood samples were tested for HEV IgG and IgM antibodies using Enzyme-Immune-Assay (EIA). We calculated weighted prevalence estimates and prevalence ratios (PRs) for possible risk factors for recent infection using multivariate Cox regression.

Results: We included 241 households (1529 participants). IgM prevalence decreased with age: 12.6% (< 5 years) to 4.3% (> 15 years). IgG prevalence increased with age: 23.5% (< 5 years) to 75.9% (> 15 years). Risk factors for recent HEV infections included: sharing the sanitation facility with other HHs (PR 1.72; 95%CI: 1.08–2.73), not systematically using soap for HW (PR 1.85; 95%CI: 1.30–2.63) and having animals sleeping inside the compound (PR 1.69; 95%CI: 1.15–2.50).

Conclusions: Evidence suggests that Am Timan was already highly endemic for HEV before the outbreak, potentially explaining the limited extent of the outbreak. Recent infection with HEV was linked to household level exposures. Future HEV outbreak response must include ensuring access to safe water, and reducing household level transmission through active hygiene and sanitation promotion activities.

Keywords: Hepatitis E virus, Chad, Seroepidemiologic studies, Risk factors, Disease outbreaks

Background

Hepatitis E virus (HEV) is a common cause of acute viral hepatitis worldwide [1]. Genotypes 1 and 2 of HEV are spread through fecal-oral transmission (from contaminated water supplies) and have been implicated in outbreaks in Asia, Africa, Latin America and the Middle East. In contrast, infection with HEV genotypes 3 and 4 are of zoonotic origin. Although the true burden of HEV globally remains unknown, it has been estimated that around 20 million of people are infected by genotype 1 and 2 annually, resulting in 3.4 million cases of symptomatic illness, 70,000 deaths and 3000 stillbirths annually [2]. The disease is usually self-limiting but severe cases can develop into fulminant hepatitis which can lead to neurological sequelae, spontaneous abortions and sometimes death. The overall case fatality rate (CFR) is estimated between 4 and 30%, but has been documented

* Correspondence: annick.lenglet@amsterdam.msf.org
†Larissa Vernier and Annick Lenglet contributed equally to this work.
[2]Médecins sans Frontières, Operational Center Amsterdam (OCA), Plantage Middenlaan 14, 1018DD Amsterdam, the Netherlands
Full list of author information is available at the end of the article

to reach up to 40% in pregnant women, particularly during the third trimester [3, 4].

Large outbreaks of HEV have been previously reported from sub-Saharan Africa, mostly in refugee and internally displaced persons (IDPs) settings in Sudan, Uganda, Kenya, South Sudan and Ethiopia [5–11]. It is known that HEV genotype 1 was implicated in the outbreaks reported from Sudan, South Sudan and Uganda [12–14]. Risk factors for HEV infection that were identified in previous outbreaks included the consumption of chlorinated surface water, handwashing in communal handwashing facilities, storing drinking water in wide-mouthed containers and having other household members previously presenting with jaundice, suggesting a level of household transmission [6, 8, 15]. There is also evidence from the outbreak in Uganda between 2007 and 2009 that person-to-person transmission was implicated in the propagation of the outbreak [16].

Chad experienced an HEV outbreak in 2004 in Goz Amer refugee camp in which 672 cases and 21 deaths of acute jaundice syndrome (AJS) were reported between June and August [17]. Between September 2016 and April 2017, a large urban outbreak of HEV genotype 1e spread in Am Timan, Chad [18]. During the course of the outbreak, 1443 cases of AJS were reported through community-based surveillance activities, and 100/250 AJS cases were confirmed as HEV infected by the Assure® Hepatitis E IgM rapid diagnostic test (RDT) from MP Diagnostics [18]. The overall AJS attack rate (AR) was estimated at 2% and three pregnant women died (2% of all pregnant women with AJS and 20% of hospitalized ones). It should be noted that active case finding for AJS was in place in this outbreak which is a very sensitive case definition, thus likely overestimating the true number of actual HEV infections. In this outbreak, risk factors for confirmed HEV infection included having at least two children below the age of 5 years living in the household, having another household member with jaundice and not always washing hands before meals, but the latter two were of limited statistical significance [18].

The Am Timan outbreak, though it was the largest documented in an urban setting in Sub-Saharan Africa, had a limited impact in terms of morbidity and mortality [18]. Previous outbreaks have reported higher ARs and more dramatic epidemic curves (particularly the refugee/IDP camp outbreaks in South Sudan and Uganda) [13, 14, 19]. In previous HEV outbreaks in sub-Saharan Africa, the CFR ranged from 1.5 to 17.8% and from 12.5 to 42.1% in overall population and pregnant women, respectively [20]. The reasons for the different epidemiological profiles of outbreaks of this genotype of HEV in sub-Saharan Africa remain unclear. Therefore, the outbreak in Am Timan, Chad, presented an opportunity to determine the seroprevalence of anti-HEV antibodies (IgM and IgG) in different age groups in March–April 2017 (the tail-end of the outbreak) and to assess the risk factors for recent HEV infections. We expected that these results would add the available evidence around HEV genotype 1 transmission in acute outbreak settings.

Methods

Study setting

The study was implemented between March 22 and April 27 2017 in Am Timan in the eastern part of the Salamat region in Chad. It is a town of approximately 65,000 residents (estimates by Médecins Sans Frontières (MSF), December 2016) and is home to a large semi-nomadic population.

Study design and sample size

We designed a cross-sectional population-based serological survey with a sample size large enough to precisely estimate seroprevalence estimates in three age groups: 0–4 years, 5–14 years and ≥ 15 years. In order to estimate a 50% level of seropositivity (IgM or IgG) with a simple random sampling (design effect = 1) and a precision of 5%, we required 382 persons per age group strata in order to have a representative sample. We estimated that the proportion of the population that represented these age groups was the following: 0–4 = 30%; 5–14 = 32%; ≥15 = 39% and the average household size was 5.5 persons. Thus, the number of households to include to reach this sample size in the least represented age group (0–4 years) was 232 households. Accounting for a refusal rate of 40%, we aimed to visit 384 households.

Participants

For the purpose of a hygiene kit distribution in December 2016, we created a comprehensive list of all, approximately 11,000, households in Am Timan. All households were assigned a unique number that consisted of a block number and house number respective to their location in the town. We used simple random sampling without replacement to select 384 households from this list using Excel 10.

The head of the household was any member of the sampled household who was 18 years or older, who could give accurate information on the household members and household exposures, who identified as the head of the household and who was present at the time of the study team visit. Household members were considered eligible for inclusion in the survey if they: were resident of that household since September 2016 (start of the outbreak), had not been absent for more than 2 weeks since September 2016, had not received blood or blood products in the 3 months before the survey, were in a health condition that would allow us to draw blood and agreed to participate.

Data collection

In each selected household, two questionnaires were administered: a household questionnaire and an individual questionnaire (Additional file 1: Household and Individual Questionnaires in French and Additional file 2: Household and Individual Questionnaires in French-English). The household questionnaire was administered to the household head and contained questions related to practices around drinking water sources, water treatment, water storage, sanitation facility, handwashing practices and animal ownership at the time of the interview. Observations of the water storage containers, sanitation facilities, handwashing practices and ownership of soap were also carried out. Additionally, the household head was asked to report any cases and deaths from AJS that had occurred in his/her family since the start of the outbreak in September 2016. The individual questionnaire included questions on sex, age and history of self-reported symptoms (including jaundice) since September 2016. It was administered to each household member older than 7 years, and to the parent/caretaker of the children younger or equal to 7 years old. Both questionnaires were completed on tablets using Open Data Kit (ODK).

Each participating individual was also asked to provide four milliliters (mL) of venous blood. Blood was drawn in sterile vacutainer tubes with ethylene diamine tetra acetic acid (EDTA) anticoagulant by professional healthcare staff. In infants difficult to handle, we collected less volume of blood or collected capillary blood from the heel in rare instances. Samples were then transported to the hospital laboratory where they were centrifuged. Serum samples were transported to Sanquin Diagnostic Service (The Netherlands) for the laboratory investigations. Transportation and storage of blood samples was done using a cold chain (2-8 °C).

Laboratory methods

All serum samples were tested for HEV IgG and IgM antibodies using Wantai Enzyme Immuno Assay (EIA) tests (Sanbio, Uden, the Netherlands) according to the instructions of the manufacturer. The IgM test is known to have a 99% specificity and a 75% sensitivity for clinical use which is the highest of the current commercial HEV serological tests available [21]. According to the manufacturer's instruction, the sensitivity for the IgG test is 100%. The specificity cannot be calculated easily as there is no gold standard test available and individuals may inverse seroconvert due to waning antibody titers. By testing samples from 2 to 3 year old children and adults the sensitivity was estimated to be 97.8% [22]. We defined a recent HEV infection as any person with detectable anti-HEV IgM. We defined a past HEV infection as any person with detectable anti-HEV IgG who did not have any detectable anti-HEV IgM.

HEV IgM positive samples were first re-tested for HEV IgG and IgM antibodies after high-speed centrifugation (10 min, 10,000×g). Samples that were repeatedly tested HEV IgM reactive were subjected to PCR using an in-house test with a 95% limit of detection of 10.3 IU/ml, as described previously [23]. Genotyping was performed for all samples with a viral load > 2000 IU/ml. ORF1 and ORF2 regions were amplified and sequenced as described previously [23].

Data analysis

Data analysis was performed using STATA version 12 and 13 (StataCorp, College Station, TX, USA). Overall and age-stratified prevalence estimates along with their 95% confidence interval (95%CI) were calculated for self-reported jaundice and HEV IgM and IgG antibodies. To infer the prevalence of the main health outcomes to the whole Am Timan population, adjusted prevalence estimates were calculated to account for clustering of cases within households. To be consistent with previous population distributions, the prevalence estimates were also weighted to account for the underrepresentation of children under 5 years (harder to get blood from) and men (more likely to be at work/absent during the interview and more likely to have travelled in the last 6 months and therefore not eligible for inclusion). Comparisons of prevalence estimates between age groups were performed by Chi-squared and Fisher's exact tests.

To determine household-level and individual exposures associated with recent HEV infections, we conducted a risk factor analysis comparing people with recent HEV infections (IgM+) to people without evidence of any HEV infection (IgM-/IgG-). Individuals with past HEV infections (IgM-/IgG+) were excluded because we could not distinguish the past infections having occurred during this outbreak from those having occurred in the more distant past. Although the presence of animals sleeping inside the compound was assessed separately for several animals i.e. chicken, dogs, cats, cows, goats, donkeys, pigeons and horses, a single variable was created to determine the association between the presence of any animals sleeping inside the compound and recent HEV infections. Using univariate Cox regression models, we estimated unadjusted prevalence ratios (PR) with their respective 95%CI for each exposure presenting enough variation among the Am Timan population (no category was included that was below 5% of total sample size). To identify risk factors and calculate adjusted PRs, we included exposures fulfilling the following three criteria in a multivariate Cox regression model: a) p-value < 0.2 in the univariate analysis, b) sufficient outcomes in each category of the exposure variable and c) sensible in terms of disease control recommendations. Variables to be kept in the final model were selected using the backward stepwise selection method (significance level < 0.05). All our models were adjusted for age and sex. All analyses accounted for the clustered and weighted survey design using Taylor-linearised adjustments to the standard errors as described in Heeringa et al. (2017) [24] and implemented using the svy commands in Stata.

Ethical considerations

The study was conducted in accordance with the Council for International Organisations of Medical Sciences (CIOMS) International Ethical Guidelines for Biomedical Research Involving Human Subjects and International Ethical Guidelines for Epidemiological Studies. The study protocol was approved by the Ethical Review Board of MSF (Study ID: 1646) and the Chadian Ministry of Health. Confidentiality and anonymity for participants were strictly respected for the duration of the study and in arising reports.

The head of the household was asked to provide informed written consent to conduct the household questionnaire and include household members in the study.

All available laboratory results were communicated back to participating individuals within 2 months after the end of data collection. All persons identified with acute infections were offered counselling and medical follow-up at the hospital if necessary.

Results

Overall findings

A total of 384 households were visited; 80 (20.8%) households were absent and 63 households (16.9%) refused to participate (Fig. 1). We included 241 HHs in the analysis (response rate: 63%). Households consisted of a median of 6 individuals (range: 1–37, mean = 7.4). Among the 1785 individuals living in the participating households, 174 (9.7%) were not eligible for inclusion in the study and 82 (4.6%) were absent on the day of the survey. We included 1529 participants in the final analysis.

The majority of the participating households (n = 143, 59.3%) relied on boreholes with or without an open tank as their source of drinking water. Most surveyed households (n = 228, 94.6%) reported that their water was chlorinated as this was being organized at all public water points as part of the HEV outbreak response. Most households (n = 184, 76.4%) used a pit latrine without a slab as their sanitation facility and of the 226

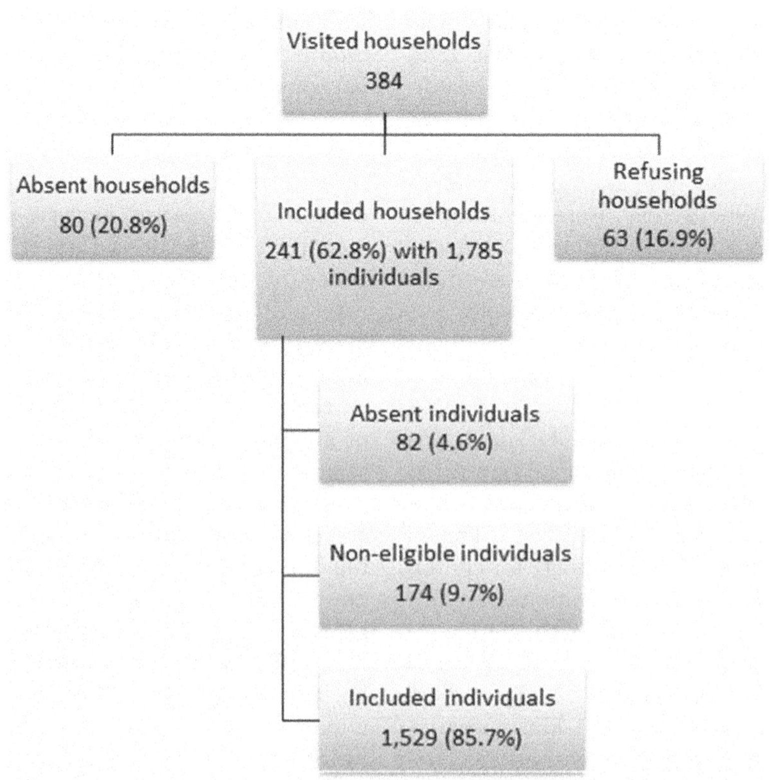

Fig. 1 Flowchart of household and study participants

latrines (99.1%) that were inspected, 69.0% ($n = 156$) were visibly dirty with feces. Thirty-seven AJS cases were reported between September 2016 and the day of the interview in 30 (12.5%) HHs. The cumulative AR for self-reported AJS during the outbreak was 2.1 per 100 persons (37/1785). Of these, two died, resulting in a AJS mortality rate and CFR of 0.1% (2/1785) and 5.4% (2/37), respectively.

Hepatitis E prevalence in Am Timan

The prevalence of recent HEV infection and past HEV infection was 7.7% (95%CI: 6.2–9.6) and 59.6% (95%CI: 56.3–62.8), respectively (Fig. 2; Additional file 3: Table S1). The prevalence of HEV recent infection was as high as 12.6% (95%CI: 8.7–17.9) among children under the age of 5 years and significantly decreased with age (Chi = 8.53; $p < 0.01$) (Fig. 2). On the contrary, the prevalence of past HEV infection significantly increased with age (Chi = 107.30; $p < 0.01$) and reached 75.9% (95%CI: 72.1–79.2) among individuals aged 15 years and older (Fig. 2). Recent infections were clustered in households with other recent infections; more than half of the recent infections ($n = 58$; 55.8%) were found in households with at least one more recent HEV infection.

The proportion of Am Timan population still susceptible to HEV was 32.7% (95%CI: 29.6–35.9). The proportion of susceptible persons significantly decreased with age (Chi = 82.18; $p < 0.01$). Among the population aged 5 years old and above, around 20% of the people were susceptible, whereas 63.9% (95%CI: 57.4–70.0) of the children under the age of 5 years old were still susceptible to HEV.

Out of 453 women aged ≥15 years, 451 (99.6%) reported about their pregnancy status; 44 (9.7%) women aged ≥15 years reported themselves as pregnant at the time of the survey. The prevalence of recent HEV infection among self-reported pregnant women was 2.3% (95%CI: 0.3–15.2).

HEV genotype

Among the 104 recent infections, 11 (10.6%) were positive for HEV RNA using PCR; 90 (86.5%) were negative and 3 (2.9%) were indeterminate. Three HEV RNA positive samples underwent genotyping which identified genotype 1e virus which was homologous to HEV isolates from Sudan and Chad.

Self-reported jaundice during outbreak and estimating HEV seroprevalence prior to the outbreak

Out of the 1527 persons included in the analysis, 30 self-reported having experienced AJS since September 2016. Of these, seven were persons with a recent infection (symptomatic rate: 7/104, 6.7%) and 19 persons had a past infection (symptomatic rate: 19/959, 2.0%). Both the IgM (Chi = 13.44, $p < 0.01$) and IgG (Chi = 4.95, $p = 0.026$) status were associated with self-reported AJS since September 2016.

The impact of the 2016–17 outbreak could not be directly inferred from our seroprevalence estimates, as past HEV infections could have occurred either early in this outbreak or before the beginning of it. However, under

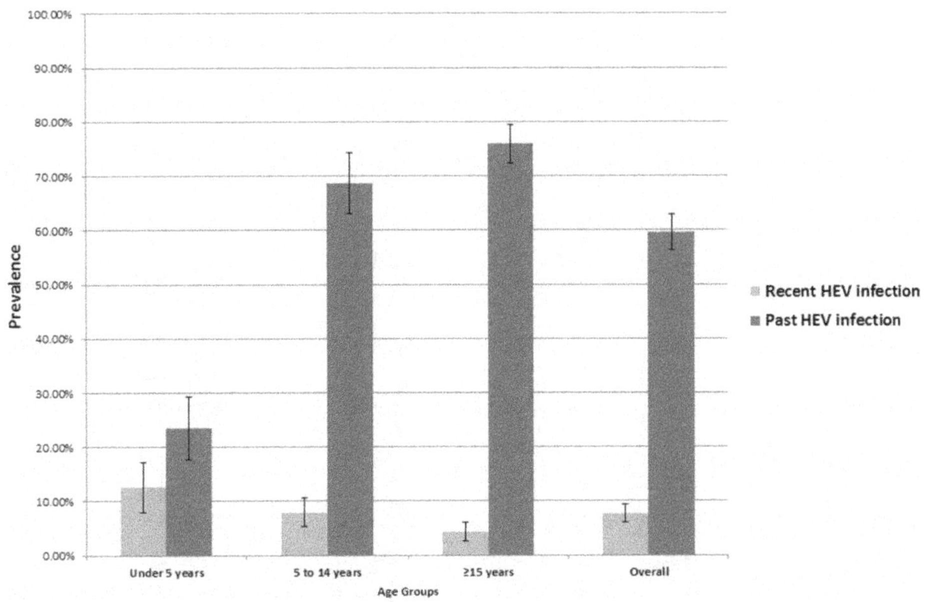

Fig. 2 Adjusted seroprevalence of recent and past HEV infection by age group ($N = 1494$)Note: Recent HEV infection = anti-HEV IgM+ / IgG ± and past HEV infection = anti-HEV IgM- / IgG+.

the assumption that 6.7% of recent infections with self-reported jaundice represent the true symptomatic rate of infection during this outbreak, we could extrapolate from the total number of jaundice cases that 388 HEV cases (104 recent infections and 284 past infections) had occurred since September 2016 (cumulative AR of 26.0% (388/1492)). In turn, this would mean that 675 past HEV infections occurred before September 2016. With this estimation, 45.2% of the population was immune before the start of this outbreak.

Risk factors associated with recent HEV infections

We compared 104 individuals with recent HEV infections and 429 persons without any HEV infection (past or recent). The unadjusted analysis indicated that having at least one child < 5 years of age in the household, not systematically using soap during handwashing and having an animal sleeping inside the compound were associated with having a recent infection of HEV (Table 1). Sex was not associated with a recent HEV infection in the unadjusted and adjusted analysis. Compared to persons older than 14 years of age, there was weak evidence that being aged 5–14 years of age was associated with recent infection of HEV. No variables around household composition were retained in the adjusted analysis. Factors that remained associated with recent infection in the adjusted analysis included: sharing the sanitation facility with other households (PR 1.72; 95%CI: 1.08–2.73), not systematically using soap for handwashing (PR 1.85; 95%CI: 1.30–2.63) and having animals sleeping inside the compound (PR 1.69; 95%CI: 1.15–2.50).

Discussion

We have determined that the prevalence of anti-HEV IgM in April 2017 in Am Timan was relatively low across all age groups considering the outbreak (including in the most susceptible group i.e. persons younger than 5 years). This can be explained by the high levels of anti-HEV IgG determined across all age groups which would reduce the number of infections and by the fact that the study was carried out during the tail-end of the outbreak as suggested by surveillance data [18].

The prevalence of anti-HEV IgG was high and increased rapidly after 5 years of age. It is possible that prior to this outbreak, the population of Am Timan was already highly exposed to HEV. The low number of susceptible persons present in the population would therefore have been low when the outbreak started. It is also possible that the outbreak infected up to 67.3% of the population over the 7–8 months of the documented outbreak but that the IgM levels had already waned for the majority of these when the study was implemented. However, this would not explain the different IgM seroprevalence between children and adults. Comparatively, 9 months after an HEV outbreak onset in an IDP camp in Kitgum, Uganda (2007–2009), 21.1% of the population tested positive for anti-HEV IgG [7]. Similar low levels of IgG levels were identified in a survey conducted 4 months after an HEV outbreak onset in a refugee

Table 1 Risk factors associated with recent HEV infections in unadjusted and adjusted Cox regression analysis

Factor	Recent infections (*N* = 104)	No infection (*N* = 429)	Unadjusted PRs		Adjusted PRs	
			PR (95%CI)	*p*-value	PR (95%CI)	*p*-value
Age group [years]				0.08		0.04
0–4	33 (31.7%)	165 (38.5%)	0.84 (0.51–1.39)		0.88 (0.53–1.46)	
5–14	42 (40.4%)	125 (29.1%)	1.46 (0.89–2.39)		1.54 (0.94–2.51)	
≥15	29 (27.9%)	139 (32.4%)	Reference		Reference	
Sex						
Female	55 (52.9%)	222 (51.8%)	1.02 (0.72–1.45)	0.89	1.07 (0.77–1.48)	0.68
Household composition						
At least one child < 5 years old	92 (88.5%)	357 (83.2%)	1.88 (1.06–3.3)	0.03	[c]	
> 6 persons	84 (80.8%)	328 (76.5%)	1.42 (0.89–2.26)	0.14	[c]	
≥ 50% of the household with past HEV infection	53 (51.0%)	179 (41.7%)	1.37 (0.90–2.07)	0.14	[c]	
Water, sanitation and hygiene						
Wide-mouthed containers owned[a]	92 (88.5%)	400 (93.5%)	0.62 (0.33–1.16)	0.13	[c]	
Shared sanitation facility[b]	82 (80.4%)	287 (70.2%)	1.67 (0.88–3.16)	0.12	1.72 (1.08–2.73)	0.02
No handwashing point next to the sanitation facility[b]	67 (65.7%)	303 (74.1%)	0.72 (0.49–1.07)	0.11	[c]	
No systematic use of soap for handwashing	42 (40.4%)	107 (24.9%)	1.68 (1.14–2.48)	0.01	1.85 (1.30–2.63)	< 0.01
Animal sleeping inside the compound	35 (33.7%)	87 (20.3%)	1.65 (1.11–2.47)	0.02	1.69 (1.15–2.50)	0.01

[a]IgM + =104 / IgM- = 428; [b] IgM + =102 / IgM- = 409; [c]Not kept in the final multivariate model

camp in Maban, South Sudan (2012–2013), where overall anti-HEV IgG prevalence was 24.1% [10]. The difference in the age-stratified prevalence estimates between Kitgum, Maban and Am Timan outbreaks supports the hypothesis that there were higher levels of immunity already present in Am Timan prior to the outbreak.

The underlying immunity for HEV infection in Am Timan before the outbreak is also evidenced in our study results which showed that the proportion of symptomatic infections was significantly lower in persons with past HEV infections compared to persons with recent infections. In addition, our calculations based on self-reported AJS estimate that 54.8% of Am Timan population was susceptible to HEV when the outbreak started. Both sets of information strengthen our hypothesis around existing high levels of HEV endemicity in Am Timan prior to this outbreak. Finally, seropositivity results for HEV in a study in Chad between 1993 and 1994 showed that 22% of hospitalized persons without acute or fulminant hepatitis had antibodies for HEV infection [25], which indicates that high levels of endemicity were reported elsewhere in the country as well.

The higher level of immunity prior the outbreak might explain the limited impact this outbreak had on the population in Am Timan in comparison to Maban or Kitgum (smaller magnitude, hospitalization rate and CFR) [20]. However, immunity levels alone cannot be the explanation. Following the Maban seroprevalence study where 54.3% of the population had been identified as still susceptible, the outbreak took hold in the refugee camps leading to a dramatic increase in cases of AJS [19]. The precise reason for this difference in outbreak dynamic is difficult to explain. A plausible reason might be that the combination of underlying population-based immunity for HEV and a reduced community-based transmission slowed the spread of the outbreak in Am Timan resulting in a less dramatic outbreak. The reduced transmission could have been facilitated by an impact of the control measures which included extensive bucket chlorination activities for most public water sources, hygiene kit distributions across all estimated 11,000 households during the outbreak and good coverage of hygiene promotion messages [26]. An alternative or complementary explanation for the reduced transmission could be the open/urban setting itself. A 2017 study by Azman, et al. showed that the risk of HEV infection in a camp was 2-fold higher than in people's home states, even though the difference was not statistically significant [27].

An interesting finding concerned the identified seroprevalence for recent infections in women who reported that they were pregnant at the time of the outbreak. Even though we anticipate that the number of self reported pregnancies was likely underestimated, the seroprevalence of recent HEV infection in this group of women was lower than that in the general population. This finding suggests that the more severe clinical course of HEV infection, which has been so frequently observed in previous outbreaks [3, 4], is not due to the higher prevalence of infection in this population group, but is due to the pathophysiological effects of HEV infection during pregnancy.

The fact that 55.8% of recent HEV cases were clustered in a household suggests that transmission might have taken place at household level. The implication of transmission of HEV at household level has also been suggested in previous HEV outbreaks [5, 8, 28], despite these being in camp settings and not open urban settings such as Am Timan. Surveillance data from Am Timan outbreak support this hypothesis as having another person with jaundice in the household and having more than five people in the household were predictive of being a confirmed HEV case [18]. This current study also identified household level factors as being associated with recent HEV infections, such as sharing a latrine with several households and not systematically using soap for handwashing. Even though we were unable to identify clear HEV transmission routes in this study, these risk factors suggest that the virus could have spread when contaminated hands came into contact with stored water, or with a communal food plates or drinking vessels. In Am Timan, cross-contamination of water or food seems plausible as the majority of households uses wide-mouthed ceramic jars to store their water [26] (which facilitates water contamination) and communal eating vessels are commonly used.

We showed that persons living in households where animals could access the family sleeping area were more at risk of having a recent HEV infection. This could either be related to high risk behaviors in animal owners that expose them to environmental contamination with HEV or it could mean that animals are involved in the transmission of the virus. Although zoonotic transmission is well-recognized for genotype 3 and 4 of HEV, it has never been demonstrated for genotype 1 and 2 [1]. However, the possibility of animal involvement in HEV genotype 1 transmission should not be excluded and further explored.

The major limitation of this study is that it was a single serological survey conducted at the tail-end of an HEV outbreak. Therefore, we were unable to document the dynamics of anti-HEV seroprevalence in this affected population. The duration and magnitude of the IgM response in infected individuals has only been well documented for genotype 3 and 4 infections and even less is known about the immune response after asymptomatic infection. The IgM level following an acute infection of HEV genotype 4 was reported to remain high for up to 2 months in most patients and to drop below detection levels after 32 weeks (8 months) [29]. Whether the immune response for genotype 1e would be similar is unknown. However, it seems likely that we missed a proportion of individuals who were infected early during the current outbreak but for whom the IgM had waned by time this study was implemented (7 to 8 months after the first outbreak alert). This is also suggested by the relatively weak IgM reactivity in most of the IgM positive samples. While samples from clinically ill HEV patients collected early during the outbreak (not as part of the study) almost always showed a saturated signal (S/CO > 15), the majority (53.5%) of the IgM positive study samples only displayed reactivity between the cutoff and 2.5 times the cutoff of the assay (Additional file 4: Figure S1). We were therefore unable to attribute past HEV infections to the outbreak or to past exposures. Consequently, the impact of this outbreak could not be assessed reliably, the underlying endemicity could only be hypothesized and risk factors could have been missed. It is also possible that we underestimated the overall seroprevalence of anti_HEV antibodies in the event that persons with acute HEV infections sought care outside of Am Timan at the time of the survey. All exposures to potential HEV infection risk factors were self-reported in this survey and thus, subjected to social-desirability bias and recall bias. Since we assessed water, sanitation and hygiene practices at the time of the interview, they might have changed during the course of the outbreak and therefore, some risk factors might have been missed. Finally, HEV outbreaks have been previously documented in semi-nomadic populations [30] and we know that part of the population in Am Timan also has this characteristic. Unfortunately, the study design was not adapted to capture these population groups and thus, we were not able to assess HEV endemicity or the risk factors associated to infection in this specific sub-population.

Conclusion

The high underlying immunity for HEV infection in the population of Am Timan before the start of the outbreak probably contributed, among other unidentified factors, to the limited impact of it (low AR, low hospitalization rate, low CFR). Therefore, we recommend implementing rapid serosurveys at the start of future outbreaks as it would facilitate risk assessment around the potential scale and impact of the outbreak. The development of better tools for simplified sample collection such as dried blood spots or oral swabs would be hugely beneficial for this. This study has again illustrated the role that household level factors play in the ongoing transmission of this virus. Based on our risk factor analysis, we recommend that control measures in future outbreaks continue to be focused on providing safe water and improving the level of personal hygiene at household level (i.e. hygiene kit/soap distributions and intensive household level hygiene promotion and education activities). In addition, we suggest considering the implementing of sanitation interventions to decrease the spread of HEV between households via latrine sharing.

Additional files

Additional file 1: (French version). Questionnaire household and individual French. Household and individual questionnaires used during the HEV seroprevalence survey in Am Timan (Chad), 2017.

Additional file 2: (English version). Questionnaire household and individual English. Household and individual questionnaires used during the HEV seroprevalence survey in Am Timan (Chad), 2017.

Additional file 3: Table S1. Adjusted seroprevalence of HEV infection stratified by age group ($N = 1494$). This is the numeric data associated with Fig. 2 in the manuscript. It shows the adjusted seroprevalence estimates by age group for recent infection (anti-HEV IgM+ / IgG±), past infection with HEV (anti-HEV IgM- / IgG+) and susceptibility for HEV infection (anti-HEV IgM- / IgG-) in Am Timan during this seroprevalence survey.

Additional file 4: Figure S1. Reactivity of IgM positive samples during the 2016–2017 outbreak in Am Timan, Chad. this figure contains reactivity data and the proportion of samples with optical density (OD) and cut-off (CO) ratios for anti-HEV IgM positive samples tested during the 2016–2017 HEV outbreak in Am Timan (Chad), which preceded the seroprevalence study discussed in this manuscript.

Abbreviations

95%CI: 95% Confidence Interval; AJS: Acute Jaundice Syndrome; AR: Attack Rate; CFR: Case Fatality Rate; EDTA: Ethylene Diamine Tetra acetic acid; EIA: Enzyme Immuo Assay; HEV: Hepatitis E Virus; IDPs: Internally Displaced Persons; IgG: Immunoglobulin G; IgM: Immunoglobulin M; MSF: Médecins Sans Frontières; ODK: Open Data Kit; PR: Prevalence Ratio; RDT: Rapid Diagnostic Test

Acknowledgements

This study would have not been possible without the dedicated 13 members of the study team who collected all the data in Am Timan. Thanks to all MSF workers in Chad (Am Timan and N'Djamena) that facilitated the different steps of the field work. We would like to acknowledge Idriss Ait-Bouziad for his support in Open Data Kit.

Funding

The implementation of the seroprevalence study described in this article was funded by MSF-OCA. We designed the study within the operational context of this outbreak of hepatitis E. MSF-OCA had no role in the study design, data collection and analysis, decision to publish or preparation of the manuscript. The authors received no specific funding for this work.

Authors' contributions

LV: collected the data, analyzed the data, interpreted the data and drafted the manuscript. AL: designed the study, interpreted the data, drafted and critically revised the manuscript. BMH: collected the data, interpreted the data, critically revised the manuscript. AMM: interpreted the data and critically revised the manuscript. CA: analyzed the data and critically revised the manuscript. SV: collected the data and critically revised the manuscript. AI: collected the data and critically revised the manuscript. PA: collected the data and critically revised the manuscript. SS: designed the study and critically revised the manuscript. CK: designed the study, interpreted the data, critically revised the manuscript. All authors read and approved the final manuscript.

Ethics approval and consent to participate
The study was conducted in accordance with the Council for International Organisations of Medical Sciences (CIOMS) International Ethical Guidelines for Biomedical Research Involving Human Subjects and International Ethical Guidelines for Epidemiological Studies. The study protocol was approved by the Ethical Review Board of MSF (Study ID: 1646) and the Chadian Ministry of Health. Each individual ≥18 years of age was asked to provide informed written consent to participate in the study. For children between 8 and 18 years of age, their caretaker was asked to provide informed written consent for study participation and the child was asked to provide written assent to participate in the study. For children < 8 years of age, only the parent/caretaker provided written informed consent for their participation.

Consent for publication
Not applicable.

Competing interests
The authors declare that they have no competing interests.

Author details
[1]Médecins sans Frontières, Operational Center Amsterdam (OCA), Quartier Aeroport, A1, Rue 1039, Porte 405, BP30, N'Djamena, Chad. [2]Médecins sans Frontières, Operational Center Amsterdam (OCA), Plantage Middenlaan 14, 1018DD Amsterdam, the Netherlands. [3]Sanquin Diagnostic Services, Department of Virology, Plesmanlaan 125, 1066 CX Amsterdam, The Netherlands. [4]Ministry of Health, BP440 N'Djamena, Chad. [5]Medical Statistics, London School of Hygiene and Tropical Medicine, Keppel Street, London WC1E7HT, UK.

References
1. Goel A, Aggarwal R. Advances in hepatitis E - II: Epidemiology, clinical manifestations, treatment and prevention. Expert Rev. Gastroenterol. Hepatol. [Internet]. 2016 [cited 2016 Oct 12];10:1065–74. Available from: http://www.ncbi.nlm.nih.gov/pubmed/27148907. Accessed 20 June 2018.
2. Rein DB, Stevens GA, Theaker J, Wittenborn JS, Wiersma ST. The global burden of hepatitis E virus genotypes 1 and 2 in 2005. Hepatology [Internet]. 2012 [cited 2016 Oct 12];55:988–97. Available from: http://www.ncbi.nlm.nih.gov/pubmed/22121109. Accessed 20 June 2018.
3. Haffar S, Bazerbachi F, Lake JR. Making the case for the development of a vaccination against hepatitis E virus. Liver Int [Internet]. 2015 [cited 2016 Oct 12];35:311–6. Available from: http://www.ncbi.nlm.nih.gov/pubmed/24836400. Accessed 20 June 2018.
4. Labrique AB, Sikder SS, Krain LJ, West KP, Christian P, Rashid M, et al. Hepatitis E, a vaccine-preventable cause of maternal deaths. Emerg Infect Dis [Internet]. 2012 [cited 2016 Oct 12];18:1401–4. Available from: http://www.ncbi.nlm.nih.gov/pubmed/22931753. Accessed 20 June 2018.
5. Mast EE, Polish LB, Favorov MO, Khudyakova NS, Collins C, Tukei PM, et al. Hepatitis E Among Refugees in Kenya: Minimal Apparent Person-to-person Transmission, Evidence for Age-dependent Disease Expression, and New Serologic Assays. Viral Hepat. Liver Dis. 1994:375–8.
6. Guthmann J-P, Klovstad H, Boccia D, Hamid N, Pinoges L, Nizou J-Y, et al. A large outbreak of hepatitis E among a displaced population in Darfur, Sudan, 2004: the role of water treatment methods. Clin Infect Dis An Off Publ Infect Dis Soc Am. 2006;42:1685–91.
7. Patel RC, Kamili S, Teshale E. Hepatitis E virus infections in children age 0-15, Uganda outbreak, 2007. J Clin Virol [Internet]. 2015 [cited 2016 Oct 12];73: 112–4. Available from: http://www.ncbi.nlm.nih.gov/pubmed/26590690. Accessed 20 June 2018.
8. Howard CM, Handzel T, Hill VR, Grytdal SP, Blanton C, Kamili S, et al. Novel risk factors associated with hepatitis E virus infection in a large outbreak in northern Uganda: results from a case-control study and environmental analysis. Am. J Trop Med Hyg [Internet]. The American Society of Tropical Medicine and Hygiene; 2010 [cited 2016 Sep 28];83:1170–3. Available from: http://www.ncbi.nlm.nih.gov/pubmed/21036857. Accessed 20 June 2018.
9. Ahmed JA, Moturi E, Spiegel P, Schilperoord M, Burton W, Kassim NH, et al. Hepatitis E outbreak, Dadaab refugee camp, Kenya, 2012. Emerg Infect Dis [Internet]. Centers for Disease Control and Prevention; 2013 [cited 2016 Sep 28];19:1010–2. Available from: http://www.ncbi.nlm.nih.gov/pubmed/23735820. Accessed 20 June 2018.
10. Centers for Disease Control and Prevention (CDC). Investigation of hepatitis E outbreak among refugees - Upper Nile, South Sudan, 2012–2013. MMWR. Morb. Mortal. Wkly. Rep. [Internet]. 2013 [cited 2016 Oct 12];62:581–6. Available from: https://www.cdc.gov/mmwr/preview/mmwrhtml/mm6229a2.htm. Accessed 20 June 2018.
11. Browne LB, Menkir Z, Kahi V, Maina G, Asnakew S, Tubman M, et al. Notes from the field: hepatitis E outbreak among refugees from South Sudan - Gambella, Ethiopia, April 2014–January 2015. MMWR Morb Mortal Wkly Rep [Internet]. 2015 [cited 2015 Oct 30];64:537. Available from: http://www.ncbi.nlm.nih.gov/pubmed/25996097. Accessed 20 June 2018.
12. Elduma A, Zein M, Karlsson M, Elkhidir I, Norder H. A single lineage of hepatitis E virus causes both outbreaks and sporadic hepatitis in Sudan. Viruses [Internet]. 2016 [cited 2017 Dec 11];8:273. Available from: http://www.mdpi.com/1999-4915/8/10/273. Accessed 20 June 2018.
13. Siddiqui MR, Cooper B, Cramond V, Thomson K, Pop-Stefanija B, de Weerdt S, et al. Unusual epidemiological characteristics of a prolonged hepatitis E outbreak in three refugee camps in South Sudan. Int. J Infect Dis [Internet]. Elsevier; 2014 [cited 2017 Dec 11];21:225. Available from: https://www.ijidonline.com/article/S1201-9712(14)00949-7/fulltext. Accessed 20 June 2018.
14. Teshale EH, Howard CM, Grytdal SP, Handzel TR, Barry V, Kamili S, et al. Hepatitis E epidemic, Uganda. Emerg Infect Dis [Internet]. 2010 [cited 2015 Oct 30];16:126–9. Available from: https://wwwnc.cdc.gov/eid/article/16/1/09-0764_article. Accessed 20 June 2018.
15. Teshale EH, Grytdal SP, Howard C, Barry V, Kamili S, Drobeniuc J, et al. Evidence of Person-to-Person Transmission of Hepatitis E Virus during a Large Outbreak in Northern Uganda. Clin. Infect. Dis. [Internet]. 2010 [cited 2015 Oct 4];50:1006–10. Available from: http://www.ncbi.nlm.nih.gov/pubmed/20178415. Accessed 20 June 2018.
16. Teshale EH, Grytdal SP, Howard C, Barry V, Kamili S, Drobeniuc J, et al. Evidence of person-to-person transmission of hepatitis E virus during a large outbreak in northern Uganda. Clin. Infect. Dis. 2010;50:1006–10.
17. Hepatitis E, Chad. Relev. Epidemiol. Hebd. [Internet]. 2004 [cited 2017 mar 14];79:313. Available from: http://www.who.int/wer/2004/wer7940.pdf?ua=1. Accessed 20 June 2018.
18. Spina A, Lenglet A, Beversluis D, de Jong M, Vernier L, Spencer C, et al. A large outbreak of hepatitis E virus genotype 1 infection in an urban setting in Chad likely linked to household level transmission factors, 2016-2017. Khudyakov YE, editor. PLoS One [Internet]. 2017 [cited 2017 Dec 13];12: e0188240. Available from: http://journals.plos.org/plosone/article?id=10.1371/journal.pone.0188240. Accessed 20 June 2018.
19. Thomson K, Dvorzak JL, Lagu J, Laku R, Dineen B, Schilperoord M,Investigation of hepatitis E outbreak among refugees - Upper Nile, South Sudan, 2012-2013. MMWR Morb Mortal Wkly Rep. 2013;62(29);581-6. Available from: https://www.cdc.gov/mmwr/preview/mmwrhtml/mm6229a2.htm. Accessed 20 June 2018.
20. Kim J-H, Nelson KE, Panzner U, Kasture Y, Labrique AB, Wierzba TF. A systematic review of the epidemiology of hepatitis E virus in Africa. BMC Infect Dis [Internet]. BioMed Central; 2014 [cited 2016 Sep 28];14:308. Available from: https://bmcinfectdis.biomedcentral.com/articles/10.1186/1471-2334-14-308. Accessed 20 June 2018.
21. Pas SD, Streefkerk RHRA, Pronk M, de Man RA, Beersma MF, Osterhaus ADME, et al. Diagnostic performance of selected commercial HEV IgM and IgG ELISAs for immunocompromised and immunocompetent patients. J Clin Virol [Internet]. 2013 [cited 2018 May 28];58:629–34. Available from: http://www.ncbi.nlm.nih.gov/pubmed/24210958. Accessed 28 May 2018.
22. Abravanel F, Chapuy-Regaud S, Lhomme S, Miedougé M, Peron J-M, Alric L, et al. Performance of anti-HEV assays for diagnosing acute hepatitis E in immunocompromised patients. J Clin Virol [Internet]. 2013 [cited 2018 May 31];58:624–8. Available from: http://www.ncbi.nlm.nih.gov/pubmed/24183927. Accessed 31 May 2018.
23. Hogema BM, Molier M, Sjerps M, de Waal M, van Swieten P, van de Laar T, et al. Incidence and duration of hepatitis E virus infection in Dutch blood

donors. Transfusion [Internet]. 2016 [cited 2017 Dec 13];56:722–8. Available from: http://www.ncbi.nlm.nih.gov/pubmed/26559806. Accessed 13 Dec 2017.

24. Heeringa S, West B, Berglund P. Applied survey data analysis. Second Edi. Chapman and Hall/CRC Press, London, United Kingdom; 2017.
25. Coursaget P, Buisson Y, N'Gawara MN, Van Cuyck-Gandre H, Roue R. Role of hepatitis E virus in sporadic cases of acute and fulminant hepatitis in an endemic area (Chad). Am. J. Trop. Med. Hyg. [Internet]. 1998 [cited 2017 Mar 14];58:330–4. Available from: http://www.ncbi.nlm.nih.gov/pubmed/9546413. Accessed 20 June 2018.
26. Spina A, Beversluis D, Irwin A, Chen A, Nassariman J-N, Ahamat A, et al. Learning from water treatment and hygiene interventions in response to a 2 hepatitis E outbreak in an open setting in Chad. J Water Health 2018; 16(2):223-32. Available from: http://jwh.iwaponline.com/content/ppiwajwh/early/2018/02/06/wh.2018.258.full.pdf.
27. Leung DT, Wamala JF, Iyer AS, Gignoux E, Gurley ES, Rumunu J, et al. High hepatitis E Seroprevalence among displaced persons in South Sudan. Am. J. Trop. Med. Hyg. [Internet]. 2017 [cited 2017 Dec 11];96:1296–301. Available from: http://www.ajtmh.org/docserver/fulltext/14761645/96/6/1296.pdf?expires=1529482680&id=id&accname=guest&checksum=91DD86C977C1DF4390398579F3BAD11C. Accessed 20 June 2018.
28. Teshale EH, Grytdal SP, Howard C, Barry V, Kamili S, Drobeniuc J, et al. Evidence of Person-to-Person Transmission of Hepatitis E Virus during a Large Outbreak in Northern Uganda. Clin Infect Dis [Internet]. 2010 [cited 2017 Dec 13];50:1006–10. Available from: https://academic.oup.com/cid/article-lookup/doi/10.1086/651077. Accessed 31 Dec 2017.
29. Huang S, Zhang X, Jiang H, Yan Q, Ai X, Wang Y, et al. Profile of acute infectious markers in sporadic hepatitis E. Rénia L, editor. PLoS One [Internet]. Public Library of Science; 2010 [cited 2017 Dec 14];5:e13560. Available from: http://dx.plos.org/https://doi.org/10.1371/journal.pone.0013560
30. Cummings MJ, Wamala JF, Komakech I, Lukwago L, Malimbo M, Omeke ME, et al. Hepatitis E in Karamoja, Uganda, 2009–2012: epidemiology and challenges to control in a setting of semi-nomadic pastoralism. Trans. R. Soc. Trop. Med. Hyg. [Internet]. 2014 [cited 2015 Oct 30];108:648–55. Available from: http://www.ncbi.nlm.nih.gov/pubmed/25092862. Accessed 20 June 2018.

Determination of hepatitis B, C and D prevalence among urban and Amerindian populations from the Eastern Brazilian Amazon

Livia Melo Villar[1*], Flavio Augusto Pádua Milagres[2], Elisabeth Lampe[1], Helena Medina Cruz[1], Leticia de Paula Scalioni[1], Monica de Avelar Figueiredo Mafra Magalhães[3], Anselmo Rocha Romão[3], Renata Gracie[3] and Vanessa Salete de Paula[4]

Abstract

Background: This study was conducted to determine the prevalence of HBV, HCV, and HDV in urban populations and Amerindians living in the state of Tocantins (Eastern Amazon).

Methods: A total of 948 individuals were recruited in Tocantinopolis city (Tocantins state) of whom 603 were Amerindians (from 6 tribes) and 345 were non-Amerindians (6 urban areas of Tocantinópolis city). Anti-HCV, HBsAg, anti-HBc, anti-HBs, anti-HBc IgM, anti-HBe, HBeAg, and anti-delta antibodies were determined using enzyme immunoassay.

Results: HBV cleared infection (both anti-HBc/anti-HBs+), chronic inactive/immune controlled HBV infection (anti-HBc + only), previous HBV vaccination (anti-HBs + only), active HBV infection (HBsAg+), individuals susceptible to HBV, and anti-HCV reactivity were found in 12.9, 1.8, 27.2, 0.5, 57.7, 1.2% in Amerindians and 12.1, 2.0, 37.1, 0.3, 55.4, 0.3% in non-Amerindians respectively. Out of 139 anti-HBc reactive individuals, 70 were anti-HBe reactive and none presented HBeAg or anti-HBc IgM. Anti-HBc prevalence was associated to older age ($p < 0.0001$). Overall anti-Delta prevalence was 0.3% and regarding anti-HBc reactive individuals, anti-delta prevalence was 3.4 and 0% in Amerindians and non-Amerindians respectively.

Conclusions: Overall low prevalence of HBV and HCV infection was found in the populations studied, but high HBV and HCV prevalence was observed in Amerindians compared to non-Amerindians suggesting that these individuals have a higher likelihood of acquiring to these infections. Anti-delta antibodies were found among Amerindians from Eastern Amazon suggesting a risk for this population. Of note is that nearly half of Amerindians had no anti-HBs, indicating a need for HBV vaccination campaigns in this population.

Keywords: Hepatitis B, Hepatitis C, Hepatitis D, Prevalence, Amerindians, Eastern Amazon, North Brazil

Background

Hepatitis B, C and D viruses, transmitted predominantly through parenteral routes, represent a considerable threat to public health. Worldwide, approximately 257 million people are chronically infected with hepatitis B virus (HBV), 71 million with chronic hepatitis C virus (HCV) and 15 million with HBV and hepatitis D virus (HDV) [1–3].

Multicenter studies conducted in several regions of Brazil have demonstrated seroprevalence rates of anti-HBc (HBV past exposure) of 11.6% and anti-HCV of 3.22% in individuals aged 10 to 69 years old from North region of Brazil [4, 5]. In the period spanning 1999 to 2016, approximately 561,000 confirmed cases of viral hepatitis were reported to health authorities in Brazil. Of these, 212.031 (37,8%) hepatitis B, 182.389

* Correspondence: liviafiocruz@gmail.com; lvillar@ioc.fiocruz.br
[1]Laboratory of Viral Hepatitis, Oswaldo Cruz Institute, FIOCRUZ, Helio and Peggy Pereira Pavillion – Ground Floor - Room B09, FIOCRUZ Av. Brasil, 4365 - Manguinhos –, Rio de Janeiro, RJ 210360-040, Brazil
Full list of author information is available at the end of the article

(32,5%) hepatitis C and 3.791 (0,7%) hepatitis D cases were identified [6].

HBV, HCV and HDV prevalence varies considerably according to geographical region of the country, where the highest HCV prevalence (3.22%) is observed in the North region [5]. The highest rates of HBV carriers and more than 70% of reported HDV cases are also observed in the Amazon Region located in the North of the country [6, 7]. HDV infection is also common in acute hepatitis B cases (29%) and fulminant hepatitis cases (74%) in the North of Brazil [8].

Some specific groups, like Amerindians, people who use drugs, beauty professionals, and military personnel are at higher risk of viral hepatitis acquisition [7, 9–12]. In 2010 the Brazilian census estimated the population of Amerindians at 896,917 individuals, corresponding to 0.47% of the general population with nearly half of them living in the Northern region of the country [13]. HBsAg prevalence varies from 0 to 20.6%, Anti-HDV from 0 to 7.7% [7] and anti-HCV from 1.4 to 1.6% [14] in the Northern Amerindian population.

Viral hepatitis is higher in the Northern areas where many Amerindians live, and even within this region prevalence varies between different areas. Most prevalence studies of viral hepatitis from the North of Brazil were conducted in Western Amazon [15–20] and there is a gap in the literature in terms of geographical variations. As a result, this information is needed to develop targeted screening programs.

This study was conducted to estimate the prevalence rates of HBV, HCV and HDV markers between Amerindians and the general population residing in the state of Tocantins (Eastern Amazon) located in the Northern region of Brazil.

Methods

A cross-sectional survey regarding hepatitis B, C and D prevalence was conducted using a non-probability sampling method among Amerindians and non-Amerindians living in Eastern Amazon. Consecutive sampling was used in which every subject meeting the criteria of inclusion is selected until the required sample size is achieved in this setting. The North Region of Brazil is comprised of seven States (Acre, Amapá, Amazonas, Pará, Rondônia, Roraima and Tocantins) that, together with Mato Grosso and Maranhão States form the Brazilian Amazon. The West Amazon region comprises the states of Amazonas, Acre, Rondônia and Roraima. The East Amazon is comprised of the states of Maranhão, Pará, Amapá, Mato Grosso and Tocantins. The study was carried out from June 2011 to June 2017 and samples were collected from 6 tribes of Amerindians and 6 urban areas of Tocantinópolis city in June 2011.

Eligibility criteria for participation of this study were: residence in the area and the provision of informed consent. Exclusion criteria were: confusion at the time of recruitment and disagreement with the terms of the informed consent.

Blood sampling and viral hepatitis detection

Each participant donated a blood sample (5 mL) by venipuncture using a vacutainer device. The sample was allowed to clot to separate the serum for analysis and was stored at – 20 °C until analysis.

Serum samples were tested for HBsAg, anti-HBc, anti-HBs, anti-HCV, using commercial enzyme immunoassay (ELISA) kits (Diasorin, Pomezia, Italy), according to the manufacturer's guidelines. HBsAg or Anti-HBc reactive samples were also assayed for anti-HBc IgM and anti-delta antibodies using ELISA kit (Diasorin), and anti-HBe and HBeAg using eletrochemiluminescence assay (ECLIA) (Roche, USA).

Samples found to be negative on preliminary screening were considered seronegative. Samples that initially tested borderline or positive were retested using ELISA to confirm the results. Indeterminate samples were excluded from the analysis.

Anti-HCV reactive samples were submitted to real time PCR (Cobas Taqman HCV 2.0, Roche, USA), which has a dynamic range of linear quantification of 20 to 1.7×10^8 IU/mL. HBsAg-reactive samples were submitted to real time PCR (Cobas Taqman HBV Test, Roche, USA), which has a dynamic range of linear quantification of 29 to 1.1×10^8 IU/mL.

Data collection and analysis

Age, gender and residential location data were obtained from each participant and entered along with serological results into (Microsoft Excel) data spreadsheets.

Prevalence was calculated for HBV, HCV and HDV markers in the studied population. Descriptive statistics were generated for the data. Chi square test for independence and exact Fisher's tests were used to compare categorical variables according to anti-HBc status. A p-value < 0.05 was considered statistically significant. All calculations were performed using the Statistical Package for the Social Sciences (SPSS for Windows, release 20.0; SPSS, Chicago, IL, USA).

The spatial representation of HBV markers analyzed was based on cartography of the digital mesh of the 2010 census, [13] and data of HBV markers according localities of the municipality of Tocantinópolis in the state of Tocantins. For the adaptation of the analyzed locations to the census tracts, the National Register of Addresses for Statistical Purposes of the IBGE was used [13]. Thematic maps of HBV markers were created using

Table 1 Hepatitis B and C virus markers among individuals from Amerindian tribes and urban areas of Tocantinopolis city ($n = 948$)

	Number Tested	HBsAg - anti-HBc + anti-HBs + (HBV cleared infection)	HBsAg - anti-HBc + anti-HBs - (Chronic inactive/immune controlled HBV infection)	HBsAg - anti-HBc – anti-HBs + (HBV Vaccination group)	HBsAg + anti-HBs – (HBV active infection)	HBsAg – anti-HBc - anti-HBs – (HBV susceptible individuals)	anti-HCV +
Total population studied	948 (100%)	120 (12.6%)	18 (1.9%)	268 (28.3%)	4 (0.4%)	538 (56.7%)	8 (0.8%)
Sex							
Female	505 (53.3%)	56 (11.1%)	9 (1.8%)	143 (28.3%)	2 (0.4%)	296 (58.6%)	1 (0.2%)
Male	443 (46.7%)	64 (14.4%)	9 (2.0%)	125 (28.2%)	2 (0.4%)	242 (54.6%)	7 (1.6%)
Age group (years)							
0–20	438 (46.2%)	9 (2.0%)	3 (0.7%)	166 (0.4%)	2 (0.4%)	258 (58.9%)	0 (0.0%)
21–40	277 (29.2%)	31 (11.2%)	0 (0.0%)	88 (31.7%)	1 (0.4%)	157 (56.6%)	4 (1.4%)
41–60	142 (14.9%)	49 (34.5%)	5 (3.5%)	9 (6.3%)	1 (0.7%)	78 (54.9%)	3 (2.1%)
> 60	91 (9.6%)	31 (34.1%)	10 (11.0%)	5 (5.5%)	0 (0.0%)	45 (49.4%)	1 (1.1%)
Location							
Amerindian tribes	603 (63.6%)	78 (12.9%)	11 (1.8%)	164 (27.2%)	3 (0.5%)	348 (57.7%)	7 (1.2%)
Prata village	53 (5.6%)	2 (3.8%)	0 (0.0%)	24 (45.3%)	0 (0.0%)	27 (50.9%)	0 (0.0%)
Girassol village	89 (9.4%)	16 (17.9%)	0 (0.0%)	14 (15.7%)	1 (1.1%)	58 (65.2%)	1 (1.1%)
Mariazinha village	206 (21.7%)	29 (14.1%)	1 (0.5%)	51 (24.7%)	1 (0.5%)	124 (60.2%)	3 (1.4%)
Riachinho village	18 (1.9%)	3 (16.6%)	0 (0.0%)	6 (33.3%)	0 (0.0%)	9 (50.0%)	0 (0.0%)
Serrinha village	66 (7.0%)	1 (1.5%)	0 (0.0%)	17 (25.7%)	0 (0.0%)	48 (72.7%)	1 (1.5%)
Folha Grossa village	171 (18.0%)	27 (15.8%)	10 (5.8%)	52 (30.4%)	1 (0.6%)	82 (0.5%)	2 (1.2%)
Non-Amerindian (Urban areas)	345 (36.4%)	42 (12.2%)	7 (2.0%)	128 (37.1%)	1 (0.3%)	191 (55.4%)	1 (0.3%)
Cacau urban area	60 (6.3%')	3 (5.0%)	1 (1.7%)	12 (20.0%)	0 (0.0%)	44 (73.3%)	1 (1.7%)
Mumbuco urban area	81 (8.5%)	9 (11.1%)	1 (1.2%)	32 (39.5%)	0 (0.0%)	39 (48.1%)	0 (0.0%)
BelaVista urban area	10 (1.0%)	2 (20.0%)	0 (0.0%)	2 (20.0%)	0 (0.0%)	6 (60.0%)	0 (0.0%)
Urban area block 18	84 (8.9%)	10 (11.2%)	3 (3.6%)	25 (29.7%)	1 (1.2%)	45 (53.6%)	0 (0.0%)
Urban area block 22	61 (6.4%)	5 (8.2%)	2 (3.3%)	21 (34.4%)	0 (0.0%)	33 (54.1%)	0 (0.0%)
Tocantinópolis Downtown	49 (5.2%)	13 (26.5%)	0 (0.0%)	36 (73.5%)	0 (0.0%)	24 (49.0%)	0 (0.0%)

the Geographic Information System (GIS) ArcGis version 10.4.

Ethical consideration

The study project was reviewed and approved by Fiocruz ethics Committee and Brazilian National Ethics Council, Brazilian Indian Foundation and local tribe leaders. For this study, authorization was solicited and obtained from the Indians' authorities at the national, regional, and local levels.

Respondents were assured about confidentiality, that their participation was voluntary and that they had full rights to withdraw from the study at any time. All participants were given a verbal explanation of the objectives and methodology of the research and were included in the study only after obtaining written signed informed consent. Parent or guardian gave written signed informed consent on behalf of any participants under the age of 18. All individuals who tested positive were sent to public health clinics to receive treatment.

Results

In the present study, 948 individuals were included aging 0 to 90 years, 569 were Amerindians and 379 were non-Amerindians. Most of them were females (53.3%) and mean age of individuals was 27.8 ± 20.6 years. The socio-demographic characteristics of the 948 individuals included in this study are shown in Table 1.

Markers of HBsAg, anti-HBc and anti-HBs were detected in 4, 138, and 388 individuals giving an overall prevalence of 0.4, 14.5, 40.9%, respectively. Among the 4 HBsAg reactive individuals, none of them presented HBeAg or anti-HBc IgM and only one presented detectable anti-HBc, anti-HBe and HBV DNA (viral load of 6469 IU/mL). Of the 138 anti-HBc-reactive individuals, 70 were anti-HBe-reactive and none presented HBeAg or anti-HBc IgM. Anti-HBc prevalence was positively associated with older age ($p < 0.0001$) in bivariate analyses (Table 2).

HBV cleared infection (both anti-HBc/anti-HBs+), chronic inactive/immune controlled HBV infection (anti-HBc + only), previous HBV vaccination (anti-HBs + only), HBV active infection (HBsAg+), individuals susceptible to HBV, and anti-HCV reactivity were found in 12.9, 1.8, 27.2, 0.5, 57.7, 1.2% in Amerindians and 12.1, 2.0, 37.1, 0.3, 55.4, 0.3% in non-Amerindians respectively.

Among HBV immune individuals ($n = 388$), 268 were previously vaccinated (only anti-HBs detected) and 120 had had a previous HBV infection (Table 1). HBV immunity was high in males and individuals aging 21 to 40 years old, but evidence of HBV vaccination (only anti-HBs detected) was more frequent in Amerindian populations, females and those less than 20 years of age.

The municipalities with the highest HBV-immune individuals were from Folha Grossa and Mariazinha villages while the lowest number of HBV-immune subjects were seen in Serrinha, Prata, Riachinho and Cacau villages (Figs. 1 and 2).

Anti-Delta was not detected in HBsAg-reactive samples, but it was present in 3 anti-HBc -reactive samples, giving an overall prevalence of 0.3%. Considering these anti-HBc-reactive samples, prevalence of anti-delta was 3.4 and 0% in Amerindians and non-Amerindians respectively. All were male, more than 60 years of age, 2 were from Folha Grossa village and 1 was from Mariazinha village.

Anti-HCV was detected in 8 individuals (7 Amerindian and 1 non-Amerindian), resulting in a prevalence of 1.2 and 0.3% in Amerindians and non-Amerindians respectively and an overall prevalence of 0.8%. High prevalence was observed in males (87.5%) and 50% of individuals aged between 21 to 40 years. HCV RNA was detected in one sample (viral load of 3552 UI/mL).

Table 2 Bivariate analysis of demographic factors associated to anti-HBc prevalence in the population studied

Variable	Total Anti-HBc		Bivariate analysis *P* Value
	Reactive $n = 138$ (%)	Non reactive $n = 810$ (%)	
Age (years)			
0–20	12 (8.7)	426 (52.6)	< 0.0001
21–40	31 (22.5)	246 (30.4)	
41–60	54 (39.1)	88 (10.9)	
> 60	41 (29.7)	50 (6.1)	
Gender			
Male	73 (52.9)	370 (45.6)	0.11
Female	65 (47.1)	440 (54.4)	
Location			
Ameridian	89 (64.5)	514 (63.5)	0.84
Non Ameridian	49 (35.5)	296 (36.5)	

Discussion

Parenterally transmitted hepatitis viruses are important threats to public health with Amerindians being potentially more exposed to these infections due to social and cultural habits. Viral hepatitis prevalence has been widely investigated in the Western Amazonian region of Brazil [15–21], but few data are available for the Eastern Amazon region [22, 23], principally in the state of Tocantins. In the present study, new data about HBV, HCV and HDV prevalence were obtained from Eastern Amazon and low prevalence of HBsAg, anti-HCV and anti-delta was observed in these individuals, showing a low risk of transmission of these viruses in this region.

Overall HBsAg prevalence was 0.4%, lower than reported in a previous study from Eastern Amazon (2.88%) [23], and hemodialysis individuals from Tocantins state (4%) [24]. HBsAg prevalence was slightly higher in Amerindians (0.3%) when compared to non-Amerindians (0.1%), but this prevalence is still lower than observed in Amerindians from other localities of the Amazon Region, such as the states of Xingu, Pará and Acre, where prevalence varies from 3.3 to 14.4% [7, 17, 22, 25]. Some authors reported that sociocultural factors such as population density, scarification, tattoos and sexual activity represent important factors in the transmission of HBV [8, 26, 27]. It is possible that the infrequency of these factors among Amerindians from Tocantins may explain their low HBV prevalence compared to other Amerindians from Amazon.

HBV cleared infection was observed in 14.5% of individuals and it was higher among Amerindians and individuals more than 40 years of age. Anti-HBc prevalence varies from 40.7 to 84.7% among Amerindians from Eastern Amazon region [7, 22, 23] and 19.7 to 95.7% among Amerindians from Western Brazilian Amazon [7, 17]. Anti-HBc prevalence was high among older individuals, in concordance

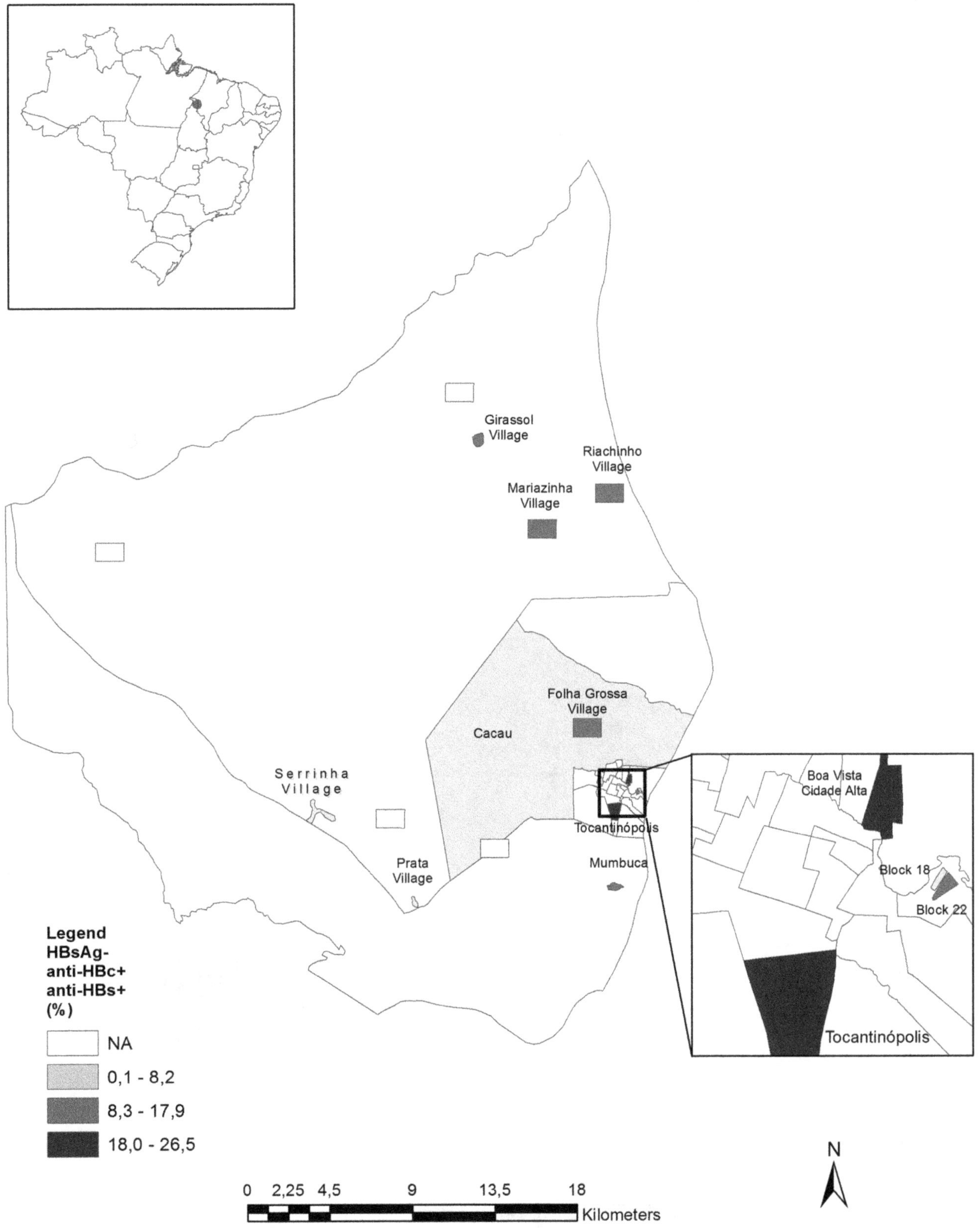

Fig. 1 Prevalence of cases of previous HBV infection (HBsAg negative/anti-HBc and anti-HBs positive) according site of recruitment in Eastern Amazon

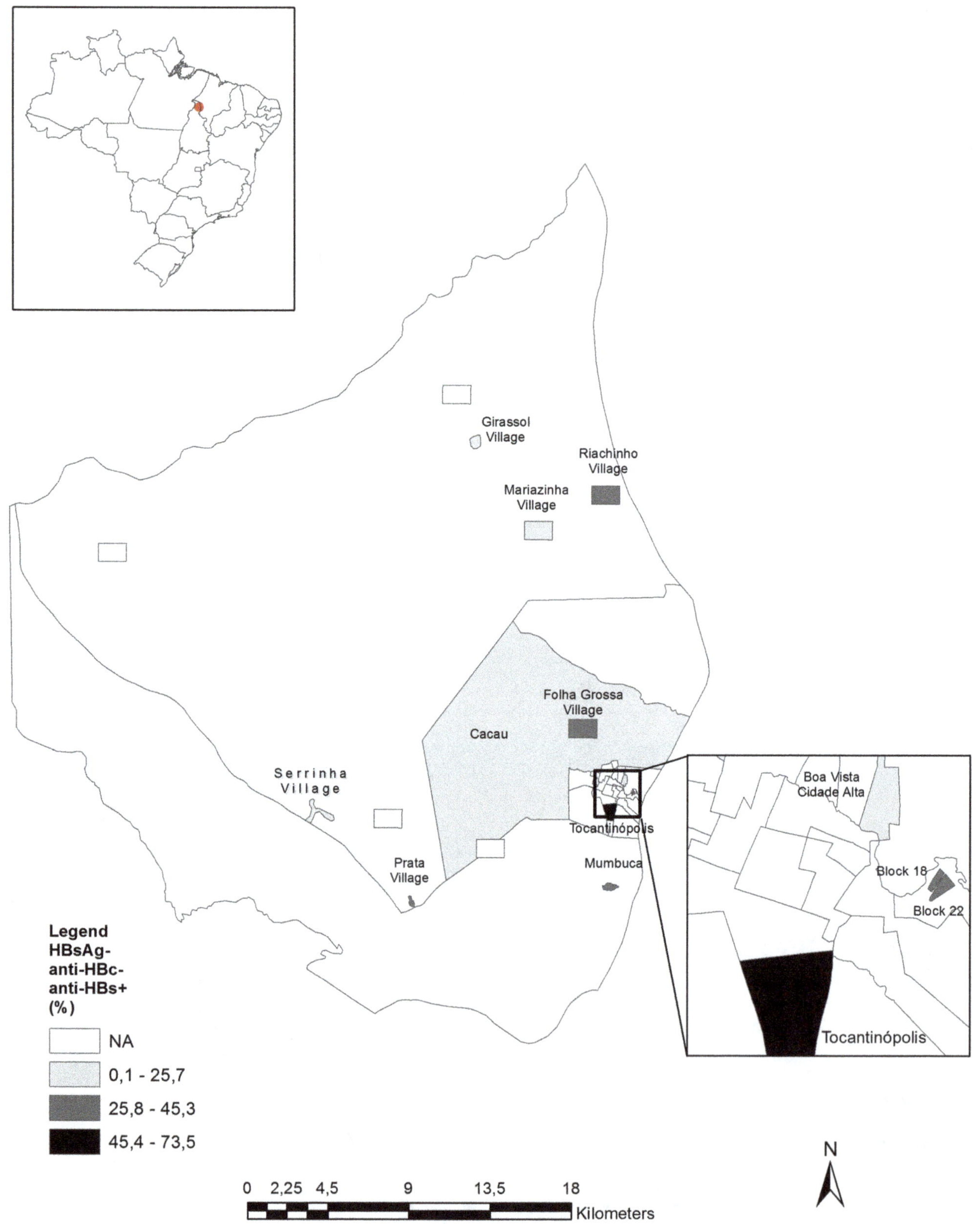

Fig. 2 Prevalence of evidence of HBV vaccination (HBsAg and anti-HBc negative/ anti-HBs positive) according site of recruitment in Eastern Amazon

with previous studies among non-Amerindians from Amazon region [16, 21, 23].

In the present study, 56.7% of subjects were susceptible to HBV infection and less than 50% were HBV immune, indicating that most individuals are not protected against HBV infection. Although Amerindians are a target group for HBV vaccination, only 27.2% of Amerindians demonstrated isolated anti-HBs reactivity, less than that observed among Amerindians from the Southern (71.0%) and Northern (39.6%) regions of Brazil [22, 28]. It is likely that the low anti-HBs reactivity could be due to poor knowledge about HBV vaccination as previously demonstrated in other groups from the Northern region [29].

Anti-HBs reactivity was irregular among distinct sites of collection where a high prevalence of HBV-immune individuals was found in downtown Tocantinopolis, Folha Grossa and Mariazinha village. This could also be explained by access to health clinics, where high HBV vaccination coverage was found in urban areas. At the time of recruitment (2011), The Brazilian Immunization Program recommended HBV vaccination for all Amerindians and for non-Amerindians newborns and children and adolescents up to 19 years of age. Additionally, the vaccination was also recommended to those at higher risk of acquiring infection such as people who use drug, health professionals, prisoners and other groups [30, 31]. In the present study, high HBV vaccine coverage was found among people aged 0–20 since HBV vaccination was implemented for this demographic.

Overall an anti-HCV prevalence of 0.8% was observed in individuals from Tocantinópolis city, lower than that observed in studies of the general population from the Eastern Amazon Region (2.2 to 5.76%) [23, 32, 33] or hemodialysis individuals from Tocantins state (13%) [24]. However, anti-HCV prevalence was high in Amerindians (1.2%) compared to non-Amerindians (0.3%) in concordance with a previous study from the Northern region (1.4%) [14].

Some studies have demonstrated that sharing cutting instruments among relatives and/or neighbors is a common habit in individuals from the Amazon region [34, 35]. These cultural habits could increase the risk of transmission of parenterally acquired viruses, such as, HCV. In addition, low knowledge about hepatitis transmission [29] and low access to treatment service could contribute to this high prevalence.

Overall anti-delta prevalence was 0.3% and all of these individuals were Amerindians, giving a prevalence of 3.4% in this group. According to the Brazilian Health Ministry, 10 confirmed cases of hepatitis D were found in Tocantins from 1999 to 2016 giving a prevalence of 0.3% in Brazil [6]. Previous studies did not find anti-delta antibodies in Amerindians from the Eastern Amazon Region, [22, 25] while an anti-delta prevalence of 2.9 to 7.3% was observed in the Western Amazon Region [15, 17, 21].

Of the residents in the northern Area of Tocantins state, approximately 4.4% are reported to be Amerindian, with 81% of the population living in urban areas [36]. In the present study, 60% of participants were Amerindian and 64% reported living rurally/in villages. The main purpose of this study is to provide new insights regarding hepatitis prevalence in Amerindians living in rural areas, so a high proportion of this group was included in the study. A major limitation of the study was the type of sampling. Consecutive sampling was used due to impossibility to conduct probability sampling in this study and since the method is very cost- and time-effective. However, it is not possible to generalize the results of the survey to the entire population and there is the possibility of under- or over-representation of the population.

Conclusions

Overall low prevalence of HBV and HCV infection was found in the population studied, but higher HBV and HCV prevalence was observed among Amerindians compared to the urban population, likely due to inadequate access to prevention or treatment services due to rural or remote location. Moreover, anti-delta antibodies were found only among Amerindians from the Eastern Amazon, suggesting a risk for infection in this population. Of note is that nearly half of Amerindians had no anti-HBs, indicating the need for HBV vaccination campaigns in this population. These findings should serve as an important baseline for future primary prevention and therapeutic intervention strategies.

Abbreviations

Anti-HBc IgM: Antibodies directed against the core antigen IgM; Anti-HBc total: Antibodies directed against the core antigen; Anti-HBe: Antibodies against HBeAg; Anti-HBs: Antibodies directed against hepatitis B surface antigen; Anti-HCV: Antibodies directed against hepatitis C virus; Anti-HDV: Antibodies directed against hepatitis D virus;
ECLIA: Electrochemiluminescence; ELISA: Enzyme immunoassay; HBeAg: HBV "e" antigen; HBsAg: Surface antigen of the hepatitis B virus; HBV: Hepatitis B virus; HCV: Hepatitis C virus; HDV: Hepatitis D virus; IBGE: Brazilian Institute of Geography and Statistics

Acknowledgements

The authors wish to thank Juliana Custódio Miguel, Elisangela Ferreira da Silva, Vanessa Alves Marques and Moyra Machado Portilho for assistance in blood analysis and Tocantins Health Secretary for the assistance in blood sample collection.

Funding

This research was supported by the Fundação de Amparo a Pesquisa do Estado do Rio de Janeiro (FAPERJ), Brazilian National Counsel of Technological and Scientific Development (CNPq) and the Oswaldo Cruz Foundation (FIOCRUZ). They had no role in designing the study and collection, analysis, and interpretation of data and in writing the manuscript.

Authors' contributions

LMV and VSP conceived the study; LMV, VSP, FAPM and EL designed the study protocol; HMC, LPS, LMV, VSP, FAPM carried out subject selection and recruitment; HMC, LPS, VSP, LMV performed the tests, analysis and interpretation of these data; ARR, RG, MAFMM performed spatial representation of HBV prevalence; LMV and VSP drafted the manuscript; ARR, RG, MAFMM, FAPM, VSP, LMV, EL critically revised the manuscript for intellectual content. All authors read and approved the final manuscript.

Ethics approval and consent to participate

This study was conducted in accordance with the ethical principles stated in the Helsinki Declaration. This study was reviewed and approved by Fiocruz ethics Committee and Brazilian National Ethics Council under the number of CAAE 32789914.6.0000.5248.

All participants were given a verbal explanation of the objectives and methodology of the research and were included in the study only after obtaining written signed informed consent. Parent or guardian gave written signed informed consent on behalf of any participants under the age of 18.

Consent for publication

Not applicable.

Competing interests

The authors declare that they have no competing interests.

Author details

[1]Laboratory of Viral Hepatitis, Oswaldo Cruz Institute, FIOCRUZ, Helio and Peggy Pereira Pavillion – Ground Floor - Room B09, FIOCRUZ Av. Brasil, 4365 - Manguinhos –, Rio de Janeiro, RJ 210360-040, Brazil. [2]Federal University of Tocantins, Tocantins, Brazil. [3]Laboratory of Information in Health, Institute of Communication and technological and scientific information in Health (ICICT), FIOCRUZ, Rio de Janeiro, Brazil. [4]Molecular Virology Laboratory, Oswaldo Cruz Institute, FIOCRUZ, Rio de Janeiro, Brazil.

References

1. World Health Organization. Hepatitis B. 2017. http://www.who.int/mediacentre/factsheets/fs204/en/. Accessed 26 Oct 2017.
2. World Health Organization. Hepatitis C. 2017. http://www.who.int/mediacentre/factsheets/fs164/en/. Accessed 26 Oct 2017.
3. World Health Organization. Hepatitis D. 2017. http://www.who.int/mediacentre/factsheets/hepatitis-d/en/. Accessed 26 Oct 2017.
4. Ximenes RA, Figueiredo GM, Cardoso MR, Stein AT, Moreira RC, Coral G, Crespo D, Dos Santos AA, Montarroyos UR, Braga MC, Pereira LM, Hepatitis Study Group. Population-based multicentric survey of hepatitis B infection and risk factors in the north, south, and southeast regions of Brazil, 10-20 years after the beginning of vaccination. Am J Trop Med Hyg. 2015;93(6):1341–8.
5. Pereira LM, Martelli CM, Moreira RC, Merchan-Hamman E, Stein AT, Cardoso MR, et al. Prevalence and risk factors of hepatitis C virus infection in Brazil, 2005 through 2009: a cross-sectional study. BMC Infect Dis. 2013;13:60.
6. Brazilian Health Ministry. Epidemiological bulletin of viral hepatitis 2017. http://www.aids.gov.br/pt-br/pub/2017/boletim-epidemiologico-de-hepatites-virais-2017. Accessed 26 Oct 2017.
7. Braga WS. Hepatitis B and D virus infection within Amerindians ethnic groups in the Brazilian Amazon: epidemiological aspects. Rev Soc Bras Med Trop. 2004;37(Suppl 2):9–13.
8. Bensabath G, Hadler SC, Soares MCP, Fields H, Dias LB, Popper H, et al. Hepatitis Delta virus infection and Labrea hepatitis. Prevalence and role in fulminant hepatitis in the Amazon basin. JAMA. 1987;258:479–83.
9. da Fonseca JC, Brasil LM. Hepatitis C virus infection in the Amazon Brazilian region. Rev Soc Bras Med Trop. 2004;37(Suppl 2):1–8.
10. Santos Cruz M, Andrade T, Bastos FI, Leal E, Bertoni N, Villar LM, et al. Key drug use, health and socio-economic characteristics of young crack users in two Brazilian cities. Int J Drug Policy. 2013;24:432–8.
11. Villar LM, de Paula VS, de Almeida AJ, do Ó KM, Miguel JC, Lampe E. Knowledge and prevalence of viral hepatitis among beauticians. J Med Virol. 2014;86:1515–21.
12. Villar LM, Ó KM, Scalioni LP, Cruz HM, Portilho MM, Mendonça AC, et al. Prevalence of hepatitis B and C virus infections among military personnel. Braz J Infect Dis. 2015;19:285–90.
13. Brazilian Geographic and Statistics Institute. IBGE. Indigenous in the 2010 population census. http://indigenas.ibge.gov.br/images/indigenas/estudos/indigena_censo2010.pdf. Accessed 26 Oct 2017.
14. Soares MC, Menezes RC, Martins SJ, Bensabath G. Epidemiology of hepatitis B, C and D viruses among indigenous Parakanã tribe in the eastern Brazilian Amazon region. Bol Oficina Sanit Panam. 1994;117:124–35.
15. de Paula VS, Arruda ME, Vitral CL, Gaspar AM. Seroprevalence of viral hepatitis in riverine communities from the western region of the Brazilian Amazon Basin. Mem Inst Oswaldo Cruz. 2001;96:1123–8.
16. Tavares-Neto J, Almeida D, Soares MC, Uchoa R, Viana S, Darub R, et al. Seroprevalence of hepatitis B and C in the western Brazilian Amazon region (Rio Branco, acre): a pilot study carried out during a hepatitis B vaccination program. Braz J Infect Dis. 2004;8:133–9.
17. Viana S, Paraná R, Moreira RC, Compri AP, Macedo V. High prevalence of hepatitis B virus and hepatitis D virus in the western Brazilian Amazon. Am J Trop Med Hyg. 2005;73:808–14.
18. Dias AL, Oliveira CM, Castilho Mda C, Silva Mdo S, Braga WS. Molecular characterization of the hepatitis B virus in autochthonous and endogenous populations in the western Brazilian Amazon. Rev Soc Bras Med Trop. 2012; 45:9–12.
19. da Costa CA, Kimura LO. Molecular epidemiology of hepatitis B virus among the indigenous population of the Curuçá and Itaquaí rivers, Javari Valley, state of Amazonas, Brazil. Rev Soc Bras Med Trop. 2012;45:457–62.
20. Vieira Gde D, Ventura CG, de Sousa CM. Occurrence and spatial distribution of hepatitis C in a western Brazilian Amazon state. Arq Gastroenterol. 2014; 51:316–9.
21. Castilho Mda C, Oliveira CM, Gimaque JB, Leão JD, Braga WS. Epidemiology and molecular characterization of hepatitis B virus infection in isolated villages in the western Brazilian Amazon. Am J Trop Med Hyg. 2012;87:768–74.
22. Azevedo RA, Silva AE, Ferraz ML, Marcopito LF, Baruzzi RG. Prevalence of serologic markers of hepatitis B and D viruses in children of the Caiabi and Txucarramãe tribes from the Indian reservation of Xingu, Central Brazil. Rev Soc Bras Med Trop. 1996;29:431–9.
23. El Khouri M, Cordeiro Q, Luz DA, Duarte LS, Gama ME, Corbett CE. Endemic hepatitis B and C virus infection in a Brazilian eastern Amazon region. Arq Gastroenterol. 2010;47:35–41.
24. Souza KP, Luz JA, Teles SA, Carneiro MA, Oliveira LA, Gomes AS, et al. Hepatitis B and C in the hemodialysis unit of Tocantins, Brazil: serological and molecular profiles. Mem Inst Oswaldo Cruz. 2003;98:599–603.
25. Nunes HM, Monteiro MR, Soares MC. Prevalence of hepatitis B and D serological markers in the Parakanã, Apyterewa Indian reservation, Pará state, Brazil. Cad Saude Publica. 2007;23:2756–66.
26. Brabin L, Brabin BJ. Cultural factors and transmission of hepatitis B virus. Am J Epidemiol. 1985;122:725–30.
27. Coimbra CEA, Santos RV, Yoshida CFY, Baptista ML, Flowers NM, Valle ACF. Hepatitis B epidemiology and cultural practices in amerindian populations of Amazonia: the Tupí-Mondé and Xavante from Brasil. Soc Sci Med. 1996; 42:1735–43.
28. Ferreira A, Greca D, Tavares E, Moriya Y, Spelling F, Boeira M, et al. Seroepidemiology of hepatitis B and C in Kaingang Indians in the south of Brazil. Rev Panam Salud Publica. 2006;20:230–5.
29. Cruz HM, de Paula VS, Villar LM. A cross-sectional study of viral hepatitis perception among residents from southeast and north regions of Brazil. Int J Environ Res Public Health. 2018;15(2):189.
30. Brazilian Health Ministry. Ordinance n. ° 1,489, July 19, 2013. http://bvsms.saude.gov.br/bvs/saudelegis/gm/2013/prt1498_19_07_2013.html. Accessed 2 Mar 2018.
31. Brazilian Health Ministry. Ordinance n. ° 1,498, July 19, 2013. 2013. http://bvsms.saude.gov.br/bvs/saudelegis/gm/2013/prt1498_19_07_2013.html. Acessed 2 Mar 2018.

32. Aquino JA, Pegado KA, Barros LP, Machado LF. Seroprevalence of hepatitis B virus and hepatitis C virus infections among individuals in the state of Pará. Rev Soc Bras Med Trop. 2008;41:334–7.
33. de Almeida MK, Dos Santos KN, Fecury AA, de Oliveira CS, Freitas AS, Quaresma JA, et al. Prevalence of viral hepatitis B and C in riverside communities of the Tucuruí dam, Pará, Brazil. J Med Virol. 2012;84:1907–12.
34. Oliveira CS, Silva AV, Dos Santos KN, Fecury AA, Almeida MK, Fernandes AP, Costa CA, Freitas AS, Corvelo TC, Martins LC. Hepatitis B and C virus infection among Brazilian Amazon riparians. Rev Soc Bras Med Trop. 2011; 44(5):546–50.
35. Valois RC, Maradei-Pereira LM, Crescente JÂ, Oliveira-Filho AB, Lemos JA. HCV infection through perforating and cutting material among candidates for blood donation in Belém, Brazilian Amazon. Rev Inst Med Trop Sao Paulo. 2014;56(6):511–5.
36. Barroso LSL. Indigenous people of Tocantins. 2016. http://www.palmas.org/tocantinsindios.htm. Accessed 30 June 2016.

Public health impact and cost effectiveness of routine childhood vaccination for hepatitis a in Jordan: a dynamic model approach

Wail A. Hayajneh[1*], Vincent J. Daniels[2], Cerise K. James[3], Muhammet Nabi Kanıbir[2], Matthew Pilsbury[2], Morgan Marks[2], Michelle G. Goveia[2], Elamin H. Elbasha[2], Erik Dasbach[2] and Camilo J. Acosta[2]

Abstract

Background: As the socioeconomic conditions in Jordan have improved over recent decades the disease and economic burden of Hepatitis A has increased. The purpose of this study is to assess the potential health and economic impact of a two-dose hepatitis A vaccine program covering one-year old children in Jordan.

Methods: We adapted an age-structured population model of hepatitis A transmission dynamics to project the epidemiologic and economic impact of vaccinating one-year old children for 50 years in Jordan. The epidemiologic model was calibrated using local data on hepatitis A in Jordan. These data included seroprevalence and incidence data from the Jordan Ministry of Health as well as hospitalization data from King Abdullah University Hospital in Irbid, Jordan. We assumed 90% of all children would be vaccinated with the two-dose regimen by two years of age. The economic evaluation adopted a societal perspective and measured benefits using the quality-adjusted life-year (QALY).

Results: The modeled vaccination program reduced the incidence of hepatitis A in Jordan by 99%, 50 years after its introduction. The model projected 4.26 million avoided hepatitis A infections, 1.42 million outpatient visits, 22,475 hospitalizations, 508 fulminant cases, 95 liver transplants, and 76 deaths over a 50 year time horizon. In addition, we found, over a 50 year time horizon, the vaccination program would gain 37,502 QALYs and save over $42.6 million in total costs. The vaccination program became cost-saving within 6 years of its introduction and was highly cost-effective during the first 5 years.

Conclusion: A vaccination program covering one-year old children is projected to be a cost-saving intervention that will significantly reduce the public health and economic burden of hepatitis A in Jordan.

Keywords: Immunization, Hepatitis a, Jordan, Impact, Cost-effectiveness analysis, Simulation, Health technology assessment, Economics

* Correspondence: wailh@just.edu.jo
[1]Department of Pediatrics, Faculty of Medicine, Jordan University of Science and Technology, PO Box 3030, Irbid 22110, Jordan
Full list of author information is available at the end of the article

Background

Hepatitis A virus (HAV) infections continue to pose significant public health issues in Jordan. Some studies over the past few decades had placed Jordan among countries with high HAV endemicity [1–3]. High endemicity is defined as seroprevalence ≥90% by age 10 years and intermediate endemicity is defined as ≥50% by age 15 years [4]. However, the most recent study conducted in 2008 [5], found that a shift in HAV infection burden from children to young adults, that is, the number of children acquiring the infection has decreased while the number of infections in adolescents and adults has increased. This epidemiological pattern among older and relatively active cohorts may lead to serious outbreaks and significant burden of disease because HAV infection in older patients is usually more symptomatic.

The World Health Organization (WHO) recommends including hepatitis A vaccination in the national immunization schedule for children ≥1 year of age when indicated, based on: incidence of acute hepatitis A; change in endemicity from high to intermediate; and consideration of cost effectiveness. According to WHO guidelines, in countries transitioning to intermediate-endemicity where the majority of the adult population will likely be susceptible to hepatitis A infection, large-scale hepatitis A vaccination programs are likely to be cost-effective and are encouraged [6].

The National Immunization Technical Advisory Group (NITAG) of Jordan has voted to introduce several vaccines: pneumococcal conjugate, rotavirus, hepatitis A and varicella to the National Immunization Program. As of December 2015, only rotavirus was introduced. In view of financial and logistic obstacles facing new vaccines introduction, cost-effectiveness and disease burden studies are expected to help decision and policy-makers determine prioritization of remaining in-plan vaccines including the hepatitis A vaccine in Jordan. The purpose of this paper is to test this evidence by assessing the potential health and economic impact of a hepatitis A vaccination program covering one-year old children in Jordan.

Methods

Modeling approach

To assess the potential health and economic impact of a two-dose hepatitis A vaccination program targeting one-year-old children in Jordan, we used a deterministic, age-structured, epidemiologic dynamic model developed previously by Dhankhar, et al. [7] and adapted for the study of HAV transmission and vaccination against HAV infection in Jordan. The model divides the population of Jordan into several distinct classes: maternal antibodies, susceptible, exposed, asymptomatic infection, outpatient, hospitalized, fulminant, patients with recent liver transplant, patients with past liver transplant, recovered, and vaccinated (Fig. 1). Each compartment was further categorized into 101 age groups (0 to < 1, 1,.. .,99, and 100 years or older). The movement of populations between compartements in the model is described in detail in Dhankhar et al. [7]

The model used in the simulations consists of 1313 coupled differential equations corresponding to the 12 epidemiological classes (see Fig. 1) and demographic equations for 101 age groups. All differential equations and details of the epidemiologic model are given in the technical supplement.

Vaccination strategies

Jordan does not have a national HAV vaccination program in place. Also, we were unable to find any data indicating signficant HAV vaccination through the private health sector. Hence, we assumed that before the start of universal vaccination no hepatitis A vaccination strategy was in place in Jordan and that, for our base case, a two-dose program covering oneyear-olds began in 2016. The program consisted of one dose at 12 months old and the second dose at 18 months old. .

In the model, the vaccination at age one year is incorporated by moving a fraction of infants from the susceptible class to the vaccination class before they are two years old. We compared routine universal vaccination of one year-olds to a no vaccine strategy.

Model parameters and data sources

We identified base case inputvalues of demographic, epidemiologic, vaccine, and economic inputs of the model through an extensive search of the published literature. The resulting input values are detailed in Table 1. Jordan specific data inputs were also identified and used where they were available.

Demographic parameters

We obtained age and gender-specific mortality from both the WHO Life Tables [8] and Jordan's IndexMundi demographic profile [9]. Population size of Jordan for 2014 was obtained from U.S. Census International Database [10] and includes Syrian refugee population.

Transmission rates and force of infection

The epidemiologic data on HAV in Jordan and the region suggest there is an ongoing shift from high endemicity to intermediate endemicity [3, 5]. The transmission of HAV in general is correlated with socioeconomic conditions and in particular sanitation and water supply infrastructure [3, 11, 12]. To account for this shift, we adjusted the age-specific force of infection by a universal (age independent) multiplier consisting of piecewise function of time that gradually reduces the force of infection. We

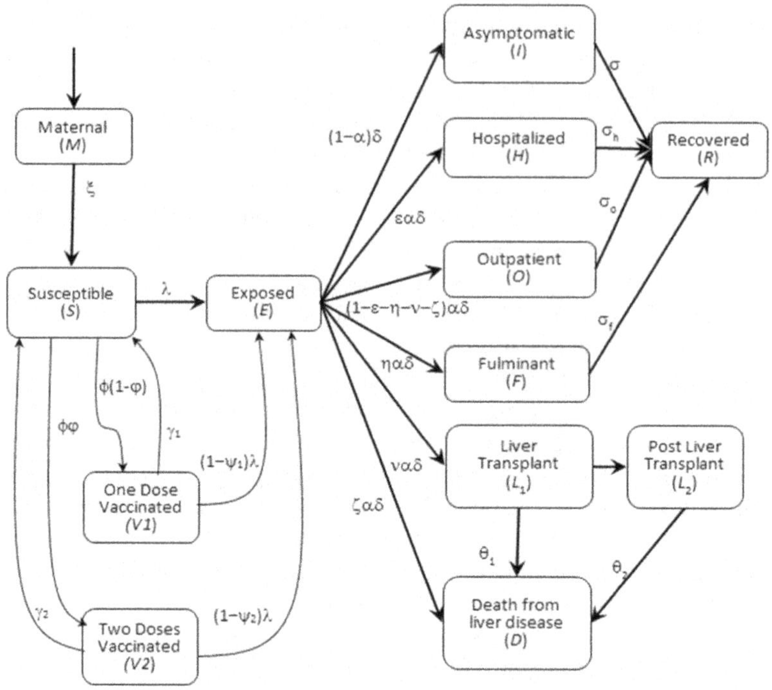

Fig. 1 Transmission model. Flow diagram of hepatitis A virus (HAV) transmission and vaccination model: newborns enter age group a = 0, and are assumed to be protected by maternal antibodies (*M*), the protection is lost over time so the children become susceptible (*S*). Upon infection, a person moves to the exposed compartment (*E*) becomes infectious after a latent period. The model distinguishes between several categories of infection and disease: Asymptomatic (*I*), Symptomatic infections are treated as outpatient (*O*), hospitalized (*H*), with fulminant disease (*F*), requiring a liver transplant (*L*), or die from Hepatitis A virus infection (*D*). Infected persons can clear their infection and move to the recovered compartment (*R*) with lifelong immunity. Susceptible individuals may be vaccinated, one dose or two and move to the appropriate Vaccinated (V1 or V2) compartment. Vaccinated individuals may move back to the susceptible (S) compartment due to waning vaccine or to the exposed compartment due to breakthrough infections. The model also applied age-specific all-cause mortality (not shown) to all persons in all epidemiologic classes

allowed for two periods of change each at a different rate. Both the dates and the magnitude of the reduction in force of infection were determined from calibration to local data. To estimate the forces of infection before the vaccination program is initiated, we used least square methods to fit the model to data on age specific sero-prevalence levels in 2008 [5] and seroprevalence in 1988 data [2]. In addition we used incidence data from Jordan Ministry of Health between 2004 and 2014 [13]. Using these data, the force of infection multiplier function indicated a 4% per year decline in force of infection between 1984 and 1999 followed by a 1% reduction for the next 10 years (see Additional file 1). The timing and magnitude of the trends are consistent with the historical socioeconmic development of Jordan as well as specific sanitation and water supply improvement efforts over the past few decades [14, 15]. Additionally, the decline in force of infections ends in about 2009 as the Syrian crisis in the region [16] begins and ultimately strains resources as a significant new population with a different level of HAV endemicity is introduced into the Jordan population [17–19].

To estimate the proportion of non-outpatient cases we used unpublished HAV hospitalization data from King Abdullah University Hospital in Jordan over the years 2003 through 2013 (see Additional file 1). The proportion of icteric HAV infections is determined using an age specific probability of developing jaundice [20].

The modeling approach does not assume that the endemic disease has reached an equilibrium state before vaccination. Thus, force of infection estimates continue to change with time during the prevaccination period. Force of infection was modeled assuming proportionate mixing, and no exogenous effects, for example, exposure during foreign travel. The force of infection is dynamically modeled so that herd effects are naturally included. Detailed description of the forces of infection are available in the supplementary material (see Additional file 1). Other parameters of the natural history of HAV infection are summarized in Table 1.

Hepatitis a virus infection parameters

We modeled several health outcomes associated with the HAV infection including outpatient visits, hospitalizations,

Table 1 Model parameters

Parameter	Base Case	Range	Distribution	Reference
Demography				
Population 2014	8,117,564	Fixed		[10]
Age Specific All-cause Mortality	Varies	Fixed		[8]
Infection				
Force of Infection		Fixed		[20, 44]
Scale parameter	0.854327	Fixed		
Shape parameter	0.00159689	Fixed		
Shape parameter	11.5766	Fixed		
Duration of Maternal Immunity (mo)	6.5	Fixed		[45]
Latency period (d)	14	Fixed		[46, 47]
Age-specific mean duration of infectiousness (wk)		Fixed		[48, 49]
0–4 y	3.5			
5–9 y	3.0			
10+ y	2.5			
Vaccine				
Vaccine efficacy, one does only (%)	100	87.3–100	Derived Distribution	[22]
Vaccine efficacy, two doses (%)	100	87.3–100	Derived Distribution	Assumed
Median duration of vaccine-derived immunity, one dose only (y)	21	20.3–21.9	Gamma (2647.1, 0.0079)	Assumed
Median duration of vaccine-derived immunity, two doses (y)	32	30.9–33.4	Gamma (2517.63,0.127)	[23]
Vaccination Strategy				
Vaccine uptake, universal strategy, first dose (%)	95%	80–97	Beta (34.37426,1.0007488)	Assumed
Vaccine adherence, probability of second dose given first dose (%)	95%	70–95	Beta (27.15759,2.49654)	Assumed
Clinical Outcomes				
Under reporting factor	11.76	Fixed		Estimated
Probability an infection is icteric	Varies	Fixed		[20]
Proportion of icteric infections hospitalized (%)				[21]
≤4 y	0.395		Dirichlet(D1)[a]	
5–14 y	1.45		Dirichlet(D2)	
15–39 y	1.91		Dirichlet(D3)	
40–59 y	1.57		Dirichlet(D4)	
60+ y	1.7		Dirichlet(D5)	
Probability of fulminant hepatitis A from an icteric infection (%)				[21]
≤4 y	0.0323		Dirichlet(D1)	
5–14 y	0.00425		Dirichlet(D2)	
15–39 y	0.0578		Dirichlet(D3)	
40–59 y	0.468		Dirichlet(D4)	
60+ y	0.68		Dirichlet(D5)	
Probability of liver transplant from an icteric infection (%)				[21]
≤4 y	0.00606		Dirichlet(D1)	
5–14 y	0.000797		Dirichlet(D2)	
15–39 y	0.0108		Dirichlet(D3)	
40–59 y	0.0877		Dirichlet(D4)	
60+ y	0.017		Dirichlet(D5)	

Table 1 Model parameters *(Continued)*

Parameter	Base Case	Range	Distribution	Reference
Probability of death from an icteric infection (%)				[21]
≤4 y	0.00468		Dirichlet(D1)	
5–14 y	0.000616		Dirichlet(D2)	
15–39 y	0.00838		Dirichlet(D3)	
40–59 y	0.0678		Dirichlet(D4)	
60+ y	0.456		Dirichlet(D5)	
Probability of death during first year of liver transplant (%)	11.6	6.0–42.0	Beta (1.14982, 8.76245)	[50]
Probability of death from year 2 and beyond after liver transplant (%)	4.4	2.4–11.0	Beta (3.80137, 82.5935)	[50]
Duration of outpatient icteric infection (d)	34.4	17–40	Gamma (34.37,1.00)	[51]
Duration of inpatient icteric infection (d)	67.8	27–78	Gamma (27.16,2.50)	[51]
Economic Parameters				
Cost of one-dose vaccine (2015 $)	10.00	8.00–14.00	Gamma (42.6844, 0.234277,1.1,3)	Estimated
Test Costs	22.55	Fixed		[26]
Cost of one-dose administration	1.91	Fixed		Estimated
outpatient cost	$15.06	10–25	Gamma (8.71228, 7.77408)	[27]
outpatient visits	3	1–4		Estimated
hospitalization cost	$ 111.5	80–150	Gamma (6.43896, 81.4262)	[26]
hospitalization duration	4.5	3–7		Estimated
fulminant cost	$35,715	32,143–39,278	Gamma (385.022, 92.7609)	[26]
annual cost of patients with liver transplant (1st year)	$70,000	50,000–90,000	Gamma (47.0596, 1487.48)	[26]
annual cost of patients with liver transplant (subsequent years)	43,203	34,563–51,843	Gamma(96.0533, 449.781)	Estimated
Public health cost of a reported infection (2013 $)	0	0–15	Gamma(1.092722,3.660584)	Estimated
work loss, outpatient (d)	15.5	7–18	Gamma(30.51056,0.508021)	[51]
work loss, inpatient (d)	33.2	10–25	Gamma(75.2776,0.4410342)	[51]
work loss, fulminant (d)	33.2	10–25	Gamma(75.2776,0.4410342)	[51]
work loss, year of transplant (d)				[25]
0–17 y	153.2	145–160	Gamma(1602.9, 0.0955766)	
18–40 y	245	238–253	Gamma (4099.41, 0.0597646)	
41–55 y	271	268–274	Gamma (31,347.9, 0.00864492)	
56–62 y	288	284–291	Gamma (26,011.2, 0.0110721)	
63+	314	306–321	Gamma (6733.62, 0.0466316)	
Labor force participation (%)				[52]
16–19 y	3.15	1–28	Beta[1.4452,44.4342]	
20–24 y	33.8	31–72	Beta[6.57547,12.8786]	
25–34 y	64.0	57–70	Beta[133.435,75.0572]	
35–44 y	59.6	51 – 71	Beta[54.5338,36.9658]	
45–54 y	47.1	35–59	Beta[30.8364,34.6337]	
55–64 y	30.7	0–62	Beta[2.30395,5.20078]	
65+	10.0	0–23	Beta[2.51432,22.6289]	
Median Monthly earnings (2014 $)				[53]
< 25 y	292	137–350	Gamma(13.6337, 21.4175)	
25+	365	250–650	Gamma(28.8788, 10.1112)	
Discount rate per year, %	3	0–5		Assumed

Table 1 Model parameters *(Continued)*

Parameter	Base Case	Range	Distribution	Reference
Utilities				
Average population norms				[31]
20–29 y	.920	0.913–0.927	Beta(5307.7008, 461.5392)	
30–39 y	.905	0.898–0.912	Beta(6099.1932,640.2468)	
40–49 y	.874	0.867–0.882	Beta(6572.4195,947.5113)	
50–59 y	.848	0.840–0.857	Beta(5810.9376,1041.5832)	
60–69 y	.824	0.812–0.836	Beta(3187.1645,680.7536)	
70–79 y	.785	0.771–0.798	Beta(2791.9027,764.6613)	
80+ y	.744	0.720–0.768	Beta(944.3511,324.9380)	
Persons with anicteric hepatitis A	.830	0.789–0.867	Beta(291.9525,59.7975)	[21]
Persons with icteric hepatitis A	.642	0.607–0.682	Beta(410.1317,228.3050)	[29]
Persons with liver transplant	.730	0.630–0.840	Beta(49.4052,18.2732)	[30]

Base-case model parameters, estimates, corresponding distributions and ranges for deterministic and probabilistic sensitivity analysis, and data source references
[a]Parameters for the Dirichlet distributions are as follows: D1 = (97.0207,0.385265,0.00456518,0.031484,0.00590325), D2 = (349.97,5.13289,0.00218903,0.0150967,0.00283064), D3 = (458.787,8.95484,0.0392421,0.270635,0.0507441), D4 = (377.566,6.07215,0.261759,1.80523,0.338481), D5 = (161.413,2.82536,0.757196,1.13014,0.0282536)

fulminant hepatitis disease, liver transplant, and death (Fig. 1). We assumed that asymptomatic hepatitis A cases do not require health care and only the management of icteric hepatitis A cases entails the use of health care resources. We further assumed that all reported and unreported icteric cases are treated and used the underreporting factor to identify the proportion of inpatient – hospitalized, fulminant hepatitis, or liver transplant – the remaining cases are assumed to receive outpatient care. Within the inpatient category the conditional probabilities shown in Table 1 are the result of dividing by the underreporting factor [7, 21].

Vaccine parameters

Vaccine efficacy for one or two doses was based on data from VAQTA [Hepatitis A Vaccine, Purified Inactivated, Merck & Co., Inc., Kenilworth, NJ] and was determined to be 100% in the base case [22]. We assumed the median duration of protection of a completed one-dose and two-dose hepatitis A vaccination in the base case was 21 and 32 years, respectively, and examined alternative assumptions in the sensitivity analysis [23]. With respect to vaccine coverage, the base case assumed that 95% of one-year-olds will receive one-dose and that 95% of those will receive the second does before they are two years old. The base case vaccination coverage was chosen based on coverage achieved in similar childhood vaccinations in the Jordanian National Immunization Program [13, 24].

Costs

We adopted a societal perspective for economic evaluation. We included both direct and indirect costs in the evaluation. The direct costs included treatment costs of HAV-associated health outcomes and vaccination. Treatment costs included costs for outpatient visits, hospitalizations, fulminant hepatitis, and liver transplantations [25–27]. Wherever possible we used Jordanian cost data, however, in some cases we used costs from similarly economically situated countries and adjusted appropriately. We use $10.00 USD per dose for the vaccine price based on estimates of current regional pricing. We assumed $1.90 for vaccine administration costs based on estimates from King Abdullah University Hospital.

Indirect costs included the costs associated with the work loss due to different health outcomes. These were estimated by multiplying the days of work loss from an HAV disease outcome by the labor force participation rate and the daily wages of the patients' age group (Table 1). We did not include public health disease control costs in the base case study as these were estimated to be very small in Jordan. However, we did include non-zero public health costs in the sensitivity analyses. All costs are reported in 2015 USD. Future costs were discounted at 3% per year. To interpret the cost-effectiveness of vaccination we used the WHO CHOICE criteria which set cost-effectiveness thresholds based on per capita GDP. According to this criteria, incremental cost-effectiveness ratio (ICER) less than one times per capita GDP is considered "very cost effective" while ICER greater than three times per capita GDP is "not cost-effective" [28].

Utilities

We calculated quality-adjusted life-years (QALYs) by applying utility weights to time spent in each health state. We assumed a weight of 0.642 for all icteric outcomes related to hepatitis A, except liver transplant [29].

For patients with liver transplants, we assumed a weight of 0.73 following transplantation [30]. We assumed the quality-of-life weight of 0.83 for persons with anicteric hepatitis A. For all other health states we used a weight of 1.0. To account for the age-specific health utilities in the general population, all utility weights were multiplied by the age-specific US population norms [31] due to a lack of Jordanian-specific data.

Implementation

The model was implemented in Mathematica 10.1 (Wolfram Research, Inc., Champaign, IL). We used the built-in function NDSolve to find numerical solutions to the system of ordinary differential equations. The built-in function NMinimize was used for model calibration. We used Mathematica for all simulations, and analyses and some figures; others were produced using Microsoft Excel 2010 (Microsoft Corp., Redmond, WA).

Analyses

Base case and sensitivity analyses

We estimated expected health outcomes (total HAV infections, symptomatic HAV infections, outpatient visits, hospitalizations, fulminant hepatitis cases, number of liver transplants, deaths, QALYs) and costs over a time horizon of 50 years.

Deterministic sensitivity analyses were performed by varying vaccination parameters (efficacy, duration of protection, cost, coverage, and adherence), cost parameters, quality-of-life weights, and discount rate.

Probabilistic sensitivity analyses (PSA) were also performed using a subset of parameters including vaccine properties and uptake, clinical outcomes, costs, and quality-of-life weights were included in a PSA as described in Table 1. The rationale for the selection of the probability distribution function for each parameter and sampling techniques used in the PSA is discussed in the technical supplement. The results are summarized using the mean of outcomes and presented using a scatter plot in the incremental cost-effectiveness plane [32]. The location of a point on the plane summarizes its cost and effectiveness. For example, all positive incremental QALYs represent health gains; negative costs represent a total cost savings for the program. If the costs are positive and the QALYs are positive then there is a threshold, the willingness to pay (WTP) for each QALY gained below which the program is considered cost-effective or cost-saving.

Model transparency and validation

To facilitate independent review and replication of our results according to industry recommendations [33] we provided a technical supplement which includes information on the model's structure, equations, inputs, outputs, and detailed description of methods of the derivation. The face validity of the model is described in Dhankhar, et al. [7] Internal validity of the model code was verified using several tests including balanced inflow and outflow between compartments and constancy of total population throughout the calculations. The predictive validity of the model was evaluated by comparing model results with epidemiologic data reported in the literature (see Additional file 1).

Results

Base case

Epidemiology results

The model predicts rapid and substantial decrease in overall incidence of Hepatitis A (Fig. 2). The model predicts a drop from 900 cases per 100,000 a year down to less than one case per 100,000 within five years of launching the vaccination program. Long-term health outcomes were predicted after the introduction of the vaccination program (Table 2). In terms of cumulative outcomes, on the 50 year time horizon there are 4.26 million infections avoided resulting in more than 1.4 million inpatient cases avoided over the 50 year time horizon.

Cost-effectiveness results

The economic impact of the vaccination program is summarized in Table 3. The results for costs and QALYs are shown for the whole population. Costs savings are achieved by 6 years after the program begins saving $46.2 million in the first 50 years.

Deterministic sensitivity analysis

The number of years to reach cost savings was most sensitive to outpatient cost, vaccine dose cost, hospitalization costs, second dose vaccine adherence, and outpatient work-loss days. The outpatient costs parameter induced the largest change. In the low cost ($10) limit, the universal vaccination program takes more than 45 years to become cost saving while in the high cost limit ($100) cost saving is attained within 4 years. The sensitivity to this factor arises from the large proportion of cases that are treated as outpatient, approximately 99% of all symptomatic cases. The next most influential parameter was the vaccine cost. The vaccine cost lower limit ($8) leads to cost savings within 4 years while the upper limit ($14) extends time to cost savings to 14 years. This sensitivity is due to the vaccine cost being the only substantial contributor to the total cost of the vaccination program.

The other factors tested lead to between − 1.4 and 1.3 years difference in reaching the cost savings threshold. For example, the lower limit of the hospitalization costs ($80) results in 6 years to cost savings while the

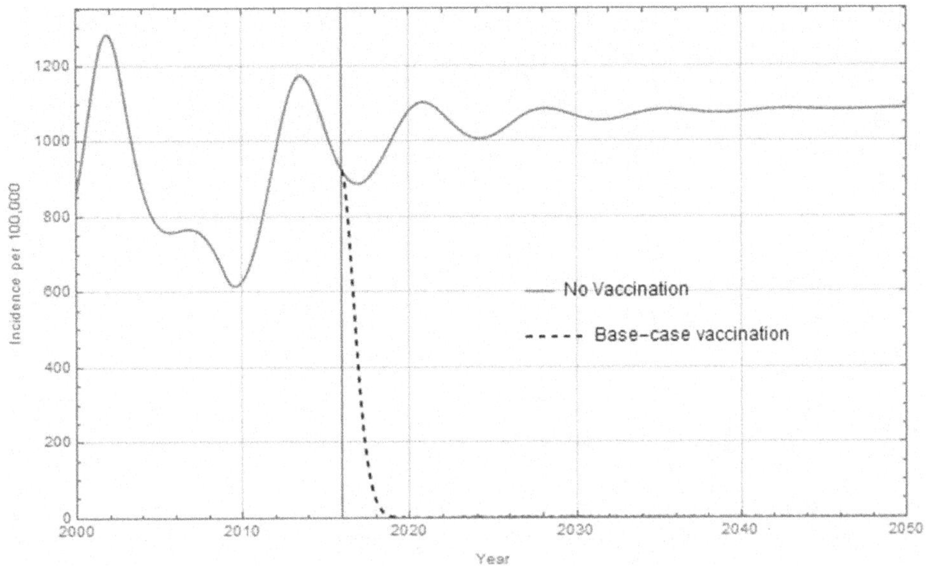

Fig. 2 hepatitis A incidence. Overall incidence of hepatitis A with no vaccine (solid line) and after vaccination (dashed line) assuming the vaccination program begins in 2016

upper limit ($150) leads to 4.6 years to cost savings. Among factors that had little effect on years-to-cost savings were the 1st dose vaccine uptake and vaccine parameters such as vaccine efficacy and duration of protection. These likewise had little effect on health outcomes. For example, with the lowest uptake, 70%, the program still reaches less than one case per 100,000 people within the five years. In fact, as long as the 1st dose uptake is > 40% this threshold will be reached. In addition, since the population has not reached endemic equilibrium by 2016, we considered a range of vaccination program start years (t_{vstart}) from 2016 through 2040. We found little qualitative difference in outcomes, for example, the time to cost savings ranged from approximately 2 to 5.4 years, with our base case, t_{vstart} = 2016, being the worst case.

The total cost savings over 50 years was most sensitive to discount rate, outpatient costs, vaccine cost, median monthly earnings 25+, probability of death after 1st year liver transplant, outpatient work loss days, and hospitalization costs in that order. Discount rate produced the largest change reducing cost savings by $9.2 million between the low (0%) and high (5%) discount rates. Outpatient costs was the second most influential parameter increasing cost savings by $7.9 million between the low and high cost values. Vaccine cost was the third most influential parameter reducing cost savings by $3.3 million between the low and high limits. All other parameters were less influential leading to changes in cost savings between -$1.3 and $1.2 million.

Table 2 Cumulative HAV cases avoided for the population of Jordan after 5, 10, 25, and 50 years of universal vaccination

Cumulative events avoided with vaccination	Universal Vaccination			
	5 years	10 years	25 years	50 years
Any Infection	326,900	748,608	1,618,125	4,260,589
Asymptomatic	225,772	509,773	1,085,502	2,813,184
Symptomatic	101,127	238,835	532,624	1,447,405
Outpatient	99,572	235,120	524,228	1,424,252
Hospitalizations	1522	3633	8195	22,475
Fulminant cases	24	61	151	508
Liver Transplants	5	11	28	95
Deaths	4	9	22	76

Table 3 Cumulative cost effectiveness/savings after 5, 10, 25, and 50 years of vaccination program. Cost savings is achieved within 6 years considering indirect costs and within 8 years if indirect costs are excluded. Values are for the entire population

Cumulative outcomes	Universal Vaccination			
	5 y	10 y	25 y	50 y
QALY's Gained[a]	4800	10,521	24,144	37,502
Vaccination Cost (millions)	$9.40	$17.52	$35.76	$52.83
Disease Cost Avoided (millions)	$8.06	$18.60	$47.78	$81.41
Indirect cost avoided (millions)	$0.99	$2.61	$8.00	$14.03
Total Cost Savings(millions, including indirect costs)	–	$3.69	$20.03	$42.60
Total Cost Savings(millions, excluding indirect cost)	–	$1.09	$12.02	$28.57
ICER[b] ($/QALY, including indirect costs)	75	Cost saving	Cost saving	Cost saving
ICER ($/QALY, excluding indirect cost)	281	Cost saving	Cost saving	Cost saving

[a]QALY, quality-adjusted life-year
[b]ICER, incremental cost-effectiveness ratio

Probabilistic sensitivity analysis (PSA)
We performed a PSA using 1024 Monte Carlo simulations. The results showed that the mean incremental cost savings for the population after 50 years was US $807,000 (95% confidence interval $41,000 to $2.1 M) with a median value of $560,000. The corresponding values for incremental QALYs gained was 460 (95% confidence interval 428 to 508) with a median value of 453. Additionally, the mean number of years to reach cost saving was 6.9 years (95% confidence interval 2.2 to 30 years) with a median value of 4.4 years.

The incremental cost-effectiveness plane shows that most (99.3%) of the PSA pairs fall in the fourth quadrant indicating they are cost saving (Fig. 3). The remaining 0.7% are in the first quadrant and are highly cost-effective. The average incremental cost-effectiveness ratio for the PSA pairs in the first quadrant is $86/QALY. The chart shows the line indicating a willingness-to-pay of $3600/QALY. This quantity is the one-times the per capita GDP of Jordan in 2014 below which therapies are considered "very cost-effective" according WHO CHOICE recommendations [28]. All of the scenarios in these analyses fell well below the $3600/QALY threshold.

Discussion

To our knowledge this is the first published modeling study of HAV in Jordan. We adapted a previously published dynamic transmission model to examine the potential impact of two-dose hepatitis A vaccination of one year-olds in Jordan. As compared with no vaccination, the model predicted that this vaccination program is cost-saving within 6 years of its introduction. The model showed the virtual elimination of HAV cases within five

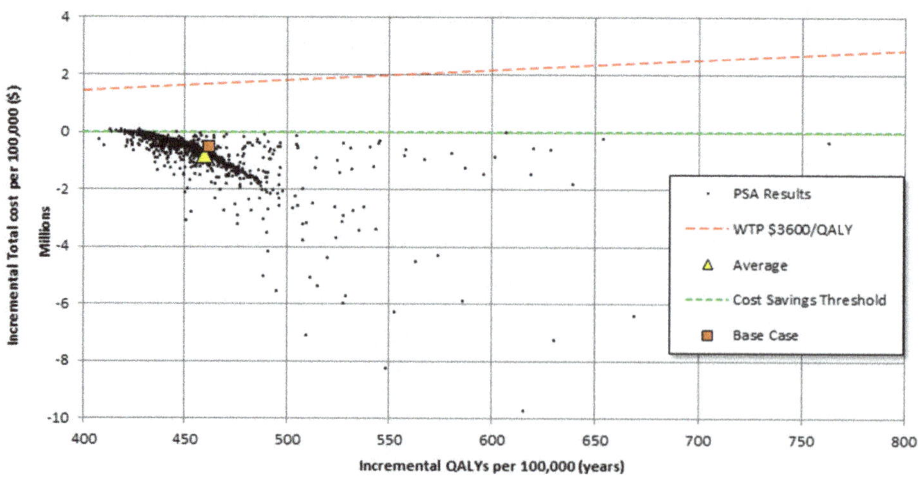

Fig. 3 Probabilistic sensitivity analysis (PSA) results. Scatter plot of the estimated joint density of incremental total costs and QALYs per 100,000 persons for vaccination program compared to no vaccination. The long dashed line represents the $3600 WTP threshold above which the program would not be very cost effective. Each black dot represents the resulting incremental cost and effectiveness of one set of parameters from the PSA. The triangle indicates the result corresponding to the average incremental cost and effectiveness. And the square represents the cost-effectiveness of the base case parameter set. All points with negative incremental cost represent cost-saving parameter sets

years of introducing a two-dose vaccination program targeting one-year olds.

Our health economic results are similar to those previously obtained from model-based analysis in other HAV intermediate endemic countries. Those analyses also support the clinical and economic value of universal mass vaccination against hepatitis A virus: > 98% reduction in incidence for toddlers and > 95% reduction for the rest of the population in the first five years in Israel [34]; a sharp disease rate decrease (88%) in Argentina [35]; total disease societal cost reduction while costing the health system <US$726 per QALY in Chile [36]; cost-saving -US $ 2.26 saved for each invested dollar- in Brazil [37, 38]; and 85 to 93% reduction for all HAV infections in Mexico [39].

Sensitivity analyses showed that outpatient costs, vaccine costs, probability of death after the 1st year of a liver transplant, were most influential in determining the time to reach cost saving. No scenarios failed to reach cost saving within 50 years. Health outcomes were not particularly sensitive to uptake or adherence. Regardless, suboptimal uptake and adherence is not expected considering consistently very high uptake levels reported by Jordanian National Immunization Program with other vaccination programs [13].

Despite similarity of overall economic value with above mentioned previous studies, their results show less optimistic health outcomes than our model's predictions [26, 36, 39, 40]. Some of the differences could be due to methodological quality variation across studies [41], but the most significant effects are likely to be due to differences in the way exogenous effects are included in the force of infection.

Our study has several limitations. First, given the lack of directly measurable data on the force of infection parameters, we had to specify a particular functional form, make simplifying assumptions, and estimate the input parameters by fitting the model to real world data. For example, when considering exogenous factors affecting the force of infection, we excluded effects due to foreign travel, or immigration. This may be a good choice for the current state, but such factors, like the ongoing influx of refugees, may become important in the future. In addition, we have assumed that ongoing and future socioeconomic changes will not have significant influence on the force of infection in the future thereby potentially overestimating the benefit of a vaccination program. Second, limited availability of reliable historical data for seroprevalence and disease incidence adds uncertainty to the model calibration. Third, we assumed that certain parameters, e.g., population size and birth rate, stay constant over the time horizon. Fourth, due to the lack of data availability for Jordan, many economic and outcomes parameters were estimated, derived, or adapted from data from other countries. Finally, we did not incorporate uncertainty in the estimated parameters of the force of infection as part of the probabilistic sensitivity analysis.

Conclusion and recommendations

This model predicted that a universal 2-dose program vaccinating one year olds against hepatitis A led to significant reductions in hepatitis A morbidity and mortality and was cost saving within 6 years and highly cost-effective during the first 5 years.

Based on the study results, the safety profile of the vaccine [42, 43] and the WHO recommendations [6], the risk-benefit profile calls for the introduction of a two-dose program of vaccinating one-year olds against hepatitis A. These two doses, at 12 and 18 months of age, could ideally be administered simultaneously with other vaccines already included in the Jordanian National Pediatric Immunization Program.

Abbreviations

GDP: Gross domestic product; HAV: Hepatitis A virus; ICER: Incremental cost-effectiveness ratio; NITAG: National Immunization Technical Advisory Group; PSA: Probabilistic sensitivity analysis; QALY: Quality-adjusted life-year; WHO: World Health Organization; WTP: Willingness to pay

Funding

Merck Sharp & Dohme Corp., a subsidiary of Merck & Co., Inc., Kenilworth, NJ, sponsored the study.

Authors' contributions

WAH: Jordan health and economic expertise, contribution to the background and conclusions. VJD: Jordan adaptation of the model, model simulations, results tabulation and analysis, contribution to methods and results sections of the manuscript and technical supplement. CKJ: acquisition of input data and reference validation. MP: model development, programing support, and contribution to the technical supplement. MM: epidemiological expertise and analysis of raw data inputs. EHE: development of the original HAV model, expertise in the model adaptation and calibration process, and contribution to the technical supplement. ED: health and economic analysis and contribution to the background section. MNK, CJA, and MG: hepatitis A subject matter experts and contribution to of the conclusions and recommendations sections [2]. All authors read and approved the final manuscript.

Consent for publication

Not applicable.

Competing interests

Several authors are employees of or are contracted by Merck & Co., Inc., which produces and markets VAQTA® (hepatitis A vaccine, inactivated).

Author details

[1]Department of Pediatrics, Faculty of Medicine, Jordan University of Science and Technology, PO Box 3030, Irbid 22110, Jordan. [2]Merck & Co., Inc., Kenilworth, NJ, USA. [3]Agile-1 for Merck & Co., Inc., Kenilworth, NJ, USA.

References

1. Battikhi MN, Battikhi EG. The seroepidemiology of hepatitis a virus in Amman, Jordan. New Microbiol. 2004;27:215–20.
2. Toukan AU, Sharaiha ZK, Abu-el-Rob OA. The seroepidemiology of hepatitis a virus infection in Jordan. Trop Gastroenterol. 1988;9:76–9.
3. Itani T, Jacobsen KH, Nguyen T, Wiktor SZ. A new method for imputing country-level estimates of hepatitis a virus endemicity levels in the eastern Mediterranean region. Vaccine. 2014;32:6067–74.
4. Jacobsen KH, Wiersma ST. Hepatitis a virus seroprevalence by age and world region, 1990 and 2005. Vaccine. 2010;28:6653–7.
5. Hayajneh WA, Balbeesi A, Faouri S. Hepatitis a virus age-specific sero-prevalence and risk factors among Jordanian children. J Med Virol. 2015;87: 569–74.
6. World Health Organization. WHO position paper on hepatitis a vaccines: June 2012 -recommendations. Vaccine. 2013;31:285–6.
7. Dhankhar P, Nwankwo C, Pillsbury M, Lauschke A, Goveia MG, Acosta CJ, et al. Public health impact and cost-effectiveness of hepatitis a vaccination in the United States: a disease transmission dynamic modeling approach. Value Heal. 2015;18:358–67.
8. World Health Organization. Global Health Observatory: Life Tables by Country Jordan. World Health Organization; 2015 [cited 2015 Nov 11]. Available from: http://apps.who.int/gho/data/?theme=main&vid=60830
9. Jordan Demographics profile 2014. 2015 [cited 2015 Nov 16]. Available from: http://www.indexmundi.com/jordan/demographics_profile.html
10. United States Census Bureau. International Database: Demographics. Jordan: United States Census Bureau; 2015. [cited 2015 Sep 24]. Available from: http://www.census.gov/population/international/data/idb/region.php?N= Results&T=13&A=separate&RT=0&Y=2010,2011,2012,2013,2014,2015&R= −1&C=JO.
11. Jacobsen KH, Koopman JS. The effects of socioeconomic development on worldwide hepatis a virus seroprevalence patterns. Int J Epidemiol. 2005;34:600–9.
12. Jacobsen KH. The global prevalence of hepatitis a virus infection and susceptibility: a systematic review. Geneva: World Heal Organ; 2009.
13. Directorate of Vital information Studies Preparation. Ministry of Health Annual Statistical Book 2014. Amman: Jordan Ministry of Health; 2015. Available from: http://www.moh.gov.jo
14. Jiries A. Water resources in Jordan. Adv Water Supply Wastewater Treat A Road to Safer Soc Environ Springer. 2011:193–9.
15. WHO & UNICEF Progress on Sanitation and Drinking Water: 2015 Update and MDG assessment. UNICEF; 2015. Available from: http://www.unicef.org/publications/index_82419.html
16. UN Refugee Agency. Syrian Regional Refugee Response: Inter-agency Information Sharing Portal. 2015. Available from: http://data.unhcr.org/syrianrefugees/country.php?id=107
17. Carrion D. Syrian refugees in Jordan: confronting difficult truths. London; 2015. Available from: https://www.chathamhouse.org/sites/files/chathamhouse/field/field_document/20150921SyrianRefugeesCarrion.pdf
18. Slaih AA. Impact of Syrian refugees on Jordan's health sector. 2013. Available from: https://data.unhcr.org/syrianrefugees/download.php?id=4345
19. UNDP. Analysis of Impact of Influx of Syrian Refugees on Host Communities. 2014. Available from: http://inform.gov.jo/en-us/By-Date/Report-Details/ArticleId/12/Analysis-of-Impact-of-Influx-of-Syrian-Refugees-on-Host-Communities
20. Armstrong GL, Bell BP. Hepatitis a virus infections in the United States: model-based estimates and implications for childhood immunization. Pediatrics. 2002;109
21. Rein DB, Hicks KA, Wirth KE, Billah K, Finelli L, Fiore AE, et al. Cost-effectiveness of routine childhood vaccination for hepatitis a in the United States. Pediatrics. 2007;119:e12–21.
22. Werzberger A, Mensch B, Kuter B, Brown L, Lewis J, Sitrin R, et al. A controlled trial of a formalin-inactivated hepatitis a vaccine in healthy children. N Engl J Med. 1992;327:453–7.
23. Wiens BL, Bohidar NR, Pigeon JG, Egan J, Hurni W, Brown L, et al. Duration of protection from clinical hepatitis a disease after vaccination with VAQTA. J Med Virol. 1996;49:235–41.
24. Nuseirat A, Qusous L, Ghanem M, editors. Jordan national drug formulary. Amman: Jordanian Food and Drug Administration; 2015. Available from: http://apps.who.int/medicinedocs/documents/s19468en/s19468en.pdf
25. Huda A, Newcomer R, Harrington C, Blegen MG, Keeffe EB. High rate of unemployment after liver transplantation: analysis of the united network for organ sharing database. Liver Transplant. 2012;18:89–99.
26. Lopez E, Debbag R, Coudeville L, Baron-Papillon F, Armoni J. The cost-effectiveness of universal vaccination of children against hepatitis a in Argentina: results of a dynamic health–economic analysis. J Gastroenterol. 2007;42:152–60.
27. World Health Organization. WHO-Choice: Estimates of Unit cost for Patient Services for Jordan. 2015 [cited 2015 Nov 19]. Available from: http://www.who.int/choice/country/jor/cost/en/
28. World Health Organization. WHO-Choice: Choosing Interventions that are cost-Effective. Geneva; 2015 [cited 2015 Dec 4]. Available from: htp://www.who.int/choice/en
29. Luyten J, Marais C, Hens N, De Schrijver K, Beutels P. Imputing QALYs from single time point health state descriptions on the EQ-5D and the SF-6D: a comparison of methods for hepatitis a patients. Value Heal. 2011;14:282–90.
30. Chong CAKY, Gulamhussein A, Heathcote EJ, Lilly L, Sherman M, Naglie G, et al. Health-state utilities and quality of life in hepatitis C patients. Am J Gastroenterol. 2003;98:630–8.
31. Hanmer J, Lawrence WF, Anderson JP, Kaplan RM, Fryback DG. Report of nationally representative values for the noninstitutionalized US adult population for 7 health-related quality-of-life scores. Med Decis Mak. 2006; 26:391–400.
32. Black WC. The CE plane a graphic representation of cost-effectiveness. Med Decis Mak. 1990;10:212–4.
33. Eddy DM, Hollingworth W, Caro JJ, Tsevat J, McDonald KM, Wong JB. Model transparency and validation a report of the ISPOR-SMDM modeling good research practices task force–7. Med Decis Mak. 2012; 32:733–43.
34. Dagan R, Leventhal A, Anis E, Slater P, Ashur Y, Shouval D. Incidence of hepatitis a in Israel following universal immunization of toddlers. JAMA. 2005;294:202–10.
35. Cervio G, Trentadue J, D'Agostino D, Luque C, Giorgi M, Armoni J, et al. Decline in HAV-associated fulminant hepatic failure and liver transplant in children in Argentina after the introduction of a universal hepatitis a vaccination program. Hepat Med. 2011;3:99–106.
36. Valenzuela MT, Jacobs RJ, Arteaga O, Navarrete MS, Meyerhoff AS, Innis BL. Cost-effectiveness of universal childhood hepatitis a vaccination in Chile. Vaccine. 2005;23:4110–9.
37. Sartori AMC, de Soárez PC, Novaes HMD, Amaku M, de Azevedo RS, Moreira RC, et al. Cost-effectiveness analysis of universal childhood hepatitis a vaccination in Brazil: regional analyses according to the endemic context. Vaccine. 2012;30:7489–97.
38. Zahdi MR, Maluf Junior I, Maluf EMCP. Hepatitis a: the costs and benefits of the disease prevention by vaccine, Paranà, Brazil. Braz J Infect Dis. 2009;13:257–61.
39. Van Effelterre TP, DeAntonio R, Cassidy A, Romano-Mazzotti L, Marano C. Model-based projections of the population-level impact of hepatitis a vaccination in Mexico. Hum Vaccin Immunother. 2012;8:1099–108.
40. Quezada A, Baron-Papillon F, Coudeville L, Maggi L. Universal vaccination of children against hepatitis a in Chile: a cost-effectiveness study. Rev Panam Salud Pública. 2008;23:303–12.
41. Anonychuk AM, Tricco AC, Bauch CT, Gilca V, Duval B, John-Baptiste A, et al. Cost-effectiveness analyses of hepatitis a vaccine. Pharmacoeconomics. 2008;26:17–32.
42. Black S, Shinefield H, Hansen J, Lewis E, Su L, Coplan P. A post-licensure evaluation of the safety of inactivated hepatitis a vaccine (VAQTA®, Merck) in children and adults. Vaccine. 2004;22:766–72.
43. Niu MT, Salive M, Krueger C, Ellenberg SS. Two-year review of hepatitis a vaccine safety: data from the vaccine adverse event reporting system (VAERS). Clin Infect Dis. 1998;26(6):1475.
44. Whitaker HJ, Farrington CP. Estimation of infections disease parameters from serological survey data: the impact of regular epidemics. Stat Med. 2004;23:2429–43.

45. Linder N, Karetnyi Y, Gidony Y, Dagan R, Ohel G, Levin E, et al. Decline of hepatitis a antibodies during the first 7 months of life in full-term and preterm infants. Infection. 1999;27:128–31.
46. Fiore AE, Wasley A, Bell BP. Prevention of hepatitis a through active or passive immunization: recommendations of the advisory committee on immunization practices (ACIP). MMWR Recomm Rep. 2006;55:1–23.
47. Leach CT. Hepatitis A in the United States. Pediatr Infect Dis J. 2004;23:551–2.
48. Amariei R, Willms AR, Bauch CT. The United States and Canada as a coupled epidemiological system: an example from hepatitis a. BMC Infect Dis. 2008;8:23.
49. Martin A, Lemon SM, Hepatitis A. Virus: from discovery to vaccines. Hepatology. 2006;43:S164–72.
50. Wolfe RA, Roys EC, Merion RM. Trends in organ donation and transplantation in the United States, 1999–2008. Am J Transplant. 2010;10:961–72.
51. Berge JJ, Drennan DP, Jacobs RJ, Jakins A, Meyerhoff AS, Stubblefield W, et al. The cost of hepatitis a infections in American adolescents and adults in 1997. Hepatology. 2000;31:469–73.
52. Mryyan N. Demographics, labor force participation, and unemployment in Jordan. In: Assaad R, editor. Jordanian Labour Mark. New Millenn. Oxford: Oxford University Press; 2014. p. 39–63.
53. Jordanian Employed Persons Age 15+ Years by Monthly Earnings Categories. Jordan Dep. Stat. 2014 [cited 2015 Nov 9]. Available from: http://jorinfo.dos.gov.jo/PXWeb2014R2/Menu.aspx?px_db=DOS+Database&px_language=en&rxid=e0c35eac-d04f-4689-ace3-8f29bf1f19da

Successful infection of BALB/c mice by a swine hepatitis E virus clone constructed with reverse genetics

Wenhai Yu[1], Chenchen Yang[2], Xianhui Hao[2], Tianwu Ma[2] and Fen Huang[2*]

Abstract

Background: Hepatitis E virus (HEV) is a leading cause of hepatitis worldwide. However, its infection biology and pathogenesis remain largely elusive. Furthermore, no proven medication is available for treating hepatitis E. Robust experimental models are urgently required to advance the research of HEV infection. Because of the lacking of a sophisticated small animal model, this study aimed to establish a mouse model of HEV infection.

Methods: We constructed a full-length swine HEV cDNA clone of genotype 4 (named as pGEM-HEV) by reverse genetics approach. And we inoculated with HEV RNA in BALB/c mice to establish small animal model for HEV infection and pathogenesis studies.

Results: The capped RNA transcripts of pGEM-HEV prepared in vitro were replication-competent in HepG2 cells. Importantly, BALB/c mice intravenously inoculated with RNA transcripts of pGEM-HEV developed an active infection as shown by shedding viruses in feces, detectable negative strand of HEV in the liver, spleen and kidney, and causing liver inflammation.

Conclusion: In this study, we successfully established of BALB/c mice-based small animal model for HEV provides an opportunity to further understand HEV pathogenesis and to develop effective antiviral medications.

Keywords: Hepatitis E virus, Infectious cDNA clone, BALB/c mice, Infectivity

Background

Hepatitis E virus (HEV) is classified in the genus *Orthohepevirus* of the family *Hepeviridae* [1]. It is a non-enveloped, single-stranded, positive-sense RNA virus, with an approximately 7.3 kb genome. The viral genome consists of three open reading frames (ORFs) flanked by short 5′ and 3′ non-translated regions, ORF1 encodes a nonstructural protein, ORF2 encodes a capsid protein and ORF3 encodes a small multifunction protein that is essential for viral infection [2–5]. A unique feature as a hepatitis virus is that HEV has a zoonotic nature and can cross-species transmit in human, swine and deer [6–10].

HEV is considered the most common cause of hepatitis worldwide [11]. It causes both endemic and epidemic forms of hepatitis E in many developing countries. It is transmitted by the fecal-oral route and waterborne transmission is most often described. In developed countries, most documented cases of acute hepatitis E are sporadic and endemic cases attributed to food consumption [11–13]. Although the infection is generally acute and self-limiting, up to about 25~30% mortality has been reported following HEV infection during pregnancy [14, 15]. However, the biology and pathogenesis of HEV infection remain largely elusive and no proven antiviral medication is available.

Robust experiment models are the most important tools for advancing fundamental and translational research of hepatitis E infection. Fortunately, several cell culture systems for propagating HEV have been recently developed [16–18]. However, the development of animal models, in particular the use of small laboratory animals, has not been well-explored. Although swine and rabbit have been used to model HEV infection [19, 20], experimental infection in mouse model, the most commonly used laboratory species, has not been established.

* Correspondence: huangfen6789@163.com
[2]Medical School, Kunming University of Science and Technology, 727 Jingming Road, Kunming, China
Full list of author information is available at the end of the article

We previously have attempted to establish BALB/c nude mice-based HEV model [21]. However, this strain lacks a thymus and is therefore unable to produce T-cells. The immunodeficient nature with a strict life condition and limited fertility has hampered the further application. To circumstance these bottlenecks, this study aimed to establish regular BALB/c mice-based HEV model. We first constructed an infectious cDNA clone of swine HEV with reverse genetics approach. We demonstrated its infectivity in cell culture and importantly also in BALB/c mice. Most interestingly, HEV provokes host response with production of anti-HEV antibodies and induction of liver inflammation, mimicking infection in human. Therefore, this model bears important implications for studying HEV infection and drug development.

Methods

Construction of a full-length cDNA clone of HEV

The full-length of swine HEV (genotype 4, KM01, GenBank No. KJ155502) was amplified with specific primers shown in Table 1 [22]. The collection of stool specimens was approved by the owner. Five overlapping fragments were amplified by PCR. The 3′ end and 5′ end of the virus were obtained using the RACE 5' or 3′ kit (Takara). The entire viral genome was ligated together at indicated restriction enzyme sites in each fragment (Fig. 1). A unique *Xba* I restriction enzyme site and a T7 RNA polymerase core promoter were introduced at the extreme 5′ terminus. Twenty-four adenosines (A) was engineered at the 3′ end of viral genome, followed by a *Cla* I restriction enzyme site for plasmid linearization (Fig. 1). PCR productions were purified and cloned into pMD-18 T vector, followed by sequencing with three clones of each fragment. The clone containing the consensus sequence was used for infectious clone assembly. One silent mutation at nucleotide (nt) 4120 (G → T) generated during the PCR amplification was retained as a genetic marker. The full-length genomic cDNA was introduced into the pGEM-7zf (+) vector (Promega) between *Xba* I and *Cla* I sites to produce a full-length HEV cDNA clone named pGEM-HEV.

In vitro transcription of capped full-length HEV genomic RNA

The full-length cDNA clones of pGEM-HEV was linearized by *Cla* I, then digested with proteinase K, and purified by phenol extraction followed by ethanol precipitation. Capped RNA transcripts from pGEM-HEV were synthesized in vitro with the T7 RiboMAX™ Express Large Scale RNA Production System (Promega, USA) according to the direction. The RNA transcripts from the cDNA clone was quantitated (1 μg /μL) and stored in – 80 °C until use.

Cell transfection and immunofluorescence assay

The human hepatoma HepG2 cells and human lung carcinoma A549 cells were incubated at 37 °C with 5% CO_2 in Dulbecco's modified eagle medium (DMEM) with 10% fetal bovine serum (FBS). To evaluate the infectivity of the pGEM-HEV clone, HepG2 (60~70% confluence) cells were transfected with the capped RNA transcripts as described previously [19]. Twenty-four hours post-transfection, the cells were fixed and stained with a HEV-specific antibody (Merck Millipore, MAB8003, German, 1:1000 dilution). Briefly, cells were fixed with 4% paraformaldehyde for 15 min at 37 °C and subsequently washed three times and incubated with HEV antibody for 60 min at 37 °C. Cells were washed three times with PBS (phosphate buffered saline) and incubated with FITC (fluorescein isothiocyanate) conjugated goat anti-mouse IgG (H + L) antibody (Promega, USA, 1:1000 dilution) for 45 min at 37 °C. Nuclei were counterstained with 4′,6-diamidino-2-phenylindole (DAPI). Cells were washed three times with PBS, and viewed under a fluorescence microscopy (Nikon Ti-E, Japan).

Inoculation of BALB/c mice with capped RNA transcripts

The protocol of animal experiments were approved by the Animal Care and Use Committee (ACUC) of Kunming University of Science and Technology. Six female, 8-week-old, SPF (specific pathogen free) BALB/c mouse purchased from SLAC laboratory animal (China), and maintained in a pathogen-free animal facility. Mice were negative to anti-HEV IgG and IgM antibodies, and HEV RNA. Six mice were randomly divided into 2 groups and each mouse was caged separately.

Group A containing Mouse 1, 2 and 3 were inoculated with RNA transcripts of the swine HEV clone pGEM-HEV (10 μg /mouse), and Group B containing mouse 4, 5 and 6 were inoculated with equal volume PBS. Feces and serum were collected every week from each mouse after inoculation. Mice were anaesthetized with pentobarbital (80 mg/kg) and euthanized by cervical dislocation at 28 days post-inoculation (dpi). Tissues, including liver, spleen, kidney and colon were collected. Animal carcasses were safely disposed by the ACUC of the Kunming University of Science and Technology (WH17037).

Detection of HEV RNA in feces, serum and tissues by nested RT-PCR and quantitative RT-PCR

Total RNA in feces, serum and tissues were extracted by Trizol (Invitrogen), according to the manufacturer's instructions. The isolated RNA was used to synthesize first-strand cDNA. The cDNA was added as the template to perform the reverse transcription nested PCR (RT-nPCR). Both positive strand and (or) negative strands

Table 1 Primers sequence

Primer ID	Sequence (5'~ 3')	Product	Length (bp)	Reference
S11	AGGCTCCTGGCRTYACTACTG	F1	1163 bp	2
S12	GCCYTGGCGAATGCTGTG			
A11	GGCCRGGAATGTAATCACG			
A12	GCGGCACTGGGCRTAAAACT			
HEV-A1	AAAGGAATGAAGAGGCTGGAG	F2	1520 bp	This study
HEV-A3	GAAAAGTCTGGCCGTGATTAC			
HEV-B2	TCCTCAGTAATAGTAAGGGC			
HEV-B4	AGGTCGATGGTTACGTTCCC			
HEV-C1	TGCCTGTTGGGCTGAGTTTTGATG	F3	1394 bp	This study
HEV-C3	GCCAGCCATAGCTTGGTTTGAAG			
D1R	AAGGTCTTGCTCCACGCAGATATC			
D3R	CTGGAAGAATGTTATACGAGACAC			
D2F	CTTGTGGAGGCCATGGTGGAGAA	F4	1243 bp	This study
D4F	ATGGTGGAGAAAGGCCAGGAT			
ER1	TCACGCCAAGCGGAGCCGAGT			
ER2	GAAGGGGTTGGTTGGATGAAT			
EF1	TTTCTGGGGTGACCGGGTTGATT	F5	1791 bp	This study
EF2	CTATATTCATCCAACCAACCCCT			
HEV31	CAGGGAGCGCGGAACGCAGAAAAGA			
HEV32	TCAATACTCCCGAGTTTTACCCACC			
5' Race-A1	GCAGTGARTARAGYGCAAYCCCHGTCT	5' RACE	501 bp	2
5' Race-A2	CGRGCCATYGCCTCNGCRACATC			
3' Race-S1	ACYACNACTGCTGCYACACGBTTYATGA	3' RACR	936 bp	2
3' Race-S2	CTYTGTTYAAYCTTGCTGAYACGCTKCTC			
T7P1	GCCTAGCTAGCTAGTCTAGATAATACGACTCACTATA	5' terminal	–	This study
PAP2	CGGTCGACCGATCGATTTTTTTTTTTTTTTTTTTTTTTTTCAGGGAGCGC	3' terminal	–	This study
HEV1	AATTATGCC(T)CAGTAC(T)CGG(A)GTTG	Positive strand of HEV RNA	348 bp	[23]
HEV2	CCCTTA(G)TCC(T)TGCTGA(C)GCATTCTC			
HEV3	GTT(A)ATGCTT(C)TGCATA(T)CATGGCT			
HEV4	AGCCGACGAAATCAATTCTGTC			
HEV6	AGCTCCTGTACCTGATGATGTTGACTC	Negative strand of HEV RNA	266 bp	[24]
HEV7	CTACAGAGCGCCAGCCTTGATTGC			
HEV8	GCTCACGTCATCTGTCGCTGCTGG			
HEV9	GGGCTGAACCAAAATCCTGACATC			
WHO-F	GGTGGTTTCTGGGGTGAC	qRT-PCR	70 bp	[25]
WHO-R	AGGGGTTGGTTGGATGAA			

of HEV in feces, serum and tissues were detected with strand-specific primers [23, 24] as described previously and shown in Table 1.

The viral titer of HEV in the feces, serum and tissues were quantified using SYBR green-based quantitative RT-PCR (qRT-PCR) with HEV-specific primers [25]. qRT-PCR was performed using the BIO-RAD CFX Connect Real-Time System under the following conditions: 95 °C for 30 s, followed by 39 cycles of 95 °C for 5 s and 60 °C for 31 s.

Determination of HEV antibodies by ELISA

The HEV IgG and IgM antibodies in serum were tested by ELISA (KHB, China) according to the manufacturer's instructions. The cutoff values for the IgG and IgM

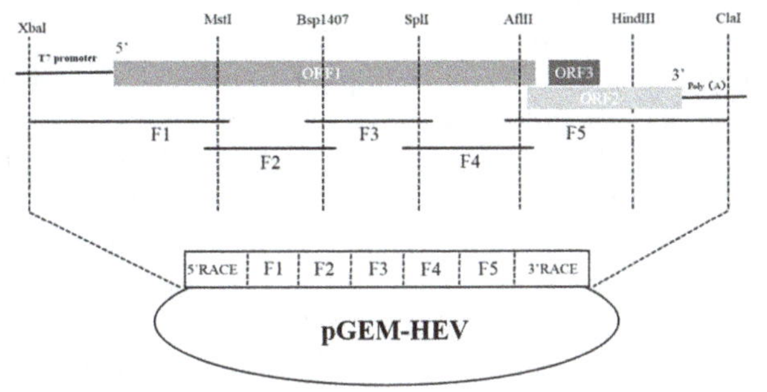

Fig. 1 A schematic diagram of the strategy used to assemble the full-length cDNA clone of swine HEV

assay were determined based on 0.22 (or 0.24 for IgM) plus the mean OD450/630 values of serum from uninfected mouse (± standard deviation, S. D.).

Profile liver biochemistry in serum

The activities of alanine aminotransferase (ALT), aspartate aminotransferase (AST) and alkaline phosphatase (ALP) in serum were measured with an automated biochemistry analyzer (Olympus 2700, Japan).

Detection of HEV ORF2 protein in tissues by Western blotting

The livers, spleens, kidneys and colons were collected and HEV capsid protein were detected in these tissues by Western blotting. Briefly, the tissues were broken in liquid nitrogen by grinding, and were lysed in RIPA buffer. Equal volumes of tissue lysates from each condition were resolved by 10% sodium dodecyl sulfate-polyacrylamide gel electrophoresis (SDS-PAGE). Analysis of protein was visualized by direct Western blotting using antibodies directed against the indicated antigens.

Infection of A549 cells with viruses recovered from mouse inoculated with capped RNA transcripts of swine HEV clones

The mouse feces were suspended into 0.1% DEPC (diethyl pyrocarbonate)-PBS. The supernatant was collected by centrifuge and microorganisms were removed by filter. A549 cells were infected with the viruses recovered from mice experimentally infected with feces supernatant. Cells were harvested at 72 h post-infection, and the HEV ORF2 protein was be detected by Western blotting.

Histopathologic examination

The liver tissues were fixed in 10% neutral buffered formalin, sectioned at a thickness of 3 μm, and stained with hematoxylin and eosin. All sections were examined using a Nikon Ti-E microscope (Japan).

Statistical analysis

Prism software (GraphPad Software) was used for statistical analysis. Data were presented as mean ± S. D..

Results

A full-length cDNA clone of swine HEV is infectious

To assess the infectivity of the pGEM-HEV cDNA clone, capped RNA transcripts were transfected into HepG2 cells. Twenty-four hours post-transfection, HEV antigens were detected by immunofluorescence assay (IFA) with an anti-HEV ORF2 monoclonal antibody. The intense fluorescent signals of HEV antigens indicating that the transfected viral RNA was replication-competent in HepG2 cells (Fig. 2). The fluorescent signal was detected in HepG2 cells transfected with the capped RNA transcripts, while no signal in non-tranfected control cells.

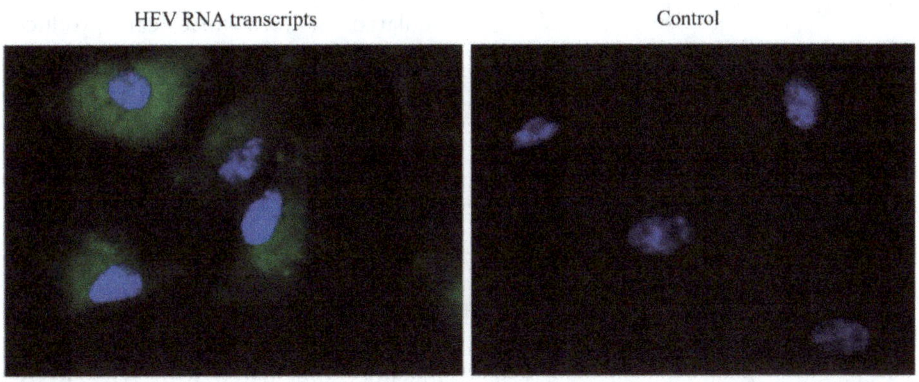

Fig. 2 Infectivity of pGEM-HEV in HepG2 cells identified by IFA. Immunofluorescence staining with anti-HEV ORF2 antibody in HepG2 cells transfected with capped full-length RNA transcripts pGEM-HEV (HEV RNA transcripts) and non-transfected control cells (Control). Nuclei were counterstained with DAPI

Capped RNA transcripts of pGEM-HEV was infectious in BALB/c mice

To further investigate whether this clone can be used to establish infection in mice, we explored the infection in BALB/c mouse model. Mice in groups A and B were intravenously injected with full-length capped RNA transcripts from pGEM-HEV (HEV RNA transcripts) and PBS (Control), respectively. HEV RNA was first detected in feces at 3 dpi in group A inoculated with RNA transcripts, and it was all detected in feces from three mice feces after 7 dpi, and lasted to the end of the experiment (Table 2). The viral titer of HEV in the feces of mice inoculated with HEV RNA transcripts was detected from 3 to 28 dpi (Fig. 3a). In the serum, HEV RNA positive-strands were all detected in mice inoculated with RNA transcripts from 7 to 28 dpi (Fig. 3b). The HEV negative-strand RNA was detected in one mouse at 7 dpi and two mice at 14 dpi in group A inoculated with RNA transcript, and all detected at 21 dpi. However, mice injected with PBS were negative to both positive and negative strands during the whole experiment.

Table 2 Detection of HEV RNA by RT-nPCR in feces, serum and tissues of mouse inoculated with capped full-length RNA transcripts of pGEM-HEV or PBS

Sample		Strand	HEV RNA transcripts	Control
Feces	0 dpi	Positive	–	–
	3 dpi	Positive	+(1/3)	+(0/3)
	4 dpi	Positive	+(2/3)	+(0/3)
	7 dpi	Positive	+(3/3)	+(0/3)
	14 dpi	Positive	+(3/3)	+(0/3)
	21 dpi	Positive	+(3/3)	+(0/3)
	28 dpi	Positive	+(3/3)	+(0/3)
Serum	0 dpi	Positive	+(0/3)	+(0/3)
		Negative	+(0/3)	+(0/3)
	7 dpi	Positive	+(3/3)	+(0/3)
		Negative	+(1/3)	+(0/3)
	14 dpi	Positive	+(3/3)	+(0/3)
		Negative	+(2/3)	+(0/3)
	21 dpi	Positive	+(3/3)	+(0/3)
		Negative	+(3/3)	+(0/3)
	28 dpi	Positive	+(3/3)	+(0/3)
		Negative	+(2/3)	+(0/3)
Tissues	Liver	Positive	+(3/3)	+(0/3)
		Negative	+(3/3)	+(0/3)
	Spleen	Positive	+(3/3)	+(0/3)
		Negative	+(3/3)	+(0/3)
	Kidney	Positive	+(2/3)	+(0/3)
		Negative	+(2/3)	+(0/3)
	Colon	Positive	+(0/3)	+(0/3)
		Negative	+(1/3)	+(0/3)

Replication of HEV in multiple tissues, including liver, spleen, kidney and colon, has been reported in both pigs and nude mice when inoculated with HEV [21, 26]. In order to further analyze the replication of HEV in different tissues, HEV genome RNA and capsid protein (ORF2) were analyzed by RT-nPCR, qRT-PCR and Western blotting, respectively. In the present study, HEV RNA was detected with a high viral titer in the liver ($6.2 \times 10^5 \pm 5.8 \times 10^4$ copies/g), spleen ($1.3 \times 10^4 \pm 3.7 \times 10^4$ copies/g), kidney ($7.1 \times 10^4 \pm 3.1 \times 10^4$ copies/g) and colon ($1.9 \times 10^4 \pm 5.8 \times 10^3$ copies/g) of mice inoculated with HEV RNA transcripts at 28 dpi (Fig. 3c). HEV RNA (both positive and negative strands) were detected in the liver and spleen in mice inoculated with HEV RNA transcripts at 28 dpi (Table 2). Although colon has been reported as a replicate site of HEV [21], only one mouse inoculated with HEV RNA transcripts at 28 dpi was found to be positive (Table 2). Meanwhile, the capsid protein of HEV (ORF2) were detected in the liver, spleen and kidney of mice inoculated with HEV RNA transcripts (Fig. 3d-g) by Western blotting. Shedding viruses in the feces, detected HEV RNA antigens in the serum and tissues indicated that HEV RNA transcripts was infectious in BALB/c mice.

BALB/c mice produce infectious HEV viruses upon inoculation of capped RNA transcripts of the swine HEV clone

To confirm whether BALB/c mice can produce infectious HEV viruses, we attempted to infect A549 cells with the recovered viruses from mice inoculated with capped RNA transcripts of the swine HEV clone. A549 cells were harvested 72 h after infection. HEV capsid protein was detected by Western blotting (Fig. 4) in cells infected with the feces of BALB/c mice inoculated with HEV RNA transcripts. This result confirmed that the inoculated BALB/c mice can produce infectious HEV, which can replicate in A549 cells.

Capped RNA transcripts of pGEM-HEV provokes humoral response in BALB/c mice

In response to HEV infection, human body develops antibodies to HEV (IgM and IgG). To investigate whether BALB/c mice provoke similar response to RNA transcripts of HEV infection, we measured serum anti-HEV IgM and IgG. An increased anti-HEV IgM and IgG levels were observed in all the mice inoculated with HEV RNA transcripts compared with the control group (Fig. 5). In the RNA transcripts inoculated group, the increased IgM level reached the pink at 21 dpi. IgG began to increase at

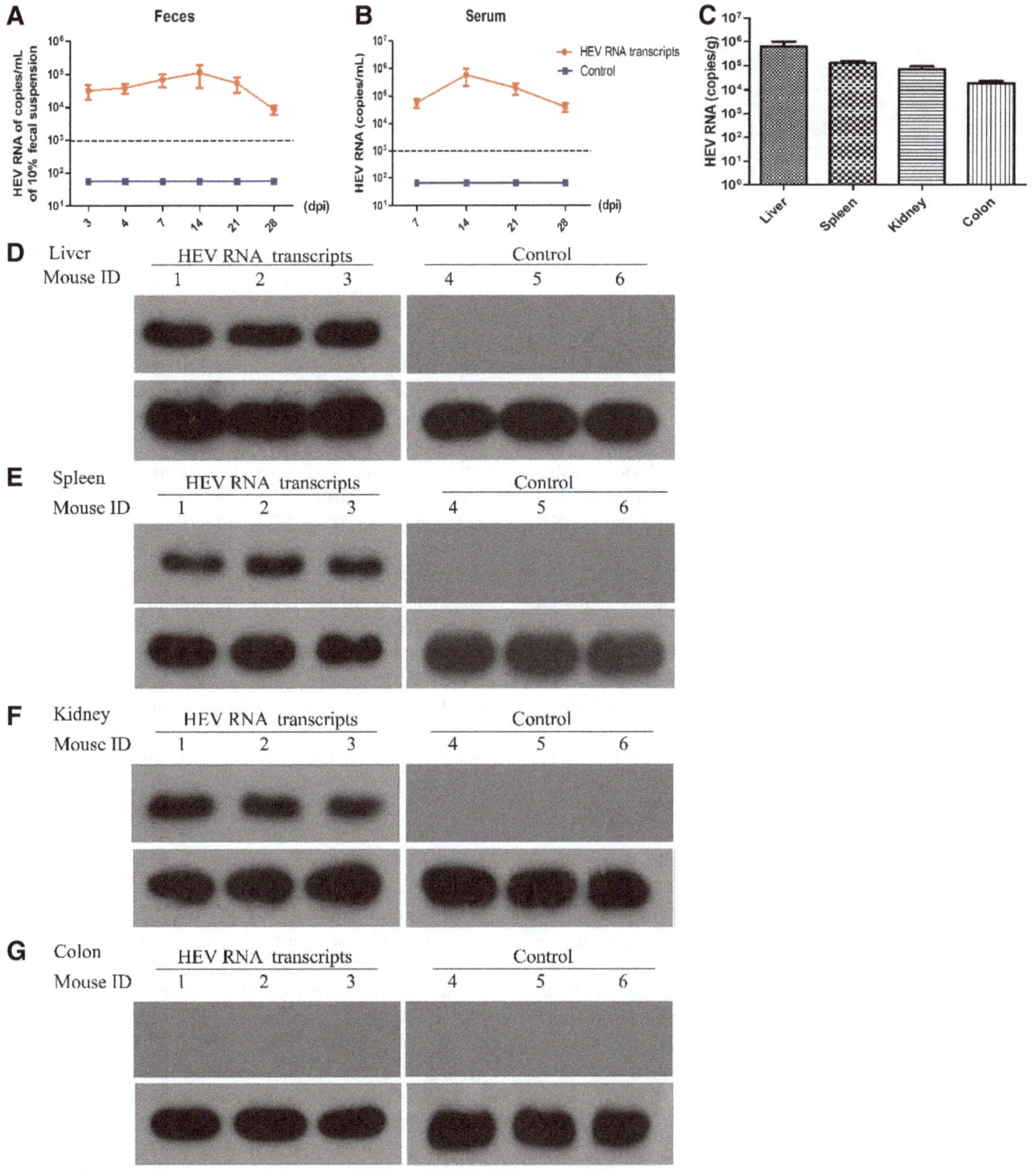

Fig. 3 HEV viral titer and HEV capsid protein detection. The viral titer of HEV in feces (**a**), serum (**b**) and tissues (**c**) were detected by qRT-PCR. HEV capsid protein was detected in different tissues of BALB/c mouse, liver (**d**), spleen (**e**), kidney (**f**) and colon (**g**) by Western blotting

21 dpi, and continued to increase until the end of the experiment. These results demonstrated that infection of the swine HEV infectious clone stimulated humoral response in BALB/c mice.

Infection of capped HEV RNA transcripts induces liver inflammation in BALB/c mice

Hepatitis is swelling and inflammation of the liver, and most commonly caused by hepatitis virus infections. To

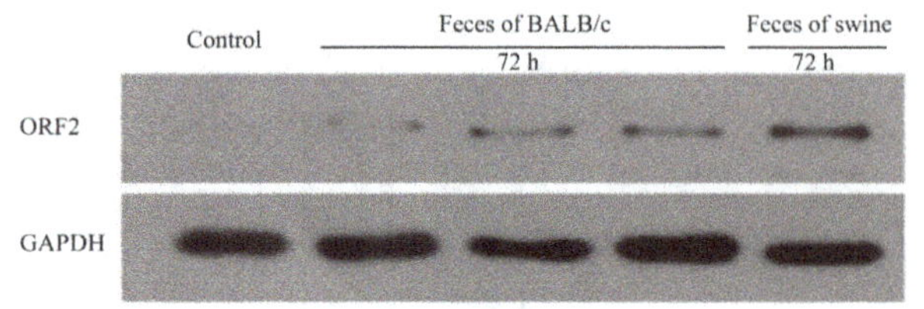

Fig. 4 BALB/c mice produce infectious HEV viruses upon inoculation of capped RNA transcripts of the swine HEV clone. A549 cells were infected with the feces suspension of BALB/c mouse inoculated with HEV RNA transcripts. Cells were harvested at 72 h post-inoculation to detect ORF2 protein by Western blotting. The feces suspension of swine HEV served as positive control. GAPDH served as a loading control

determine whether infection of capped HEV RNA transcripts can also cause liver injury/inflammation in BALB/c mice, we first tested the widely used liver enzymes for detecting liver damage. The levels/activities were characterized using an automated biochemistry analyzer. To our surprise, the elevated ALT, AST and ALP levels/activities in BALB/c inoculated with HEV RNA transcripts was very similar to the clinical feature of HEV infected patients (Fig. 6a, b and c).

Furthermore, histopathologic examination showed swelling of liver cells and liver capsules were filled with inflammatory exudates and liver hemorrhage in mice inoculated with RNA transcripts of HEV (Fig. 6d). Increased infiltrating lymphocytes and macrophages were observed in these mice. In contrast, no damage was observed in any of the control tissues. These results indicate that infection of swine HEV RNA transcripts triggered liver inflammation in BALB/c mice.

Discussions

Lessons from the research of hepatitis B and C viruses have taught us the importance of developing robust experimental models for understanding their infection biology, pathogenesis, as well as antiviral drug development. However, the restricted tropism of host and cell type for hepatitis virus infection has always challenged the development of experimental

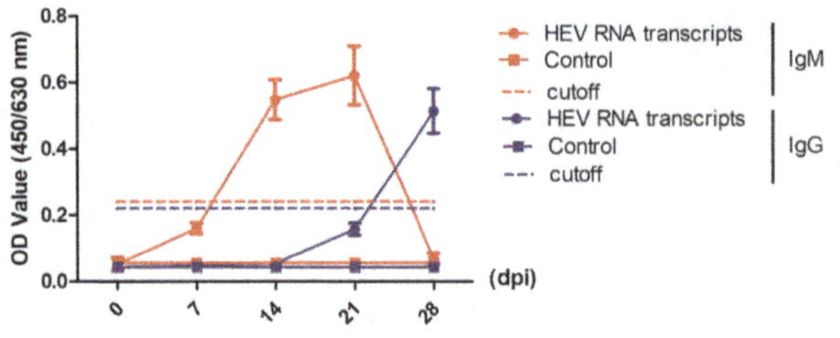

Fig. 5 Anti-HEV IgM and IgG antibodies in BALB/c mouse were tested by ELISA. Anti-HEV IgM and IgG antibodies in BALB/c mouse inoculated with HEV RNA transcripts or PBS were tested by ELISA

models. Despite the recent establishment of several cell culture systems of HEV [27], animal models are urgently need for studying HEV pathogenicity and antiviral drug development.

Non-human primates have been successfully employed for HEV research in early days [28, 29], but non-human primates are not available for research anymore, because of the ethics. Although swine is the mainly reservoir of HEV, it is not suitable as an experimental model for HEV because of its large body size. In contrast, mice are the most commonly used small animal for research purpose. This study, we reported the successful establishment of HEV infection in BALB/c mice with an infectious swine HEV clone generated by reverse genetics approach.

In fact, we have previously attempted to establish HEV mouse model using BALB/c nude mice [21]. Because nude mice lack the thymus and are therefore unable to produce T-cells. We thought that the immunodeficient nature of these mice could be an advantage of permitting HEV infection. Indeed, we have succeeded the infection in BALB/c nude mice with genotype 4 swine HEV strain [21]. However, the immunodeficient property in turn hampered the study of HEV pathogenesis. Because hepatitis is an inflammatory process mainly mediated by host immune response. Furthermore, these mice have a strict life condition and limited fertility, which also hampers the further application. To circumstance these limitations, we now have succeeded with infecting the regular BALB/c mice, which have a competent immune system. In the present study, the RNA transcripts of infectious cDNA clone of swine HEV was successfully infected BALB/c mice. HEV RNA was detected at 3 dpi in feces, which is similar to our genotype 4 swine HEV strain inoculated into BALB/c nude mice [21], but earlier than that inoculated pigs with genotype 4 swine HEV RNA transcripts (7 dpi) [20] and *Sprague-Dawley* rat (SD rat) inoculated with genotype 4 swine HEV RNA transcripts [30]. HEV produces an intermediate negative-strand RNA when it replicates. The negative-strand of HEV was detectable at 7 dpi in serum of all mice inoculated with RNA transcripts. Furthermore, the negative-strand was found in the HEV replicated sites, including liver (3/3), spleen (3/3), kidney (2/3) and colon (1/3). Moreover, HEV RNA was detected in the feces, serum and tissues (liver, spleen, kidney and colon). Shedding HEV in feces, and detection of negative-strand RNA in liver, spleen and kidney firmly demonstrated the infectivity of the genotype 4 swine HEV pGEM-HEV cDNA clone is infectious in BALB/c mice, although previous study reported that C57BL/6 mice is not permissive for HEV infection [31]. More interestingly, we observed

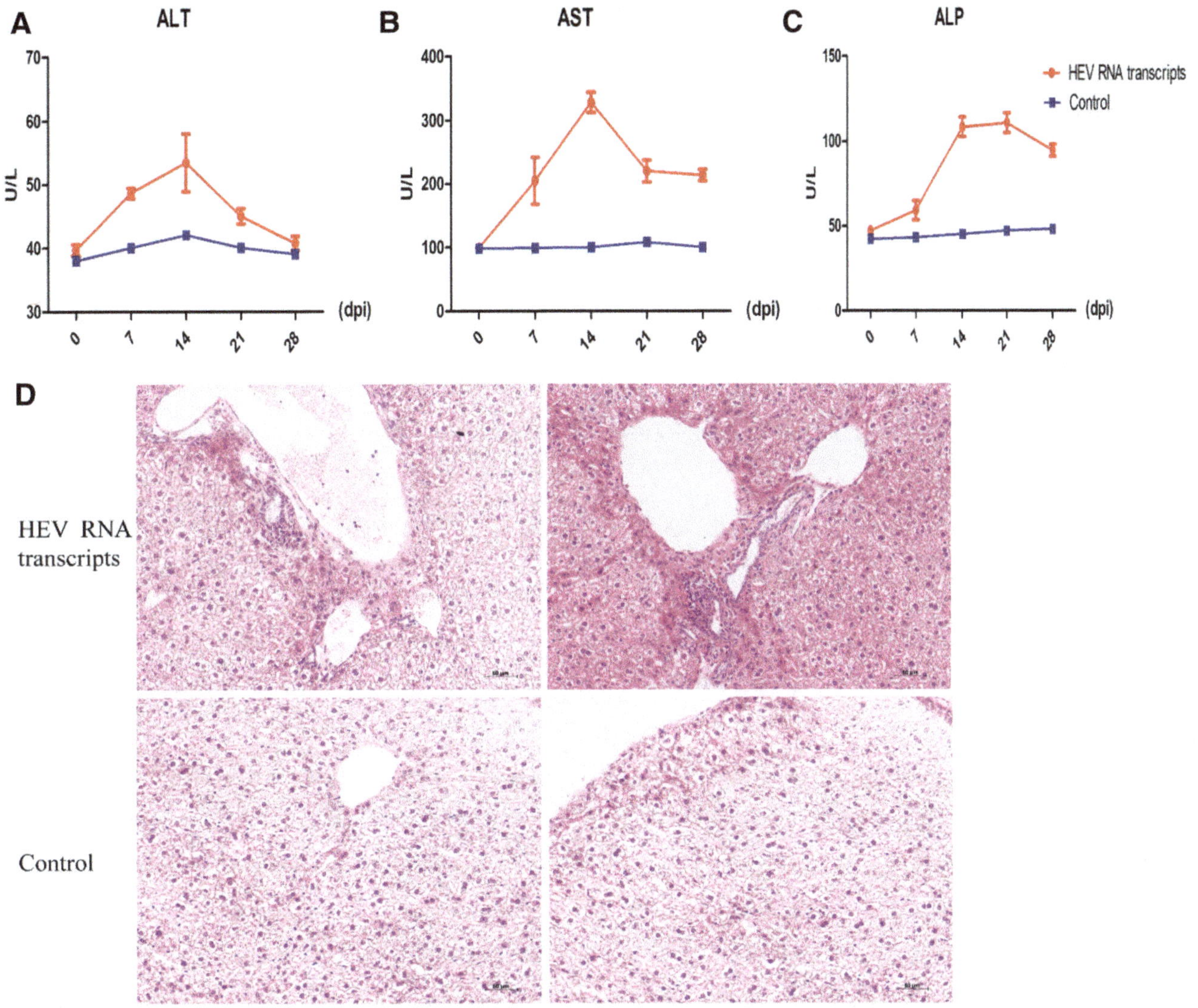

Fig. 6 The activities of liver-specific enzymes and the pathological changes in BALB/c mouse inoculated with HEV RNA transcripts of pGEM-HEV. The level/activity of ALT (**a**), AST (**b**) and ALP (**c**) were determined in BALB/c mouse inoculated with HEV RNA transcripts or PBS. Histopathological analyses of the liver of BALB/c mice inoculated with HEV RNA transcripts of pGEM-HEV (HEV RNA transcripts) or PBS (Control) stained with H&E (**d**)

humoral response and liver injury in infected BALB/c mice, indicating that this model is promising for studying HEV pathogenesis.

Although HEV infects BALB/c mice has been successfully established, key parameters should be determined in the future, such as identification of infected cell populations, observation of inflammatory manifestation, and then explicit comparisons with HEV infected patients to assess potential for clinical relevance. The establishment of HEV infection based on BALB/c mice is benefit to screen anti-HEV drugs and develop vaccines in vivo.

Conclusion

In this study, we successfully established BALB/c mice-based animal model with an infectious cDNA clone of genotype 4 swine HEV constructed by reverse genetics approach. This swine HEV clone strain is capable of modeling HEV infection, and studying host response and pathogenesis. Furthermore, this model also bears importantly implications for future anti-HEV drug development.

Abbreviations

A549 cells: Human lung carcinoma cell line; ACUC: Animal Care and Use Committee; ALP: Alkaline phosphatase; ALT: Alanine aminotransferase; AST: Aspartate aminotransferase; ATCC: American Type Culture Collection; DAPI: 4′,6-diamidino-2-phenylindole; DEPC: Diethyl pyrocarbonate; DMEM: Dulbecco's modified eagle medium; dpi: days post-inoculation; ELISA: Enzyme-linked immunosorbent assay; FBS: Fetal bovine serum; FITC: Fluorescein isothiocyanate; HepG2 cells : Human hepatocellular carcinoma cell line; HEV: Hepatitis E virus; IFA: Immunofluorescence assay; IgG: Immunoglobulin G; IgM: Immunoglobulin M; ORFs: Open reading frames; PBS: Phosphate buffered saline; qRT-PCR: quantitative real time PCR; RACE: Rapid Amplification of cDNA Ends; RT-nPCR: Reverse transcription nested PCR; S.

D.: Standard deviation; SD rat: *Sprague-Dawley* rat; SDS-PAGE: Sodium dodecyl sulfate-polyacrylamide gel electrophoresis; SPF: Specific pathogen free

Acknowledgements
Authors thank Xiancheng Zhao for her contribution on HEV full-length genome amplification, and Ping Yan for his contribution on sample collection.

Funding
This study was supported by National Natural Science Foundation of China (grant number 31360619 and 81660338 to Fen Huang), Natural Science Foundation of Yunnan province (grant number 2017FA036 to Fen Huang and 2018FB132 to Wenhai Yu), Fundamental Research Funds for the Central Universities (grant number 2016ZX310179) and PUMC Youth Fund (grant number 2017310038) to Wenhai Yu. The funders had no role in study design, data collection and analysis, decision to publish, or preparation of the manuscript.

Authors' contributions
WY, CY, XH and TM performed the experiment; FH, CY and WY wrote the manuscript. All authors contributed to the analysis and interpretation of data. All authors have read and approved the manuscript, and ensure that this is the case.

Consent for publication
Not applicable

Competing interests
The authors declare that they have no competing interests.

Author details
[1]Institute of Medical Biology, Chinese Academy of Medical Sciences and Peking Union Medical College, 935 Jiaoling Road, Kunming, China. [2]Medical School, Kunming University of Science and Technology, 727 Jingming Road, Kunming, China.

References

1. Smith DB, Simmonds P, Jameel S, Emerson SU, Harrison TJ, Meng XJ, Okamoto H, Van der Poel WH, Purdy MA. Consensus proposals for classification of the family Hepeviridae. J Gen Virol. 2014;95(Pt 10):2223–32.
2. Billam P, Sun ZF, Meng XJ. Analysis of the complete genomic sequence of an apparently avirulent strain of avian hepatitis E virus (avian HEV) identified major genetic differences compared with the prototype pathogenic strain of avian HEV. J Gen Virol. 2007;88(Pt 5):1538–44.
3. Panda SK, Nanda SK, Zafrullah M, Ansari IH, Ozdener MH, Jameel S. An Indian strain of hepatitis E virus (HEV): cloning, sequence, and expression of structural region and antibody responses in sera from individuals from an area of high-level HEV endemicity. J Clin Microbiol. 1995;33(10):2653–9.
4. Huang YW, Opriessnig T, Halbur PG, Meng XJ. Initiation at the third in-frame AUG codon of open reading frame 3 of the hepatitis E virus is essential for viral infectivity in vivo. J Virol. 2007;81(6):3018–26.
5. Tam AW, Smith MM, Guerra ME, Huang CC, Bradley DW, Fry KE, Reyes GR. Hepatitis E virus (HEV): molecular cloning and sequencing of the full-length viral genome. Virology. 1991;185(1):120–31.
6. Meng XJ, Purcell RH, Halbur PG, Lehman JR, Webb DM, Tsareva TS, Haynes JS, Thacker BJ, Emerson SU. A novel virus in swine is closely related to the human hepatitis E virus. Proc Natl Acad Sci U S A. 1997; 94(18):9860–5.
7. Hsieh SY, Meng XJ, Wu YH, Liu ST, Tam AW, Lin DY, Liaw YF. Identity of a novel swine hepatitis E virus in Taiwan forming a monophyletic group with Taiwan isolates of human hepatitis E virus. J Clin Microbiol. 1999;37(12):3828–34.
8. Feagins AR, Opriessnig T, Huang YW, Halbur PG, Meng XJ. Cross-species infection of specific-pathogen-free pigs by a genotype 4 strain of human hepatitis E virus. J Med Virol. 2008;80(8):1379–86.
9. Feagins AR, Opriessnig T, Guenette DK, Halbur PG, Meng XJ. Detection and characterization of infectious hepatitis E virus from commercial pig livers sold in local grocery stores in the USA. J Gen Virol. 2007;88(Pt 3):912–7.
10. Tei S, Kitajima N, Takahashi K, Mishiro S. Zoonotic transmission of hepatitis E virus from deer to human beings. Lancet. 2003;362(9381):371–3.
11. Rein DB, Stevens GA, Theaker J, Wittenborn JS, Wiersma ST. The global burden of hepatitis E virus genotypes 1 and 2 in 2005. Hepatology. 2012; 55(4):988–97.
12. Dalton HR, Bendall R, Ijaz S, Banks M. Hepatitis E: an emerging infection in developed countries. Lancet Infect Dis. 2008;8(11):698–709.
13. Aggarwal R, Krawczynski K. Hepatitis E: an overview and recent advances in clinical and laboratory research. J Gastroenterol Hepatol. 2000;15(1):9–20.
14. Khuroo MS, Kamili S. Aetiology, clinical course and outcome of sporadic acute viral hepatitis in pregnancy. J Viral Hepat. 2003;10(1):61–9.
15. Kumar A, Beniwal M, Kar P, Sharma JB, Murthy NS. Hepatitis E in pregnancy. Int J Gynaecol Obstet. 2004;85(3):240–4.
16. Shukla P, Nguyen HT, Torian U, Engle RE, Faulk K, Dalton HR, Bendall RP, Keane FE, Purcell RH, Emerson SU. Cross-species infections of cultured cells by hepatitis E virus and discovery of an infectious virus-host recombinant. Proc Natl Acad Sci U S A. 2011;108(6):2438–43.
17. Shukla P, Nguyen HT, Faulk K, Mather K, Torian U, Engle RE, Emerson SU. Adaptation of a genotype 3 hepatitis E virus to efficient growth in cell culture depends on an inserted human gene segment acquired by recombination. J Virol. 2012;86(10):5697–707.
18. Tanaka T, Takahashi M, Takahashi H, Ichiyama K, Hoshino Y, Nagashima S, Mizuo H, Okamoto H. Development and characterization of a genotype 4 hepatitis E virus cell culture system using a HE-JF5/15F strain recovered from a fulminant hepatitis patient. J Clin Microbiol. 2009;47(6):1906–10.
19. Huang YW, Haqshenas G, Kasorndorkbua C, Halbur PG, Emerson SU, Meng XJ. Capped RNA transcripts of full-length cDNA clones of swine hepatitis E virus are replication competent when transfected into Huh7 cells and infectious when intrahepatically inoculated into pigs. J Virol. 2005;79(3):1552–8.
20. Cordoba L, Feagins AR, Opriessnig T, Cossaboom CM, Dryman BA, Huang YW, Meng XJ. Rescue of a genotype 4 human hepatitis E virus from cloned cDNA and characterization of intergenotypic chimeric viruses in cultured human liver cells and in pigs. J Gen Virol. 2012;93(Pt 10):2183–94.
21. Huang F, Zhang W, Gong G, Yuan C, Yan Y, Yang S, Cui L, Zhu J, Yang Z, Hua X. Experimental infection of Balb/c nude mice with hepatitis E virus. BMC Infect Dis. 2009;9:93.
22. Fu H, Wang L, Zhu Y, Geng J, Li L, Wang X, Bu Q, Zhuang H. Analysing complete genome sequence of swine hepatitis E virus (HEV), strain CHN-XJSW13 isolated from Xinjiang, China: putative host range, and disease severity determinants in HEV. Infect Genet Evol. 2011;11(3):618–23.
23. Huang FF, Haqshenas G, Guenette DK, Halbur PG, Schommer SK, Pierson FW, Toth TE, Meng XJ. Detection by reverse transcription-PCR and genetic characterization of field isolates of swine hepatitis E virus from pigs in different geographic regions of the United States. J Clin Microbiol. 2002; 40(4):1326–32.
24. Nanda SK, Panda SK, Durgapal H, Jameel S. Detection of the negative strand of hepatitis E virus RNA in the livers of experimentally infected rhesus monkeys: evidence for viral replication. J Med Virol. 1994;42(3): 237–40.
25. Baylis SA, Blumel J, Mizusawa S, Matsubayashi K, Sakata H, Okada Y, Nubling CM, Hanschmann KM. World Health Organization international standard to harmonize assays for detection of hepatitis E virus RNA. Emerg Infect Dis. 2013;19(5):729–35.
26. Huang F, Hua X, Yang S, Yuan C, Zhang W. Effective inhibition of hepatitis E virus replication in A549 cells and piglets by RNA interference (RNAi) targeting RNA-dependent RNA polymerase. Antivir Res. 2009;83(3):274–81.

27. Okamoto H. Hepatitis E virus cell culture models. Virus Res. 2011;161(1): 65–77.
28. Aggarwal R, Kamili S, Spelbring J, Krawczynski K. Experimental studies on subclinical hepatitis E virus infection in cynomolgus macaques. J Infect Dis. 2001;184(11):1380–5.
29. Panda SK, Ansari IH, Durgapal H, Agrawal S, Jameel S. The in vitro-synthesized RNA from a cDNA clone of hepatitis E virus is infectious. J Virol. 2000;74(5):2430–7.
30. Zhu Y, Yu X, Zhang Y, Ni Y, Si F, Yu R, Dong S, Huang Y, Li Z. Infectivity of a genotype 4 hepatitis E virus cDNA clone by intrahepatic inoculation of laboratory rats. Vet Microbiol. 2013;166(3–4):405–11.
31. Li TC, Suzaki Y, Ami Y, Tsunemitsu H, Miyamura T, Takeda N. Mice are not susceptible to hepatitis E virus infection. J Vet Med Sci. 2008;70(12): 1359–62.

24

Prevalence and associated knowledge of hepatitis B infection among healthcare workers in Freetown, Sierra Leone

Yu-Ling Qin[1†], Bo Li[1†], Yue-Su Zhou[1†], Xin Zhang[1], Lei Li[1], Bing Song[1], Peng Liu[1], Yue Yuan[1], Zhong-Peng Zhao[2], Jun Jiao[2], Jing Li[2], Yi Sun[2], Stephen Sevalie[3], Joseph E. Kanu[3], Ya-Jun Song[2], Jia-Fu Jiang[2*], Foday Sahr[3,4*], Tian-Jun Jiang[1*] and Chinese Military Medical Experts Group in Sierra Leone

Abstract

Background: Hepatitis B virus (HBV) is considered highly prevalent in West Africa. However, major gaps in surveillance exist in Sierra Leone. Although healthcare workers (HCWs) are at high risk for HBV infection, little is known about the prevalence and knowledge of hepatitis B among HCWs in Sierra Leone.

Methods: A cross-sectional study of all HCWs at the No. 34 Military Hospital located in Freetown, Sierra Leone, was conducted from March 20 to April 10, 2017. Whole blood was collected and screened for HBV markers using a one-step rapid immunochromatographic test with positive samples tested for HBV DNA. Additionally, questionnaires assessing self-reported knowledge of HBV infections were administered to all participants. Data were processed and analyzed using SPSS (version 17.0) software.

Results: A total of 211 HCWs were included in this study with a median age of 39.0 years (range: 18–59). Of the participating HCWs, 172 (81.5%) participants were susceptible (all markers negative), 21(10.0%) were current HBV (HBsAg positive) and nine (4.3%) were considered immune because of past infection (HBsAg negative and anti-HBc positive; anti-HBs positive). Additionally, nine (4.3%) participants displayed immunity to the virus as a result of prior hepatitis B vaccination (only anti-HBs positive). Of the 21 HCWs with positive HBsAg, 13 (61.9%) had detectable HBV DNA. There was a significantly lower risk for current HBV infection among HCWs older than 39 years (OR 0.337, $p =$ 0.046). In addition, only 14 (6.6%), 73 (34.6%) and 82 (38.9%) participants in this survey had adequate knowledge about the clinical outcome, routes of transmission, and correct preventive measures of HBV infection, respectively.

Conclusions: HCWs in Sierra Leone lacked adequate knowledge of the hepatitis B virus. Additionally, the low coverage rate of hepatitis B vaccination among HCWs fails to meet WHO recommendations, leaving many of the sampled HCWs susceptible to infection. This study reaffirms the need for more intensive training for HCWs in addition to strengthening vaccination programmes to protect HCWs against HBV in Sierra Leone.

Keywords: Hepatitis B virus, Healthcare workers, Prevalence, Sierra Leone

* Correspondence: jiangjf2008@gmail.com; fodaysahr1@gmail.com; aba302@163.com
[†]Yu-Ling Qin, Bo Li and Yue-Su Zhou contributed equally to this work.
[2]Beijing Institute of Microbiology and Epidemiology, Beijing, China
[3]No. 34 Military Hospital, Wilberforce, Freetown, Sierra Leone
[1]Beijing 302 Hospital, Beijing, China
Full list of author information is available at the end of the article

Background

Hepatitis B virus (HBV) infection is a major threat to public health globally. According to the World Health Organization (WHO), approximately 257 million people are infected with chronic HBV [1]. Infection with HBV can increase the risk of death from liver cirrhosis and hepatocellular carcinoma, which is the sixth most common cancer and the third cause of cancer death worldwide [2]. The WHO reported that hepatitis B prevalence is the highest in the western Pacific region and Africa, where 6.2 and 6.1% of the adult population are infected, respectively [1]. Sierra Leone, located in West Africa, is considered a high-endemic area. A study conducted among primary school children, in 1998, detected HBsAg in 18% of the children tested [3]. In 2005, a study showed a 6.2% seroprevalence of hepatitis B among pregnant women of middle and high socio-economic class in Sierra Leone [4]. Recently, a study screening blood donor candidates for blood-borne pathogens found a HBsAg prevalence of 15% in men and 13% in women from a single hospital in Tonkolili Province, Sierra Leone [5]. These results illustrate the serious public health risks that hepatitis B poses in Sierra Leone. In addition, HBV continues to be an understudied topic in Sierra Leone. Due to limited resources, little has been done to combat hepatitis B in Sierra Leone despite the suspected high burden of disease. Although the hepatitis B vaccine was introduced for 6 to 14 week-old children, there are currently no active programs administering the vaccine at birth. Furthermore no coordinated HBV vaccination program been put in place to prevent infection among the adult population [6].

Healthcare workers (HCWs) are considered a high-risk group for HBV infection due to occupational exposure to blood-borne pathogens. Previous studies in Africa found high HBV infection and exposure rates (roughly 10%) in HCWs in South Africa and Nigeria. Worldwide, approximately 2 million HCWs are infected with HBV through sharp injury [7–9]. This study was designed to evaluate the prevalence of HBV markers in HCWs as well as to assess their knowledge of HBV infection and prevention in Sierra Leone.

Methods

Study area and sample population

A cross-sectional study was conducted at the No. 34 Military Hospital in Freetown, Sierra Leone from March 20 to April 10, 2017. This hospital serves as a medical center for the Republic of Sierra Leone Armed Forces in addition to also being a teaching and general hospital. A total of HCWs, including medical doctors, nurses and other non-clinical health workers, were studied and written, informed consent was obtained from each subject.

Laboratory detection of hepatitis B virus

Blood samples were drawn from the antecubital vein of the 211 participants by phlebotomists of the No. 34 Military Hospital clinical laboratory then centrifuged for 5 min at 12,000 g at room temperature. Serological tests were performed to detect five markers including HBsAg, anti-HBs, HBeAg, anti-HBe and anti-HBc, by using a one-step rapid immunochromatographic test (Shanghai Kehua Bio-engineering Co., Ltd., Shanghai, China). Test results were interpreted and reported as positive or negative based on the manufacturer's instructions.

Viral deoxyribonucleic acid (DNA) was extracted using the QIAamp DNA Blood Mini Kit (QIAGEN, Germantown, MD, USA) according to the manufacturer's instructions. HBV DNA was amplified using real-time PCR (qPCR) (Light Cycler Software Version 4.1, Roche Diagnostics, Penzburg, Germany) HBV DNA assay kits (Sansure Biotech, Changsha, China) in all HBsAg positive samples.

Design and administration of the questionnaire

Data were collected using a self-administered questionnaire, which was developed after reviewing relevant research [10–12]. The survey had questions on socio-demographic characteristics, knowledge of HBV clinical outcome, route of transmission and preventive measures against hepatitis B infection, previous infection, and previous vaccination history. No vaccinations were offered to HCWs as part of this study. Seventeen questions had binary (yes or no) responses, and three multi-items questions focusing on the clinical outcome of HBV infection, route of transmission and proper preventive measures had only one correct answer. Each study participant was expected to complete the questionnaire.

Statistical analysis

The data obtained from the questionnaire and the results of the laboratory test were analyzed using SPSS (version 17.0, SPSS Inc. Chicago, IL). The response for each question was given a score of one and zero indicating a right or wrong answer was provided, respectively. Then we summed and graded the total scores as 'poor', 'intermediate' or 'adequate' level for each study participant based on the distribution located in the tri-sectional quantiles of the grouped data array. The Pearson Chi-square test was used to determine the relationships between participant characteristics and HBV marker detection rates. Multivariable factor analysis for current HBV infection was

Table 1 Prevalence of five hepatitis B virus serological markers by socio-demographic characteristics of the study participants

Characteristic	Tested no. (%)	HBsAg (+) no. (%)	*P* value	HBsAb (+) no. (%)	*P* value	HBeAg (+) no. (%)	*P* value	HBeAb (+) no. (%)	*P* value	HBcAb (+) no. (%)	*P* value
Age (y)											
≥ 39y	112 (53.1)	6 (5.4)	0.021*	7 (6.3)	0.342	0 (0.0)	0.469	7 (6.3)	0.027*	10 (8.9)	0.066
< 39y	99 (46.9)	15 (15.2)		3 (3.0)		1 (1.0)		16 (16.2)		18 (18.2)	
Gender											
Male	108 (51.2)	10 (9.3)	0.820	7 (6.5)	0.333	0 (0.0)	0.488	11 (10.2)	0.826	13 (12.0)	0.686
Female	103 (48.8)	11 (10.7)		3 (2.9)		1 (1.0)		12 (11.7)		15 (14.6)	
Working experience											
≥ 9y	113 (53.6)	8 (7.1)	0.168	7 (6.2)	0.345	0 (0.0)	0.464	8 (7.1)	0.076	10 (8.8)	0.066
< 9y	98 (46.4)	13 (13.3)		3 (3.1)		1 (1.0)		15 (15.3)		18 (18.4)	
Education level											
High school	39 (18.5)	6 (15.4)	0.365	1 (2.6)	0.645	0 (0.0)	0.873	5 (12.8)	0.807	7 (17.9)	0.601
Diploma certificate	166 (78.7)	14 (8.4)		9 (5.4)		1 (0.6)		17 (10.2)		20 (12.0)	
Bachelor's degree or higher	6 (2.8)	1 (16.7)		0 (0.0)		0 (0.0)		1 (16.7)		1 (16.7)	
Occupation											
Medical doctor	7 (3.3)	2 (28.5)		0 (0.0)		0 (0.0)		3 (42.9)		3 (42.9)	
Nurse	169 (80.1)	17 (10.1)	0.182	9 (5.3)	0.687	1 (0.6)	0.883	18 (10.7)	0.015*	23 (13.6)	0.029*
Others staff	35 (16.6)	2 (5.7)		1 (2.9)		0 (0.0)		2 (5.7)		2 (5.7)	
Department											
Internal Medicine	21 (10.0)	1 (4.8)	0.560	1 (4.8)	0.071	0 (0.0)	0.338	2 (9.5)	0.637	2 (9.5)	0.384
Surgical Department	47 (22.3)	8 (17.0)		1 (2.1)		0 (0.0)		8 (17.0)		9 (19.1)	
Emergency Department	16 (7.6)	1 (6.3)		1 (6.3)		0 (0.0)		1 (6.3)		1 (6.3)	
Paediatric	19 (9.0)	2 (10.5)		0 (0.0)		1 (5.3)		2 (10.5)		4 (21.1)	
Obstetrics and Gynecology	9 (4.3)	0 (0.0)		0 (0.0)		0 (0.0)		0 (0.0)		0 (0.0)	
Under Fives Clinic	6 (2.8)	0 (0.0)		1 (16.7)		0 (0.0)		0 (0.0)		0 (0.0)	
Laboratory	16 (7.6)	0 (0.0)		0 (0.0)		0 (0.0)		0 (0.0)		0 (0.0)	
OP Theatre	22 (10.4)	2 (9.0)		1 (4.5)		0 (0.0)		2 (9.0)		2 (9.0)	
Pharmacy	5 (2.4)	1 (20.0)		2 (40.0)		0 (0.0)		1 (20.0)		1 (20.0)	
Others	50 (23.7)	6 (12.0)		3 (6.0)		0 (0.0)		7 (14.0)		9 (18.0)	
Hepatitis history											
YES	14 (6.6)	2 (14.3)	0.268	1 (7.1)	0.908	0 (0.0)	0.905	2 (14.3)	0.391	3 (21.4)	0.429
NO	176 (83.4)	15 (8.5)		8 (4.5)		1 (0.6)		17 (9.7)		21 (11.9)	
Unknown	21 (10.0)	4 (19.0)		1 (4.8)		0 (0.0)		4 (19.0)		4 (19.0)	
HBV vaccination											
YES	37 (17.5)	1 (2.7)	0.135	6 (16.2)	0.002*	0 (0.0)	1.000	1 (2.7)	0.087	1 (2.7)	0.034*
NO	174 (82.5)	20 (11.5)		4 (2.3)		1 (0.6)		22 (12.6)		27 (15.5)	
Sharps injury											
Never	110 (52.1)	11 (10.0)	0.955	5 (4.5)	0.739	1 (1.0)	0.630	14 (12.7)	0.586	15 (13.6)	0.962
Once	36 (17.1)	4 (11.1)		1 (2.8)		0 (0.0)		4 (11.1)		5 (13.9)	
More than once	65 (30.8)	6 (9.2)		4 (6.2)		0 (0.0)		5 (7.7)		8 (12.3)	
Total	211 (100)	21 (10.0)		10 (4.7)		1 (0.5)		23 (10.9)		28 (13.3)	

*Statistically significant at $P < 0.05$

carried out for seven possible risk factors, including age, gender, working experience years, education background, occupation, vaccination, and sharp injury history. Differences were considered statistically significant when the p value was < 0.05.

Results

Demographic characteristics among HCWs

The median age of the 211 HCWs who participated in the study was 39.0 years (range:18–59). Roughly half of participants were male (51.2%), over the age of 39 (46.9%), and had spent less than 9 years in their current job (46.4%). The majority of HCWs had a middle education level (Diploma Certificate, 78.7%) (Table 1).

Prevalence of HBV

Of the 211 HCWs, the positive detection rates of the five markers HBsAg, anti-HBs, HBeAg, anti-HBe and anti-HBc were 10.0, 4.7, 0.5, 10.9 and 13.3%, respectively (Table 1). Twenty-one of the (10.0%) HCWs tested positive for current HBV infections (HBsAg positive, anti-HBc positive) (Table 2), nine (4.3%) were considered immune due to past infection (HBsAg negative and anti-HBc positive; anti-HBs positive), and nine (4.3%) participants were immune due to hepatitis B vaccination (only anti-HBs positive). In total, 172 (81.5%) participants were considered susceptible (all markers negative) (Table 2). Among 21 participants who were HBsAg positive, 13 (61.9%) were HBV DNA positive. Twelve of them were determined very low-level HBV DNA (< 10^3) and one had a DNA concentration of 5.6 × 10^3 copies/mL.

Table 2 Summary of hepatitis B virus infection status among HCWs in the hospital, Sierra Leone

HBV infection classification	Number (%) ($n = 211$)
Susceptible	172 (81.5)
All markers negative	172 (81.5)
Acute or chronic infection	21 (10.0)
HBsAg (+), HBeAb (+), HBcAb (+)	19 (9.0)
HBsAg (+), HBeAb (+)	1 (0.5)
HBsAg (+), HBcAb (+)	1 (0.5)
Immune due to hepatitis B vaccination	9 (4.0)
Only HBsAb (+)	9 (4.3)
Immune due to natural infection	9 (4.0)
Only HBcAb (+)	5 (2.4)
HBeAb (+), HBcAb (+)	2 (0.9)
HBsAb (+), HBeAb (+)	1 (0.5)
HBeAg (+), HBcAb (+)	1 (0.5)

Anti-HBs positive rate of participants who reported receiving a HB vaccine significantly increased. This was in comparison to participants who had not received vaccination (16.2% vs. 1.7%, $p = 0.001$) (Table 2). Of the 211 participants, only 14 (6.6%) participants had clear HBV infection history, out of which 4 tested positive for serological markers (Table 2). The prevalence of the "current infection" group was significantly higher in HCWs < 39 years old ($p = 0.018$) (Table 3). Multivariable factor analysis for risk for current HBV infection showed that there was a significantly lower risk for current HBV infection among those HCWs aged > 39 years (OR = 0.337; 95% CI:0.116–0.980; $p = 0.046$) (Table 4).

Knowledge of HBV infection and associated factors

According to participants' responses, 77.3% (163/211) of staff were not aware of clinical outcomes of HBV infection, while 63 (29.9%) and 93(44.1%) had a poor knowledge on transmission routes and preventive measures of HBV, respectively. The survey also revealed that working experience was associated with greater knowledge of preventive measures for HBV($p = 0.017$) and medical doctors were more knowledgeable about the consequences of HBV infection ($p = 0.05$) (Table 5).

Discussion

The global prevalence of hepatitis B is among the highest in parts of Africa, containing an estimated 50 million chronic carriers of HBV [13, 14]. Previous studies have shown HBsAg positive rates above 10% in African countries such as Burkina Faso, the Central African Republic, and Nigeria [15–17]. While in Sierra Leone reported HBsAg prevalence varied with different populations and times. Reports indicated a prevalence of 18% among children at a primary school in capital in 1998 [3], 6.2% among pregnant women of middle and high socio-economic status in 2005 [4], and 13–15% among blood donor candidates in Tonkolili District in 2017 [5]. In our present study, the sero-prevalence of HBsAg in HCWs was 10.0%, which is similar to rates observed in Uganda [18], but higher than those in Nigeria (1.5%) [19] and drastically higher than the developed European Region [20]. However, our study also found that the prevalence of anti-HBs was only 4.7% as compared to a South African report which detected a 19.9% anti-HBs positive rate in HCWs [21]. These results, especially the high prevalence of HBsAg and current HBV infection, suggest that hepatitis B is a very serious health concern in Sierra Leone. Our study also showed that the HBeAg positivity was low, but HBV DNA positivity was quite high (62%). This may be indicative of the effects of HBV pre-C mutation in the study

Table 3 Prevalence of four hepatitis B virus infection status by socio-demographic characteristics of the study participants

Characteristic	Tested no. (%)	Susceptible no. (%)	*P* value	Current infection no. (%)	*P* value	Past infection no. (%)	*P* value	Immune due to vaccination no. (%)	*P* value
Age (y)			0.337		0.018*		0.506		0.506
≥ 39y	112 (53.1)	94 (83.9)		6 (5.4)		6 (5.4)		6 (5.4)	
< 39y	99 (46.9)	78 (78.8)		15 (15.2)		3 (3.0)		3 (3.0)	
Gender			0.989		0.730		0.744		0.499
Male	108 (51.2)	88 (81.5)		10 (9.3)		4 (3.7)		6 (5.6)	
Female	103 (48.8)	84 (81.6)		11 (10.7)		5 (4.9)		3 (2.9)	
Working experience			0.452		0.419		0.509		0.736
≥ 9y	113 (53.6)	90 (79.6)		13 (11.5)		6 (5.3)		4 (3.5)	
< 9y	98 (46.4)	82 (83.7)		8 (8.2)		3 (3.1)		5 (5.1)	
Education level			0.933		0.365		0.716		0.716
High school	39 (18.5)	31 (79.5)		6 (15.4)		1 (2.6)		1 (2.6)	
Diploma certificate	166 (78.7)	136 (81.9)		14 (8.4)		8 (4.8)		8 (4.8)	
Bachelor's degree or higher	6 (2.8)	5 (83.3)		1 (16.7)		0 (0.0)		0 (0.0)	
Occupation			0.736		0.894		0.311		0.780
Medical doctor	7 (3.3)	6 (85.7)		1 (14.3)		0 (0.0)		0 (0.0)	
Nurse	169 (80.1)	136 (80.5)		17 (10.1)		9 (5.3)		7 (4.1)	
Other staff	35 (16.6)	30 (85.7)		3 (8.6)		0 (0.0)		2 (5.7)	
Department			0.000*		0.560		0.738		0.007*
Internal medicine	21 (10.0)	18 (85.7)		1 (4.8)		1 (4.8)		1 (4.8)	
Surgical Department	47 (22.3)	36 (76.6)		8 (17.0)		3 (6.4)		0 (0.0)	
Emergency Department	16 (7.6)	14 (87.5)		1 (6.3)		0 (0.0)		1 (6.3)	
Pediatric	19 (9.0)	15 (78.9)		2 (10.5)		2 (10.5)		0 (0.0)	
Obstetrics and Gynecology	9 (4.3)	0 (0.0)		0 (0.0)		0 (0.0)		0 (0.0)	
Under Fives Clinic	6 (2.8)	5 (83.3)		0 (0.0)		0 (0.0)		1 (16.7)	
Laboratory	16 (7.6)	16 (100.0)		0 (0.0)		0 (0.0)		0 (0.0)	
OP Theatre	22 (10.4)	19 (40.9)		2 (9.0)		0 (0.0)		1 (4.5)	
Pharmacy	5 (2.4)	2 (40.0)		1 (20.0)		0 (0.0)		2 (40.0)	
Others	50 (23.7)	38 (76.0)		6 (12.0)		3 (6.0)		3 (6.0)	
Hepatitis history			0.355		0.854		0.110		0.393
YES	14 (6.6)	10 (71.4)		2 (14.3)		2 (14.3)		0 (0.0)	
NO	176 (83.4)	143 (81.3)		17 (9.7)		7 (4.0)		9 (5.1)	
Unknown	21 (10.0)	19 (90.5)		2 (9.5)		0 (0.0)		0 (0.0)	
HBV vaccination			0.588		0.135		1.000		0.001*
YES	37 (17.5)	29 (78.4)		1 (2.7)		1 (2.7)		6 (16.2)	
NO	174 (82.5)	143 (82.2)		20 (11.5)		8 (4.6)		3 (1.7)	
Sharps injury			0.025*		0.351		0.670		0.063
Never	110 (52.1)	82 (74.5)		14 (12.7)		6 (5.5)		8 (7.3)	
Once	36 (17.1)	32 (88.9)		2 (5.6)		1 (2.8)		1 (2.8)	
More than once	65 (30.8)	58 (89.2)		5 (7.7)		2 (3.1)		0 (0.0)	
Total	211 (100)	172 (81.5)		21 (10.0)		9 (4.3)		9 (4.3)	

*Statistically significant at $P < 0.05$

Table 4 Multivariable analysis of possible risk factors for current HBV infection

Variables	Category	Frequency	OR	95% CI for OR	*P* Value
Age	≥39y	6/112	0.337	0.116–0.980	0.046*
	<39y	15/99			
Gender	Male	10/108	1.304	0.471–3.609	0.609
	Female	11/103			
Working experience	≥9y	13/113	1.334	0.502–3.547	0.563
	<9y	8/98			
Education background	Low	6/39	0.401	0.104–1.547	0.185
	Mid	14/166			
	High	1/6			
Occupation	Doctors	1/7	2.114	0.496–9.018	0.312
	Nurses	17/169			
	Others	3/35			
Vaccination	Yes	1/37	0.291	0.036–2.383	0.250
	No	20/174			
Sharps injury	Never	14/110	0.692	0.391–1.225	0.207
	Once	2/36			
	More than once	5/65			

*Statistically significant at $P < 0.05$

population, another issues which requires further investigation.

A significant difference in current infection rate between participants younger than 39 years old ($p = 0.018$) was observed in this study. Additionally, multivariable analysis of possible risk factors suggests a lower risk for current HBV infection among those HCWs aged > 39 years (OR = 0.337; 95% CI:0.116–0.980; $p = 0.046$). This finding may be due to differences in lifestyle or behavior between the two groups, however a larger sample size is needed to adequately study this risk factor. As expected, we also found that HBV vaccination was a protective factor for anti-HBs positive (immune status due to vaccination), as demonstrated elsewhere [22]. Before the vaccination program was launched in 1995, HBsAg carriage in the African population was very high [23]. In Sierra Leone, the hepatitis B vaccine is not available for the entire population because of limited resources. Our study found that only 17.5% HCWs reported previous HBV vaccination history, which is higher than those in the Democratic Republic of Congo (3.6%) [10] and Ethiopia (5.4%) [24]. However, only 16.2% of those vaccinated produced protective antibodies against HBV. This may have resulted from receiving a vaccination many years ago thereby resulting in waning immunity. In addition, there were three individuals who did not report previous HBV vaccination, but had similar

Table 5 Responses of the study participants to basic hepatitis B knowledge

Characteristic	The consequences of infection				Route of transmission				Preventive measures			
	no. (%)			*P* value	no. (%)			*P* value	no. (%)			*P* value
	Poor	Intermed	Good		Poor	Intermed	Good		Poor	Intermed	Good	
Age (y)												
< 39y	77 (77.8)	15 (15.2)	7 (7.1)	0.920	31 (31.3)	35 (35.4)	33 (33.3)	0.896	41 (41.4)	17 (17.2)	41 (41.4)	0.736
≥ 39y	86 (76.8)	19 (16.9)	7 (6.3)		32 (28.6)	40 (35.7)	40 (35.7)		52 (46.4)	19 (16.9)	41 (36.7)	
Gender												
Female	75 (72.8)	20 (19.4)	8 (7.8)	0.322	26 (25.4)	42 (40.8)	35 (33.9)	0.222	42 (41.7)	19 (18.5)	42 (40.8)	0.634
Male	88 (81.5)	14 (12.9)	6 (5.6)		37 (34.3)	33 (30.6)	38 (35.2)		51 (47.2)	17 (15.7)	40 (37.0)	
Working experience												
< 9y	74 (75.5)	19 (19.4)	5 (5.1)	0.380	27 (27.6)	35 (35.7)	36 (36.7)	0.752	33 (33.7)	19 (19.4)	46 (46.9)	0.017*
≥ 9y	89 (78.8)	15 (13.3)	9 (7.9)		36 (31.9)	40 (35.4)	37 (32.7)		60 (53.1)	17 (15.0)	36 (31.9)	
Education level												
High school	25 (65.8)	9 (23.7)	4 (10.5)	0.324	9 (20.5)	16 (41.0)	13 (33.3)	0.378	15 (38.5)	9 (23.1)	14 (35.9)	0.324
Diploma certificate	133 (79.6)	24 (14.4)	10 (5.9)		51 (31.7)	58 (35.4)	58 (35.4)		75 (45.7)	26 (15.9)	66 (40.2)	
Bachelor's degree or higher	5 (83.3)	1 (16.7)	0 (0.0)		3 (37.5)	1 (12.5)	2 (25.0)		3 (50.0)	1 (16.7)	2 (33.3)	
Occupation												
Medical doctor	4 (57.1)	2 (28.6)	1 (14.3)	0.050*	0 (0.0)	3 (42.9)	4 (57.1)	0.196	2 (28.6)	1 (14.3)	4 (57.1)	0.221
Nurse	137 (81.1)	21 (12.4)	11 (6.5)		56 (33.1)	59 (34.9)	54 (31.9)		80 (47.3)	30 (17.8)	59 (34.9)	
Other staff	22 (62.9)	11 (31.4)	2 (5.7)		7 (20.0)	13 (37.1)	15 (42.9)		11 (31.4)	5 (14.3)	19 (54.3)	
Total	163 (77.3)	34 (16.1)	14 (6.6)		63 (29.9)	75 (35.5)	73 (34.6)		93 (44.1)	36 (17.1)	82 (38.9)	

*Statistically significant at $P < 0.05$

immunological results to those who had been vaccinated, which was likely a result of recall bias. Vaccination of HCWs for HBV has been recommended by the WHO. However, even in South Africa, where there is a stronger healthcare system, only 30.6–52.4% of HCWs had protective levels of anti-HBs [7]. In addition, 81.5% HCWs in Sierra Leone tested negative for all markers, indicating susceptibility to HBV infection. Thus, there is an urgent need to expand vaccination coverage rates among HCWs in Sierra Leone.

The present study also found that there was poor knowledge of HBV, including the clinical outcome of infection, route of transmission and preventive measures of HBV, among HCWs. Therefore, HCWs in Sierra Leone will continue to be at risk of HBV infections until training and vaccination programs are strengthened. Our study also demonstrates that HCWs with longer working experience had more knowledge about preventive measures as compared to those with less work experience ($p = 0.007$). Furthermore, medical doctors had more knowledge of the consequences of HBV infection ($p = 0.05$), as expected compared to other occupations. It is generally assumed that education level and departments correlate with overall knowledge levels of the infection. However, this was not the case as these factors were not significant across all categories of knowledge, which is likely due to the small sample size of specific departments and education levels.

Limitations

The data presented in this study comes from a single hospital, which may not be representative of other healthcare facilities in Sierra Leone. It would be premature to draw broader conclusions regarding the prevalence and knowledge of hepatitis B across all HCWs in Sierra Leone.

Conclusions

HCWs in Sierra Leone lacked adequate knowledge of the hepatitis B virus.. Additionally, there were low coverage rates of hepatitis B vaccination that does not seem to be able to meet the WHO recommendations, leaving many HCWs susceptible to hepatitis B infection in the sampled population. Local health authorities need to make a coordinated effort to increase vaccination uptake considering the cost-effectiveness of broad immunization against hepatitis B and incorporate more intensive training against blood-borne pathogens for HCWs in Sierra Leone.

Abbreviations

DNA: Deoxyribonucleic acid; HBV: Hepatitis B virus; HCWs: Healthcare workers; WHO: World Health Organization

Acknowledgements

We are thankful to all healthcare workers who volunteered their valuable information and to the Public Health Department for their great assistance in organization this investigation and collecting the data. The authors also express gratitude to Dr. Michael E. von Fricken from George Mason University for editing the manuscript. Chinese Military Medical Experts Group in Sierra Leone: Yu-Ling Qin, Bo Li, Yue Yuan, Yi Sun, Jing Li, Zhong-Peng Zhao, Jun Jiao, Ya-Jun Song, Tian-Jun Jiang, Jia-Fu Jiang.

Funding

This project was supported by a training grant by Beijing 302 Hospital, of which YLQ and JFJ were coprincipal investigators.

Authors' contributions

YLQ, BL XZ, and TJJ conceived the survey. YLQ, BL, YY, YSZ, SB, LL, PL and TJJ designed and created the questionnaire. BL, YJS, YY, JL, ZPZ, JJ, SS, YS, JEK and TJJ conducted the survey. JFJ, BL, YLQ and YY executed data collection and managing and statistical analysis. BL and JJF drafted the manuscript. FS supervised this work. All authors critically revised the article and approved the final version of the manuscript.

Consent for publication

Not applicable.

Competing interests

The authors declare that they have no competing interests.

Author details

Beijing 302 Hospital, Beijing, China. [2]Beijing Institute of Microbiology and Epidemiology, Beijing, China. [3]No. 34 Military Hospital, Wilberforce, Freetown, Sierra Leone. [4]College of Medicine and Allied Health Sciences, Freetown, Sierra Leone.

References

1. World Health Organization. Global Hepatitis Report. 2017. Available at: http://apps.who.int/iris/bitstream/10665/255016/1/9789241565455-eng.pdf?ua=1.
2. Turati F, Edefonti V, Talamini R, Ferraroni M, Malvezzi M, Bravi F, et al. Family history of liver cancer and hepatocellular carcinoma. Hepatology. 2012;55(5):1416–25.
3. Hodges M, Sanders E, Aitken C. Seroprevalence of hepatitis markers; HAV, HBV, HCV and HEV amongst primary school children in Freetown, Sierra Leone. West Afr J Med. 1998;17:36–7.
4. Wurie IM, Wurie AT, Gevao SM. Sero-prevalence of hepatitis B virus among middle to high socio-economic antenatal population in Sierra Leone. West Afr J Med. 2005;24(1):18–20.
5. Garcia-Tardon N, Gresnigt TM, Fofanah AB, Grobusch MP. Hepatitis B and C in Tonkolili Province, Sierra Leone. Lancet. 2017;390(10101):1485.
6. World Health Organization. Preventing perinatal hepatitis B virus transmission: a guide for introducing and strengthening hepatitis B birth dose vaccination. Geneva: World Health Organization; 2015.
7. Sondlane TH, Mawela L, Razwiedani LL, Selabe SG, Lebelo RL, Nare Rakgole J, et al. High prevalence of active and occult hepatitis B virus infections in healthcare workers from two provinces of South Africa. Vaccine. 2016;34(33):3835–9.
8. Alese OO, Alese MO, Ohunakin A, Oluyide PO. Seroprevalence of hepatitis B surface antigen and occupational risk factors among health care workers in Ekiti state. Nigeria J Clin Diagn Res. 2016;10(2):LC16–8.
9. Coppola N, De Pascalis S, Onorato L, Calò F, Sagnelli C, Sagnelli E. Hepatitis B virus and hepatitis C virus infection in healthcare workers. World J Hepatol. 2016;8(5):273–81.
10. Shindano TA, Bahizire E, Fiasse R, Horsmans Y. Knowledge, attitudes, and practices of health-care workers about viral hepatitis B and C in south Kivu. Am J Trop Med Hyg. 2017;96(2):400–4.
11. Topuridze M, Butsashvili M, Kamkamidze G, Kajaia M, Morse D, McNutt LA. Barriers to hepatitis B vaccine coverage among healthcare workers in the republic of Georgia: an international perspective. Infect Control Hosp Epidemiol. 2010;31(2):158–64.

12. Winchester SA, Tomkins S, Cliffe S, Batty L, Ncube F, Zuckerman M. Healthcare workers' perceptions of occupational exposure to blood-borne viruses and reporting barriers: a questionnaire-based study. J Hosp Infect. 2012;82(1):36–9.
13. Ott JJ, Stevens GA, Groeger J, Wiersma ST. Global epidemiology of hepatitis B virus infection: new estimates of age-specific HBsAg seroprevalence and endemicity. Vaccine. 2012;30:2212–9.
14. Aba HO, Aminu M. Seroprevalence of hepatitis B virus serological markers among pregnant Nigerian women. Ann Afr Med. 2016;15(1):20–7.
15. Komas NP, Vickos U, Hubschen JM, Bere A, Manirakiza A, Muller CP, et al. Cross-sectional study of hepatitis B virus infection in rural communities, Central African Republic. BMC Infect Dis. 2013;13:286.
16. Tao I, Compaore TR, Diarra B, Djigma F, Zohoncon TM, Assih M, et al. Seroepidemiology of hepatitis B and C viruses in the general population of Burkina Faso. Hepat Res Treat. 2014:781843.
17. Musa BM, Bussell S, Borodo MM, Samaila AA, Femi OL. Prevalence of hepatitis B virus infection in Nigeria, 2000-2013: a systematic review and meta-analysis. Niger J Clin Pract. 2015;18:163–72.
18. Ziraba AK, Bwogi J, Namale A, Wainaina CW, Mayanja-Kizza H. Sero-prevalence and risk factors for hepatitis B virus infection among health care workers in a tertiary hospital in Uganda. BMC Infect Dis. 2010;29(10):191.
19. Abiola AH, Agunbiade AB, Badmos KB, Lesi AO, Lawal AO, Alli QO. Prevalence of HBsAg, knowledge, and vaccination practice against viral hepatitis B infection among doctors and nurses in a secondary health care facility in Lagos state, South-Western Nigeria. Pan Afri Med J. 2016;23:160.
20. Hope VD, Eramova I, Capurro D, Donoghoe MC. Prevalence and estimation of hepatitis B and C infections in the WHO European region: a review of data focusing on the countries outside the European Union and the European free trade association. Epidemiol Infect. 2014;142:270–86.
21. Burnett RJ, François G, Mphahlele MJG, Africa PN, Satekge MM, et al. Hepatitis B vaccination coverage in healthcare workers in Gauteng Province, South Africa. Vaccine. 2011;29(25):4293–7.
22. Ghadir MR, Belbasi M, Heidari A, et al. Distribution and risk factors of hepatitis B virus infection in the general population of Central Iran. Hepat Mon. 2012;12:112–7.
23. Burnett RJ, François G, Kew MC, Leroux-Roels G, Meheus A, Hoosen AA, et al. Hepatitis B virus and human immunodeficiency virus co-infection in sub-Saharan Africa: a call for further investigation. Liver Int. 2005;25(2):201–13.
24. Abeje G, Azage M. Hepatitis B vaccine knowledge and vaccination status among health care workers of Bahir Dar City Administration, Northwest Ethiopia: a cross sectional study. BMC Infect Dis. 2015;15:30.

Hepatitis A surveillance: sensitivity of two information sources

Gloria Carmona[1*], Marta Vilaró[2,3], Pilar Ciruela[1,3], Mireia Jané[1,3], Lluis Giralt[3], Laura Ruiz[1], Sergi Hernández[1,2], Àngela Domínguez[2,3], Working Group of the Epidemiological Surveillance Network of Catalonia and Working Group of the Microbiological Reporting System of Catalonia

Abstract

Background: The frequency of mild forms of hepatitis A, especially in children, could lead to underreporting. The objective of the study was to investigate the sensitivity of two surveillance systems, mandatory Statutory Disease Reports and the Microbiological Reporting System of Catalonia, using capture-recapture techniques.

Methods: The study was conducted in Catalonia between 2011 and 2015. Hepatitis A cases reported to two independent surveillance systems were included: Statutory Disease Reports (SDR) and Microbiological Reporting System of Catalonia (MRS). The variables collected were: age, sex, year of declaration, size of municipality (< 10,000 and ≥ 10,000), country of birth (Spain or abroad), reporting centre (primary care/hospital) and notification method (electronic or paper). The capture-recapture analysis and the estimate of 95% confidence intervals were made using the Chapman formula for comparison of two sources, both for the estimate of the total number of cases and the stratification according to variables. Multinomial logistic regression was performed to obtain an adjusted estimate.

Results: The SDR had a greater overall sensitivity than the MRS (48.8%; 43.5–55.6 vs. 19.3%; 17.2–21.9). In cases aged < 15 years the sensitivity of both systems was higher (76.6%; 72.7–81 vs. 25.2%; 20.9–29.5) than in cases aged > 15 years (25.5%; 22.8–28.3 vs. 12.1%; 10–14.2). For those born in Spain, the sensitivity was 57.2% (49.6–67.4) in the SDR and 27.1% (23.5–31.9) in the MRS, lower than that for foreign-born patients (58%; 51.2–66.8 vs. 49.1%; 43.4–56.6). In electronically-reported cases, the sensitivity was much higher in the SDR than in the MRS (47.2%; 42.3–52.1 vs. 9.4%; 6.5–12.3). No differences were observed according to sex, size of municipality, and year of declaration or reporting centre. The estimated total number of cases using the Chapman formula was very similar to the adjusted estimate (1121; 985–1258 vs. 1120; 876–1525), indicating the robustness of the results.

Conclusions: The sensitivity of the SDR was greater than that of MRS, especially in patients aged < 15 years, although for patients born abroad the difference in sensitivity was lower. Reinforced surveillance combining the SDR and MRS improves the efficiency in the detection of cases.

Keywords: Hepatitis A, Capture-recapture, Estimated incidence

Background

The Statutory Disease Reporting System (SDR) is a passive surveillance system through which health professionals declare all infectious diseases subject to surveillance in Catalonia (Spain): the reporting systems and procedures are regulated by a Decree that must be complied with [1, 2]. Suspicion is sufficient to notify the SDR. The reporting physician may have the suspicion or confirmation of hepatitis A and, when reporting, should declare whether the notification is due to suspicion or laboratory confirmation.

The Microbiological Reporting System of Catalonia (MRS) is a surveillance system based on microbiologists reporting microorganisms that cause acute infectious diseases in Catalonia [3]. The MRS is based on reporting only laboratory-confirmed cases and does not notify cases ruled out (negative and false positive IgM).

* Correspondence: gloria.carmona@gencat.cat
[1]Public Health Agency of Catalonia (ASPCAT), Roc Boronat 81-95, 08005 Barcelona, Spain
Full list of author information is available at the end of the article

The SDR and MRS are complementary and their integrated management constitutes a reinforced surveillance system capable of improving the detection of cases of diseases under surveillance.

Although all public or private health professionals are required to report any suspicion of any disease covered by the SDR, in practice there is underreporting by some professionals and, in consequence, the real incidence of the disease is underestimated. Among the main causes of underreporting are not knowing the obligation to report the disease, not appreciating the importance of doing so, and the pressures on health care [4].

Knowledge of the real incidence of diseases is also affected by underdetection. In the case of hepatitis A in children aged < 6 years, the infection is asymptomatic (without jaundice) in approximately 70% of children, which leads to underdetection. However, in adolescents and adults, 70% of cases are symptomatic [5]. The resources allocated by public health services to surveillance systems are limited, and periodic evaluation contributes to maximizing their efficiency [6].

The capture-recapture method is a statistical method for estimating the real incidence of diseases in a given population. It consists of studying, for two or more information sources, the number of cases detected by one source and the number of cases detected in the two or more sources used (coincident cases) to estimate cases not detected by the different sources used [7]. This method has the advantage of being much cheaper than others based on an active search for cases and allows similar results to be obtained [8]. The conditions for application of the capture-recapture methodology are [7, 8]: a) the population under study has to be closed, i.e., there should be no changes during the time in which the capture of cases occurs in the systems compared; b) there must be a method of determining whether an individual identified by one source is the same as an individual identified in the other system; c) each individual must have the same probability of being captured by either system; d) the systems must be independent. The aim of this study was to investigate the sensitivity of two surveillance systems using the capture-recapture method: the SDR and the MRS in Catalonia.

Methods

Information sources

The SDR is based on physicians reporting suspected cases of diseases deemed to be of mandatory report. One of the main functions of the SDR is epidemiological surveillance and control of these diseases and outbreaks of any aetiology considered as a priority for control in Catalonia, a Spanish region with 7.5 million inhabitants, which includes hepatitis A. The mere suspicion of hepatitis A by a physician means it must be reported as a suspected case. The reporting physician may have a suspicion or a confirmed case of hepatitis A and the report must state whether the case is suspected or laboratory confirmed (in which case the method of confirmation must be stated).

In Catalonia, there are definitions for suspected and confirmed cases of hepatitis A. Cases included in the SDR must meet one of the following definitions:

Suspected case

A case that meets the clinical case definition.

Clinical case definition

Person with discrete onset of symptoms (malaise, abdominal pain, anorexia, diarrhoea, nausea, intermittent vomiting, arthralgia) and one of the following three symptoms: fever, jaundice or elevated serum aminotransferase levels.

Confirmed case

(1) A case that meets the clinical case definition and is confirmed by laboratory tests: positive IgM against hepatitis A (anti-HAV positive), or (2) A case that meets the clinical case definition and is epidemiologically-linked to a confirmed case.

All cases reported to the SDR are reviewed to verify that they meet the definition of a suspected or confirmed case. Cases that do not meet the definition of suspected cases are classified as "non-cases" and are excluded.

This study only includes cases that met the case definition and were laboratory confirmed or were epidemiologically-linked to a confirmed case: suspected cases were excluded.

The MRS is a basic information system that belongs to the epidemiological surveillance network of Catalonia. The MRS collects information on microorganisms causing infectious diseases detected by laboratories participating in the system. The main objectives of the MRS are to provide information on certain diseases through the identification of the microorganisms involved and to determine trends and changes in the epidemiological patterns of microorganisms and microbiological resistance. Until 2015, the MRS was a voluntary surveillance system which covered 82% of acute hospital beds [2].

At the end of 2015, Catalonia drafted new legislation to harmonize the list of diseases to be subject to monitoring in accordance with the European norm. Under this new regulation, the MRS went from a voluntary reporting system to a system of obligatory declaration.

In the years included in the study (2011–2015), the laboratories participating in the MRS did so voluntarily. Professionals working in the Microbiology services of Catalonia involved in the system reported detections of specific anti-HAV IgM, providing data to identify the case (name).

Notification data in both the SDR and MRS are contained in an application in which data exploitation and analysis can be managed. The SDR and MRS are interconnected, since the two systems are complementary for communicable disease surveillance, but the independence of the sources is maintained. Cases that meet the clinical case definition and are epidemiologically linked to a confirmed case are not declared to the MRS because, by definition, they do not require confirmation, and are detected by the SDR.

Data collection

MRS: We extracted all records coded for hepatitis A (confirmed cases) reported from January 2011 to December 2015 from the MRS. Likewise, we extracted all hepatitis records from the SDR dataset for the same study period. We then linked the databases using the personal identification code (PIC). When the PIC was not available, the date of report, age and sex were used to identify duplicates between the two sources. In cases with inconclusive/unclear matching, the hospital was used as a fifth matching criterion. The variables recorded for each case were age, sex, year of report, size of municipality (< 10,000 and ≥ 10,000), country of birth, type of report (electronic or paper) and centre of report (hospital or primary care centre).

SDR: Confirmed cases reported to the SDR according to the confirmed case definition were selected. Confirmed case: case that meets the clinical case definition and is laboratory-confirmed (specific anti-HAV IgM), or a case that meets the clinical case definition and is epidemiologically-linked to a confirmed case.

The study was not submitted for research ethics approval as the activities described were conducted as part of the legislated mandate of the Health Department of Catalonia, the competent authority for the surveillance of communicable diseases, which is officially authorized to receive, treat and temporarily store personal data on cases of infectious disease according to Decree 203/2015 of the 15 September which created the epidemiological surveillance network [2]. Therefore, all study activities formed part of public health surveillance and were thus exempt from institutional board review and did not require informed consent.

Personal data were used only for evaluation during the matching process. All the necessary measures to protect the confidentiality of personal data were taken during the whole evaluation (access to the data restricted to the personnel involved in data analysis and removal of personal data from the datasets after matching).

Statistical methods

The total number of hepatitis A cases was estimated using the two-source capture-recapture method that uses Chapman's formula [9] to reduce bias due to small samples:

$$N = \frac{(L1+1)(L2+1)}{a+1} - 1$$

$$95\%\mathrm{CI} = \mathrm{N} \pm 1.96\sqrt{\frac{(\mathrm{L1}+1)(\mathrm{L2}+1)(\mathrm{L1}-\mathrm{a})(\mathrm{L2}-\mathrm{a})}{(\mathrm{a}+1)^2(\mathrm{a}+2)}}$$

where L1 is the number of cases in the SDR dataset, L2 is the number of cases reported to the MRS, and a is the number of cases captured by both systems. The sensitivity (Se) of case ascertainment by the two sources is calculated as the proportion of true cases detected by each source, i.e. Se(1) = L1/N for source 1 and Se(2) = L2/N for source 2. Sensitivity for the two sources when they are combined was calculated as the proportion of cases detected by one of the two sources or both, i.e. Se(1,2) = (L1 + L2-a)/N.

Estimates were made for the entire 5-year period and additionally stratified by age group, sex, year of report, size of municipality, country of birth, centre of report and type of report. (electronic or paper).

The independence of the sources was considered when applying the capture-recapture method [10, 11]. In the two-by-two table, where a represents cases reported by two sources or combinations of sources, b and c cases reported exclusively by either of the two sources, and x the estimated cases not reported by either of the sources, the odds ratio (OR = ax/bc) should not significantly differ from one.

A multinomial logit model [12, 13] was used to evaluate patient characteristics to the probability of capture, which allows more precise estimates of the number of estimated cases [14]. This identifies patient characteristics related to the probability of capture by the different sources. We used a backwards stepwise procedure (using likelihood ratio tests, with a p-value of > 0.2 as the criterion for removing variables from the model) [15, 16] to eliminate covariates, starting with a full model including all potential covariates and using the parameter estimates from the model to estimate the sizes of population subgroups and calculate the estimated incidence. We also derived confidence intervals which allow for the uncertainty in estimating the total number of cases. All analyses were made using R software version 3.0.1.

Results

The distribution of patient characteristics by source is shown in Table 1. The mean age was 20.6 years in the SDR and 27.5 years in the MRS; 55% of patients were aged < 15 years in the SDR and 46% in the MRS. The male-female percentage was 56% vs.44% in the SDR, and

Table 1 Hepatitis A patient characteristics by source, Catalonia 2011–2015

	SDR (*n* = 547)	MRS (*n* = 216)
Age at report, years		
Mean (SD)	20.6 (18.6)	27.5 (23.1)
Median (IQR)	10 (29)	25 (40)
< 2 years, n (%)	29 (5.3%)	8 (3.7%)
2–4 years, n (%)	77 (14.1%)	26 (12.0%)
5–14 years, n (%)	196 (35.8%)	65 (30.1%)
15–24 years, n (%)	21 (3.8%)	8 (3.7%)
25–34 years, n (%)	92 (16.8%)	22 (10.2%)
35–44 years, n (%)	68 (12.4%)	28 (13.0%)
45–54 years, n (%)	33 (6.0%)	29 (13.4%)
> 55 years, n (%)	31 (5.7%)	29 (13.4%)
NAs	0 (0.0%)	1 (0.5%)
Sex, n (%)		
Male	308 (56.3%)	126 (58.3%)
Female	239 (43.7%)	90 (41.7%)
NAs	0 (0.0%)	0 (0.0%)
Year of report, n (%)		
Year 2011	134 (24.5%)	18 (8.3%)
Year 2012	127 (23.2%)	50 (23.1%)
Year 2013	107 (19.6%)	31 (14.3%)
Year 2014	101 (18.5%)	62 (28.7%)
Year 2015	74 (13.5%)	55 (25.5%)
NAs	4 (0.7%)	0 (0.0%)
Size of municipality, n (%)		
< 10,000 people	115 (21.0%)	75 (34.7%)
≥ 10,000 people	430 (78.6%)	127 (58.8%)
NAs	2 (0.4%)	14 (6.5%)
Country of birth, n (%)		
Spain	186 (34.0%)	88 (40.7%)
Other countries	92 (16.8%)	78 (36.1%)
NAs	269 (49.2%)	50 (23.1%)
Type of report, n (%)		
Electronic	184 (33.6%)	37 (17.1%)
Paper	363 (66.4%)	179 (82.9%)
NAs	0 (0.0%)	0 (0.0%)
Centre of report, n (%)		
Primary healthcare centre	184 (33.6%)	65 (30.1%)
Hospital	182 (33.3%)	151 (69.9%)
NAs	181 (33.1%)	0 (0.0%)

NAs Not available

58% vs. 42% in the MRS. The number of Spanish-born patients was 34% in the SDR and 41% in the MRS and, in both cases was higher than the number of foreign-born patients. Paper was the main form of report (66% in the SDR and 83% in the MRS). The centre of report was 34% primary healthcare and 33% hospital in the SDR and 70% hospital reports and 30% primary healthcare in the MRS.

Capture-recapture analysis

The odds ratio (OR) to verify the independence of the two sources was 0.99 (95% CI 0.69–1.29), reinforcing the independence of the sources.

From 2011 to 2015, 547 cases were reported to the SDR (503 laboratory-confirmed and 44 without laboratory confirmation but epidemiologically-linked to a laboratory-confirmed case) and 216 to the MRS, 105 cases were included in both sources. The estimated total number of case reports expected during the whole period was 1121 (95% CI 985–1258) (Table 2). A decrease in the number of reported cases was observed between 2011 (134 cases) and 2015 (74 cases) and no outbreak was detected during the study period. The sensitivity was 48.8% (95%CI 43.5–55.6%) for the SDR and 19.3% (95%CI 17.2–21.9%) for the MRS (Table 3). The estimated total number of cases was statistically significant (p-value< 0.001) which means there were differences between the sensitivity of the two sources. Sensitivity increased to 58.7% (95%CI 54.9–62.4%) when the datasets were combined.

Table 3 shows the unreported cases, the estimated number of cases and the sensitivity for both sources stratified by the characteristics considered.

The sensitivity was 76.6% (95%CI 72.7–81.0) for the SDR and 25.2% (95%CI 20.9–29.5) for the MRS in the < 15 years age group, and 25.5% (95%CI 22.8–28.3) for the SDR and 12.1% (95%CI 10.0–14.2) for the MRS in the ≥15 years age group: the differences were statistically significant (p-value< 0.001). The 2–4 years age group had the highest sensitivity in both the SDR and MRS: 81.3% (95%CI 70.7–95.7) in the SDR and 27.5% (95%CI 23.8–32.3) in the MRS (Fig. 1). The sensitivity of the two sources was very similar between males (SDR 46.4%; 95%CI 39.8–55.7% and MRS 19.0%; 95%CI 16.3–22.8) and females (SDR 52.6%; 95%CI 44.9–63.6 and MRS 19.8 95%CI 16.9–24.0), without significant differences.

Table 2 Capture-recapture analysis of two datasets to estimate the total number of hepatitis A cases, Catalonia 2011–2015

		SDR		Total
		Identified	Not identified	
MRS	Identified	105	111	216
	Not identified	442	463	905
	Total	547	574	1121

SDR Statutory Disease Reporting
MRS Microbiological Reporting System of Catalonia

Table 3 Capture–recapture analysis of all hepatitis A cases and of subgroups, Catalonia 2011 to 2015

	No. records in SDR	No. records in MRS	Matched records	Calculated unreported cases	Estimated total no. of cases (95% CI)	SDR Sensitivity (%) (95% CI)	MRS Sensitivity (%) (95% CI)	Difference in sensitivity of the two sources	*p*-value
All cases	547	216	105	463	1121 (985–1258)	48.8 (43.5–55.6)	19.3 (17.2–21.9)	29.5%	< 0.001
Age at notification, years									
< 15 years	302	99	76	68	393 (357–430)	76.6 (72.7–81.0)	25.2 (20.9–29.5)	51.4%	< 0.001
> = 15 years	245	116	29	627	959 (687–1232)	25.5 (22.8–28.3)	12.1 (10.0–14.2)	13.4%	
Sex									0.667
Male	308	126	58	288	664 (554–775)	46.4 (39.8–55.7)	19.0 (16.3–22.8)	27.4%	
Female	239	90	47	172	454 (376–533)	52.6 (44.9–63.6)	19.8 (16.9–24.0)	32.8%	
Year of declaration									
Year 2011	134	18	9	155	268 (168–369)	50.0 (36.4–79.9)	6.7 (4.9–10.7)	43.3%	Ref
Year 2012	127	50	34	44	187 (158–216)	68.0 (58.8–80.6)	26.8 (23.2–31.7)	41.2%	< 0.001
Year 2013	107	31	21	41	158 (126–190)	67.7 (56.3–85.5)	19.6 (16.3–24.6)	48.1%	0.005
Year 2014	101	62	22	144	285 (207–364)	35.5 (27.8–48.9)	21.8 (17.1–30.1)	13.7%	0.015
Year 2015	74	55	19	104	214 (153–276)	34.6 (26.8–48.5)	25.7 (19.9–36.1)	8.9%	0.008
Size of municipality									0.070
< 10,000 people	115	75	33	102	259 (205–312)	44.5 (38.5–50.6)	29.0 (23.5–34.6)	15.5%	
> =10,000 people	430	127	72	270	755 (652–858)	57.0 (53.5–60.5)	16.8 (14.2–19.5)	40.2%	
Country of birth									< 0.001
Spain	186	88	50	101	325 (376–375)	57.2 (49.6–67.4)	27.1 (23.5–31.9)	30.1%	
Other countries	92	78	45	34	159 (138–180)	58.0 (51.2–66.8)	49.1 (43.4–56.6)	8.9%	
Type of notification									< 0.001
Electronic	184	37	17	186	390 (269–511)	47.2 (36.0–68.5)	9.5 (7.3–13.8)	37.8%	
Paper	363	179	88	281	735 (642–830)	49.4 (43.8–56.6)	24.4 (21.6–27.9)	15.8%	
Centre of notification									0.704
Primary health care centre	184	65	29	186	406 (310–503)	45.3 (36.6–59.5)	16.0 (12.9–21.0)	45.1%	
Hospital	182	151	76	103	360 (318–404)	50.5 (45.2–57.3)	41.9 (37.5–47.6)	5.6%	

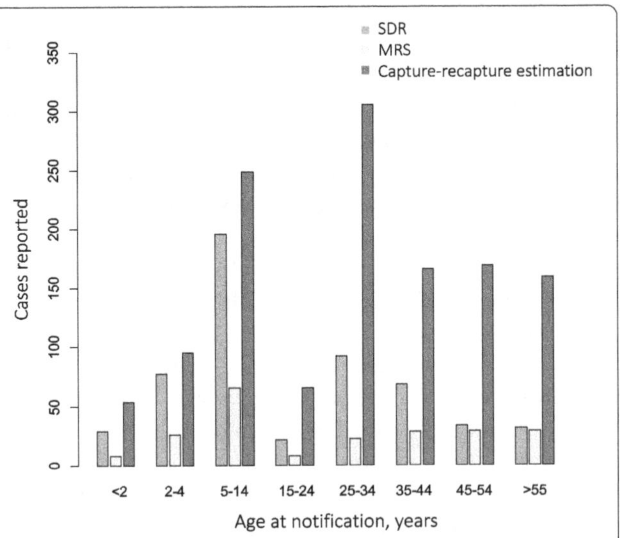

Fig. 1 Cases by age groups reported to MRS and SDR systems and estimation cases by capture-recapture method

No differences were observed according to the size of the municipality.

Comparing sensitivities by country of birth was statistically significant (p-value< 0.001) due mainly to the sensitivity of the MRS, with 27.1% (95%CI 23.5–31.9) for Spanish-born people and 49.1% (95%CI 43.4–56.6%) for foreign-born people. Paper reports were the most used by the two sources and the sensitivity for the SDR was similar, but electronic report had a sensitivity of 9.4% (95%CI 6.5–12.3%) while on paper it was 15.3% (95%CI 13.2–17.4%; $p < 0.001$). There were no significant differences in sensitivity according to the type of centre for either source: the sensitivity was 32.8% (95% CI 27.5–40.6%) in the SDR and 27.2% (95%CI 22.8–33.7) in the MRS for hospitals and 69.6 (95%CI61.2–80.6%) and 24.5% (21.6–28.5%) for primary healthcare.

The final multinomial logit model obtained after the stepwise procedure shows the characteristics that explain the identification of cases by the two sources and, therefore, the sensitivity of the two sources in identifying hepatitis A cases in Catalonia. The results of the multinomial logit model are shown in Table 4. In the final multivariate model, the variables considered statistically significant in defining the sensitivity of the two sources were the age at report (< 15 vs. > = 15 years), the country of birth and the type of report. Other variables that were also important in explaining the sensitivity of the two sources were the year of report (2011 to 2013 vs.2014 to 2015) and the centre of report. The odds of being identified by one of the two sources for the ≥15 years age group was 0.44 times (95%CI 0.26–0.74) that of the < 15 years age group; the odds for people born in Spain were 0.25 times (95% CI 0.15–0.43) that for foreign-born people; and the odds for paper reporting were 0.36 times (95%CI 0.21–0.64) that for electronic reporting. With these variables in the model, the adjusted estimate of the total number of cases was 1120 (95%CI 876–1525). This estimate was similar to that obtained by Chapman's formula, suggesting the results were consistent and robust.

Table 4 Variables defining the sensitivity of the sources in detecting hepatitis A. Multinomial Logit model

	OR (95%CI)	p-value
Age at notification (≥ 15 years)	0.44 (0.26, 0.74)	0.002
Year of declaration (2014–2015)	0.65 (0.40, 1.07)	0.089
Country of birth (Spain)	0.25 (0.15, 0.43)	< 0.001
Type of notification (Paper)	0.36 (0.21, 0.64)	< 0.001
Centre of notification (Hospital)	1.59 (0.92, 2.76)	0.099

OR odds ratio

Discussion

The results of this study provide robust estimates due to the fact that the sources studied are independent and because the assumption of independence was confirmed. Various authors have employed capture-recapture methods using independent sources that are the same or very similar to those we used to assess the sensitivity of different sources of the surveillance system for hepatitis A and other diseases. Overhage et al. [17] used two sources to assess hepatitis A surveillance completeness: a) automated electronic laboratory reports and b) spontaneous reporting by physicians: Durosoy et al. [18] also used two sources of hepatitis A surveillance: a) laboratory results and b) notifications by physicians. Matin et al. [19], in a study that assessed how many cases of hepatitis A are not reported, used three data sources: a) the Laboratory Reporting System, b) the Local Health Protection Unit and c) data derived from a specific project on hepatitis A genotyping.

The sensitivity of the SDR was greater than that of the MRS in both the global and the subgroup analyses. This may be because the SDR system is compulsory and has 100% coverage throughout Catalonia while, in the years analysed, the MRS system was voluntary and encompassed around 80% of Catalonia healthcare services. In addition, the SDR also includes a few clinically-compatible but not laboratory-confirmed cases which were epidemiologically-linked to a laboratory-confirmed case.

The new Decree [2] has established the obligatory nature of report to the MRS system by public and private hospital and primary healthcare microbiology laboratories in Catalonia. Future studies are required to determine whether this change affects the completeness of reporting from this source and, if so, to quantify the changes.

Other factors that contribute to the lower sensitivity of the MRS with respect to hepatitis A are that the serological tests necessary for the diagnosis of hepatitis A are not performed in all reporting microbiology laboratories, so some hospitals do not report cases. In addition, 70% of reports to the MRS are hospital-based and hepatitis A is detected mainly in primary healthcare centres.

Although the real incidence of clinical cases of hepatitis A is difficult to ascertain due to underreporting, evaluating the sensitivity of the sources used for disease surveillance is of interest because it may help to improve the detection of cases and the adoption of appropriate control measures [16, 20].

Our study underlines the importance of integrating information from different sources to monitor, prevent and control outbreaks [21].

Reviews of hepatitis A only or of foodborne diseases including hepatitis A in developed countries [22, 23] have found that hepatitis A is frequently underreported, as did the results of the study by Simmons et al. [24], who assessed the completeness of the notification system by comparing notifications with laboratory-confirmed cases of hepatitis A and other foodborne illnesses.

A meta-analysis of the completeness of the reporting of hepatitis A cases between 1997 and 2015 obtained heterogeneous results, ranging from 4 to 97%. Differences were attributed to factors such as the type of source used for case detection, reporting mechanisms (automatic methods, other methods) and staffing infrastructure [22].

A Turkish study by Durosoy et al. to determine the completeness of two sources (reporting and laboratory) for various diseases (hepatitis, brucellosis, syphilis, measles and HIV/AIDS) found that only 31.6% of cases of hepatitis A reported by the laboratory had been notified to the surveillance system. The incidence rates calculated from the cases reported to the surveillance system placed the region at the level of low incidence for hepatitis A, whereas if the cases identified by the laboratory were added, the incidence level increased and placed the region in the intermediate incidence zone [18]. A 2006 capture-recapture study conducted in England found high underreporting of hepatitis A cases, with a completeness of 27.8% (95% CI 19–38.7% [19].

In the present study, the sensitivity was significantly greater in cases in children aged < 15 years than in those aged ≥15 years, both for the SDR (76.6%, 72.7–81) and the MRS (25.2%, 20.9–29.5). The 2–4 years age group had the greatest sensitivity for both sources (81.3% for the SDR system versus 27.5% for the MRS). The sensitivity fell with increasing age, especially in the SDR, and from 45 years of age upwards was slightly below 20% for both sources. Although most capture-recapture studies do not analyse the sensitivity of the different sources across different age groups [23], the New Zealand study by Simmons et al. of foodborne diseases also showed a greater sensitivity for reporting hepatitis A in younger people [24]. It is difficult to find a simple explanation for the fact that more cases were reported in children than in adults, especially because hepatitis A is clinically more florid in adults. In any case, our results suggest the advisability of targeting health professionals to reinforce the reporting of cases in adults.

The sensitivity of the MRS was lower than that of the SDR throughout the study years, although it increased in more recent years, and was 25.7% (95% CI 19.9–36.1) in 2015. The improvement in the MRS results in recent years coincides with increased coverage of reporting to the MRS, especially in primary healthcare.

According to the country of birth, the notification of cases of hepatitis A in foreign-born people was more sensitive (p value < 0.001) than that in people born in Spain for the two sources. The country of origin is of great relevance for the surveillance of communicable diseases [25], and our results suggest that there is a greater concern on the part of respondents to report cases occurring in foreign-born people than those occurring in the native population. It may be that health professionals have a greater suspicion of hepatitis A in people born in countries where the disease is endemic than in people born in Spain which, in recent years, has seen a significant decrease in the disease incidence.

Although there were no significant differences in the results obtained in the two sources according to the type of centre, the SDR had greater sensitivity in cases reported by primary healthcare centres (69.6%) than in cases reported by hospitals (32.8%). In contrast, in the MRS, the sensitivity was slightly higher in hospitals (27.2%) than in primary healthcare centres (24.5%). The SDR results may be due to the fact that a percentage of hepatitis A cases, especially in children, do not present complications, and therefore are not hospitalized, with primary healthcare professionals detecting and reporting the disease.

In our study, the sensitivity of electronic reporting was higher than that obtained by paper-based reports for the SDR (47.2% vs. 31.1%), whereas the comparable figures for the MRS were 9.4% vs. 15.3%, with the differences being statistically significant. The greater implementation of electronic reporting in the SDR may explain these results.

Notification by electronic procedures that must be validated by epidemiological surveillance unit technicians is increasing and adds opportunities for disease reporting to the surveillance system. In a study carried out in Andalusia, Spain, it was estimated that the verification process of reports received electronically accounted for approximately 10% of the activity of the personnel responsible for the surveillance of communicable diseases

[26], but this not inconsiderable time is justified if, as our data suggest, it serves to increase the sensitivity of the system. Difficulties in the electronic transportability of the data generated in hospitals may explain why the sensitivity was lower for the cases reported electronically to the MRS in our study, a limitation also reported by other authors [27]. Overhage et al. [17] found that electronic data transmission from the laboratory increased paper-based reporting by more than four-fold.

This study has strengths and limitations. The main strength is that 91% of the cases reported to the two sources had reported the PIC. The detection of coincident cases (cases declared to both sources) was made through the PIC when this data was available. In cases in which the PIC was not available, the study of coincident cases was made by comparing the name and surname, age, sex, hospital or primary healthcare centre and the date of report of the case.

One limitation is that, as noted above, MRS coverage is not universal, unlike the SDR, which is. However, since both sources should be used for the monitoring and control of hepatitis A, we believe that this does not invalidate the assessment of the results obtained.

The sensitivity of the sources studied for the surveillance of hepatitis A cannot be generalized to other diseases because physicians' perceptions of the importance of hepatitis A for public health differs from that of other diseases and because laboratory confirmation methods may be more complex for some diseases than for others [28]. In the aforementioned New Zealand study, among food-borne transmissible diseases, hepatitis A was the disease for which the reporting of cases by physicians showed the lowest sensitivity [23].

Conclusion

In conclusion, the sensitivity of enhanced surveillance by combining two information sources (compulsory reporting by physicians and voluntary reporting by microbiology laboratories) was 59%, improving the sensitivity of each source separately and helping to improve the quality of epidemiological surveillance necessary for adequate control of hepatitis A.

The resources allocated by public health services to surveillance systems are limited, and periodic evaluation contributes to maximizing their efficiency. Capture-recapture methods may contribute knowledge of the true incidence rates of communicable diseases.

Acknowledgements

To the Working Group of the Epidemiological Surveillance Network of Catalonia and Working Group of the Microbiological Reporting System of Catalonia.

The Working Group of the Epidemiological Surveillance Network of Catalonia is composed of: C. Arias, J. Álvarez, I. Barrabeig, N. Camps, M. Company, M. Carol, P. Godoy, A. Martínez, S. Minguell, I. Parron, MR. Sala-Farré, J. Torres, A. Rovira, S. Manzanares (Agència de Salut Pública de Barcelona).

The Working Group of the Microbiological Reporting System of Catalonia is composed of: F.Ballester; I. Pujol (Hospital Universitari de Sant Joan de Reus); MÁ. Benítez, A. Cebollero (Consorci de Laboratoris Intercomarcal de l'Alt Penedès); J. Costa, J. Vila (Hospital Clínic-Casa de la Maternitat); A. Calderón (Hospital Municipal de Badalona); M. Curriu (Hospital Comarcal de Sant Bernabé); M Á. Domínguez, L. Calatayud (Hospital Universitari de Bellvitge); EM. Dopico (Laboratori Clínic de l'Hospitalet); MJ. Ferri (Hospital Universitari de Girona Dr. Josep Trueta); PJ. Ayala (Clínica de Terres de l'Ebre); J. Massa, D. Saenz, C. Gallés (Hospital Comarcal Calella-Blanes); P. Gassiot (Hospital de Figueres); F. Gómez, C. Molina (Hospital Universitari Joan XXIII de Tarragona); A.González-Cuevas (Hospital General del Parc Sanitari Sant Joan de Déu); C. Guardia (CAP Doctor Robert); M. Juanpere (Hospital Móra d'Ebre); M. Monsonis (Hospital Sant Joan de Déu. Esplugues de Llobregat); C. Martí (Hospital General de Granollers); N. Margall (Hospital de la Santa Creu i Sant Pau); L. Matas (Hospital Universitari Germans Trias i Pujol); M. Morta (Hospital Sant Joan de Déu. Manresa-Fundació Althaia); S. Noguer (Hospital del Vendrell); M. Olsina (Hospital General de Catalunya); P. Pérez (Catlab-Centre Analítiques Terrassa); E. Padilla, M. Micó (Laboratori de referència de Catalunya, Prat de Llobregat); MO.Pérez-Moreno (Hospital Verge de la Cinta de Tortosa); T. Pumarola, F. Rodriguez-Frias (Hospital Universitari Vall d'Hebron); X. Raga (Hospital de Sant Pau i Santa Tecla); M. Ribelles (Hospital Universitari Arnau de Vilanova de Lleida); E. Sanfeliu (Hospital d'Olot Comarcal de la Garrotxa); G. Sauca (Hospital de Mataró); G. Solé (Hospital de Sabadell-Centre Sanitari Parc Taulí) and A. Vilamala (Hospital Universitari de Vic).

Funding

This work was partially funded by CIBER of Epidemiology and Public Health (CIBERESP) Carlos III Health Institute and the Catalan Agency for the Management of Grants for University Research (AGAUR Grant Number 2017/SGR 1342). The funding sources played no part in the design of the study and collection, analysis, and interpretation of data and in writing the manuscript.

Authors' contributions

LR and SH prepared databases, monitored and validated data and reviewed the article for important intellectual content. LG and MV conducted the statistical analysis (capture-recapture methodology) and reviewed the article for important intellectual content. GC is the first author and has written and led the article. PC, MJ and AD critically reviewed data and the final article. All authors gave final approval of the version to be published and agreed to be accountable for all aspects of the work in ensuring that questions related to the accuracy or integrity of any part of the work are appropriately investigated and resolved.

Ethics approval and consent to participate

The study was not submitted for research ethics approval as the activities described were conducted as part of the legislated mandate of the Health Department of Catalonia, the competent authority for the surveillance of communicable diseases, which is officially authorized to receive, treat and temporarily store personal data on cases of infectious disease according to Decree 203/2015 of the 15 September which created the epidemiological surveillance network. Therefore, all study activities formed part of public health surveillance and were thus exempt from institutional board review and did not require informed consent.

Consent for publication

Not applicable.

Competing interests

The authors declare they have no competing interests.

Author details
[1]Public Health Agency of Catalonia (ASPCAT), Roc Boronat 81-95, 08005 Barcelona, Spain. [2]Departament de Medicina, Universitat de Barcelona, Barcelona, Spain. [3]CIBER Epidemiología y Salud Pública (CIBERESP), Barcelona, Spain.

References

1. Generalitat de Catalunya. Manual de notificació per als declarants al sistema de notificació de les Malalties de Declaració Obligatòria (MDO), 2016. http://canalsalut.gencat.cat/ca/professionals/vigilanciaepidemiologica/malalties-de-delaracio-obligatoria-i-brots-epidemics/.
2. Generalitat de Catalunya. Decret 203/2015, de 15 de setembre, pel qual es crea la Xarxa de Vigilància Epidemiològica i es regulen els sistemes de notificació de malalties de declaració obligatòria i els brots epidèmics. DOGC 2015; núm 6958:1-19
3. Generalitat de Catalunya. Manual de procediment de notificació microbiològica obligatòria (SNMC), 2016. http://canalsalut.gencat.cat/ca/professionals/vigilanciaepidemiologica/sistema-de-notificacio-microbiologica-de-catalunya-snmc/.
4. Keramarou M, Evans MR. Completeness of infectious disease notification in the United Kingdom: a systematic review. J Inf Secur. 2012;64:555–64.
5. Murphy TD, Denniston MM, Hill HA, Mc Donald M, Klevens MR, Elam-Evans LD, Nelson NP, Iskander J, Ward JD. Progress toward eliminating hepatitis a disease in the United States. MMWR. 2016;65:29–41.
6. Iqbal K, Klevens RM, Jiles R. Comparison of acute viral hepatitis data quality using two methodologies, 2005-2007. Public Health Rep. 2012;127:591–7.
7. Freixa Blanxart M, Guàrdia Olmos J, Honrubia Serrano ML, Peró Cebollero M. Validation of the capture-recapture method. Psicothema. 2000;12(Suppl 2): 231–5.
8. Laska EM. The use of capture-recapture methods in public health. Bull World Health Organ. 2002;80:845.
9. Chapman DG. Some properties of the hypergeometric distribution with applications to zoological censuses. University of California Publications in Statistics 1. 1951;131-60.
10. Ballivet S, Salmi LR, Dubourdieu D. Capture-recapture method to determine the best design of surveillance system. Application to a thyroid cancer registry. Eur J Epidemiol. 2000;16:147–53.
11. Tilling K, Sterne JAC, Wolfe CDA. Estimation of the incidence of stroke using a capture-recapture model including covariates. Int J Epidemiol. 2001;30: 1351–9.
12. Alho JM. Logistic regression in capture-recapture models. Biometrics. 1999; 149:392–400.
13. Tilling K, Sterne JAC. Capture-recapture models including covariate effects. Am J Epidemiol. 1999;149:392–40.
14. Maldonado G, Greenland S. Simulation study of confounder-selection strategies. Am J Epidemiol. 1993;138:923.
15. LaPorte RE, Dearwater SR, Chang Y-F, et al. Efficiency and accuracy of disease monitoring systems: applications of capture-recapture methods to injury monitoring. Am J Epidemiol. 1995;142:1069–77.
16. Amstrong GK, Bell BP. Hepatitis a virus infections in the United States: model-based estimates and implications for childhood immunization. Pediatrics. 2002;109:839–45.
17. Overhage JM, Grannis S, McDonald CJ. A comparison of the completeness and timeliness of automated electronic laboratory reporting and spontaneous reporting of notifiable conditions. Am J Public Health. 2008;98: 344–50.
18. Durusoy R, Karababa AO. Completeness of hepatitis, brucellosis, syphilis, measles and HIV/AIDS surveillance in Izmir, Turkey. BMC Public Health. 2010;10:71.
19. Matin M, Grant A, Granerod J, Crowcroft N. Hepatitis a surveillance in England - how many cases are not reported and does it really matter? Epidemiol Infect. 2006;134:1299–302.
20. Oviedo M, Muñoz P, Domínguez A, Borrás E, Carmona G. A statistical model to estimate the impact of hepatitis a vaccination programme. Vaccine. 2008; 26:6157–64.
21. Tavoschi L, Severi E, Niskanen T, Boelaert F, Rizzi V, Liebana E, Gomes Dias J, Nichols G, Takkinen J, Coulombier D. Food-borne diseases associated with frozen berries consumption: a historical perspective, European Union, 1983 to 2013. Euro Surveill. 2015;20(29):21193.
22. Savage RD, Rosella LC, Brown KA, Khan K, Crowcroft NS. Underreporting of hepatitis a in non-endemic countries: a systematic review and meta-analysis. BMC Infect Dis. 2016;16:281.
23. Simmons G, Whittaker R, Boyle K, Morris AJ, Upton A, Calder L. Could laboratory-based notification improve the control of foodborne illness in New Zeland? NZ Med J. 2002;115:237–40.
24. Neave PN, Heywood AE, Gibney KB, Leder K. Imported infections: what information should be collected by surveillance systems to inform public health policy? Trav Med Infect Dis. 2016;14:350–9.
25. Onieva-García MA, López-Hernández B, Molina-Rueda MJ, Cabrera-Castro N, Mochón-Ochoa MM. Contribution of electronic health record in surveillance of notifiable diseases. Rev Esp Salud Pública. 2015;89:515–22.
26. Backer HD, Bisell SR, Vugia DJ. Disease reporting from an automated laboratory-based reporting system to a state health department via local county health departments. Public Health Rep. 2001;116:257–65.
27. Sickbert-Bennett EE, Poole DJW, MacDonald PDM, Maillard JM. Completeness of communicable disease reporting, North Caroline, USA, 1995-1997 and 2000-2006. Emerg Infect Dis. 2011;17:23–9.
28. World Health Organization. Technical considerations and case definitions to improve surveillance for viral hepatitis. Policy brief. Geneva: WHO Press; 2016.

26

Uptake of hepatitis B vaccination and its determinants among health care workers in a tertiary health facility in Enugu, South-East, Nigeria

I. B. Omotowo[1*], I. A. Meka[3], U. N. Ijoma[2], V. E. Okoli[1], O. Obienu[2], T. Nwagha[4], A. C. Ndu[1], D. O. Onodugo[2], L. C. Onyekonwu[5] and E. O. Ugwu[6]

Abstract

Background: Hepatitis B vaccination is the most effective method of prevention for hepatitis B virus infection. It is a major public health problem in Nigeria, and health workers are at increased risk. This study determined the uptake of hepatitis B vaccination and assessed its determinants among health care workers (HCWs).

Methods: A hospital-based cross-sectional study was conducted between July and August, 2016 using self-administered structured questionnaires among 3132 HCWs in University of Nigeria Teaching Hospital, Enugu, South-East, Nigeria. Data was analysed using SPSS version 22. Binary logistic regression analysis was used to identify factors that influenced uptake of vaccination. Ethical clearance was obtained from the Research Ethics Committee of the health facility.

Results: The uptake of hepatitis B vaccination was 14.2% ($n = 445$). The number of doses received were: 3 doses (218/3132, 48.9%), 2 doses (71/3132, 16.0%), and one dose (156/3132, 35.1%). The reasons for non-uptake of vaccination included: cost of vaccine 48 (10.8%), 'did not believe they could be infected' 28 (6.6%), long vaccination schedule, and lack of time 150 (35.1%). The Odds for uptake of hepatitis B vaccination were 22% lower among nurses compared to doctors (AOR = 0.78, 95% CI = 0.54–0.98, $P = 0.037$). It increased with increasing age (AOR = 1.30, 95% CI = 1.08–1.59, $P < 0.001$), increasing duration of work in the hospital (AOR = 1.19, 95% CI = 1.09–1.32, $P = 0.032$), and was about twice higher among those that had tertiary education than others that had less education (AOR = 1.96, 95 CI = 0.76–5.07, $P = 0.164$).

Conclusions: The uptake of hepatitis B vaccination was low among HCWs in Enugu, Nigeria. Age, staff category, and duration of work in the hospital, were independently associated with hepatitis B vaccination. Provision of adequate hepatitis B surface antigen screening facilities and vaccination sites where the cost of vaccination is subsidized for all HCWs is recommended.

Keywords: Health care workers, Hepatitis B, Hepatitis B vaccine, Nigeria

* Correspondence: babatundeomotowo@yahoo.com
[1]Department of Community Medicine, College of Medicine, University of Nigeria, Enugu Campus, Nigeria
Full list of author information is available at the end of the article

Background

Hepatitis B is spread through contact with blood and body fluids of an infected person. It is a major public health problem in Nigeria and health care workers (HCWs) including general physicians, surgeons, dental surgeons, nurses and other medical staff. These HCWs are at increased risk of acquiring the disease due to occupational exposure to blood and body fluids [1, 2]. Hepatitis B is a life-threatening liver infection caused by Hepatitis B Virus (HBV). It can cause chronic and often fatal liver diseases, such as liver cirrhosis and cancer. Globally, about a billion individuals have been infected with HBV at some point in their lifetime and almost 350 million people are chronically infected with HBV, out of which more than a million die annually from its related causes [3]. Majority of the infected cases are living in sub-Saharan Africa [4].

World Health Organization (WHO) reported that about two million health care workers risk occupational exposure to HBV each year and vaccination coverage is low among them [5]. The Department of Health and Human Services, Centers for Disease Control and Prevention (CDC) reported in United States that "the risk of being infected is dependent on the prevalence of the HBV carriers and frequency of exposure of HCWs to blood and body fluids and the infectivity of the virus" [6]. Health care workers in Nigeria are particularly at a greater risk because Nigeria is a holoendemic area, with HBV carrier rate of 15–37% [7]. The risk of acquiring HBV in some cadres of HCWs is four times greater than that of the general population [8].

Hepatitis B vaccination is the mainstay of HBV prevention and has been reported to reduce the risk of acquiring the infection virtually to zero [9, 10]. It is recommended for exposed HCWs as part of the universal precautions policy for protection of HCWs [6]. HCWs who are HBV negative after screening should take hepatitis B vaccination, while those who are HBV positive should be treated. However, vaccination among HCWs remains a challenge for many countries [11]. Some studies reported that all HCWs including administrative staff in a hospital can receive the hepatitis B vaccine [11]. The mode of transmission of HBV in health care settings is most often by needle prick injuries and poor adherence to universal precautions [12]. The prevention of occupational hazards requires a thorough knowledge of the risks and practical measures to be taken, and the need for HCWs workers to familiarize themselves with universal work precautions [13]. It is estimated that about a million HCWs had cut and puncture injuries per year [14].

There is wide implementation of policy and uptake of the hepatitis B vaccine in some countries such as UK, USA, and Israel [10]. In 2016, Nigeria developed a national guideline for prevention, care and treatment of HBV and hepatitis C virus (HCV) infections, and vaccination of HCWs was included as one of the preventive methods in health care settings. However, to the best of the authors' knowledge, there is no policy or implementation of any policies that makes uptake of Hepatitis B vaccination compulsory to all HCWs in Nigeria. This study was conducted to evaluate the uptake of hepatitis B vaccination and its determinants among HCWs in a tertiary health facility in South-East, Nigeria.

Methods

Study area

This study was conducted between July and August 2016 among HCWs in University of Nigeria Teaching Hospital (UNTH), Enugu, South-East Nigeria. The UNTH is a tertiary health facility, and the national cardiothoracic center of excellence. The facility attends to patients from all over Nigeria.

Study design and sampling technique

This was a hospital-based cross-sectional study. It was conducted prior to the free HBV and HCV screening programmes organised by Roche Products Limited in collaboration with the hospital's Management. To the best of the authors' knowledge, it was the first free HBV and HCV screening programme ever organized for all the hospital's HCWs.

Data collection

Data was collected using pre-tested self-administered structured questionnaires designed to collect information on socio-demographic characteristics, knowledge of transmission and risk factors of HBV, HBV status, uptake of hepatitis B vaccination, doses of vaccine received, and reasons for non-uptake of the vaccine by the participants.

Participants in the study

Figure 1 shows the respondents' flow chart. The first stage showed that 3132 out of 3422 HCWs completed the questionnaires correctly given a response rate of 91.2%. In the second stage, 893 (28.5%) out of 3132 knew their HBV status. Third stage showed that 872 (97.6%) out of 893 participants that knew their HBV status were HBV negative, while 21 (2.4%) were HBV positive. The fourth stage showed the participants who have received hepatitis B vaccination and the doses received.

Data analysis

Data collected were analysed using SPSS version 22 (SPSS Inc., Chicago, Illinois, USA). Descriptive analyses were expressed as percentages. Socio-demographic characteristics of the respondents (age, sex, marital status, level of education, and duration of work in the hospital)

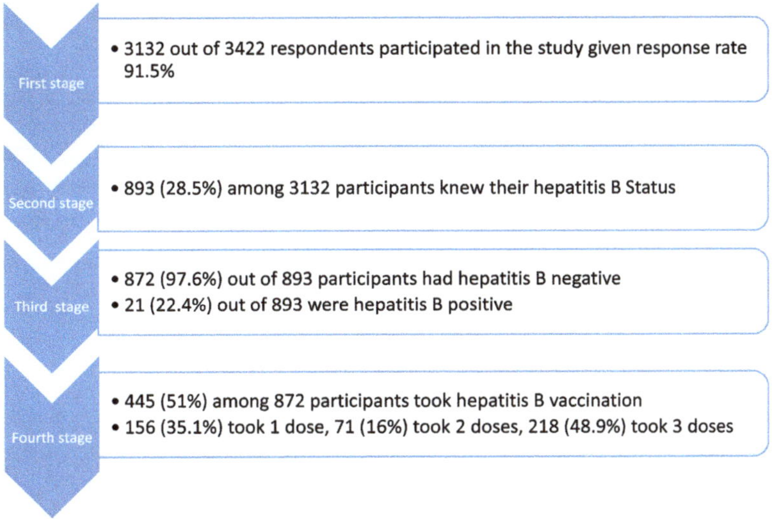

Fig. 1 Participants flow chart

and how it affected the uptake of hepatitis B vaccination was determined. The relationship between the factors and uptake of hepatitis B vaccination was calculated using Chi-square test to determine significance at $p < 0.05$. Binary logistic regression analysis was performed to determine socio-demographic characteristics of respondents associated with uptake of hepatitis B vaccination and the number of doses received. Variables with statistical significance of $P \leq 0.2$ in the bivariate models were included in the multivariate analysis. Strength of association was expressed using Odds ratio and statistical significance presented using *P*-values and 95% confidence intervals for odds ratio. For all analyses, P-values of < 0.05 were considered statistically significant.

Operational definitions

Uptake of hepatitis B vaccination referred to respondents who have received at least one dose of the hepatitis B vaccine. HBV negative referred to absence of hepatitis B surface antigen (HBsAg), while presence of HBsAg was referred as HBV positive. 'Knew their hepatitis B status' referred to respondents who have been screened in the past and had prior knowledge of their hepatitis B status, whether positive or negative. Full hepatitis B vaccination referred to respondents who have received 3 doses of the vaccine.

Ethical approval

Ethical approval was obtained from Health Research Ethics Committee of the tertiary health facility, and informed written consent was obtained from all the participants.

Results

Socio-demographic characteristics of the participants

The mean age of the participants was 39.4 ± 9.6 (range: 18–75) years. Majority 1151(36.7%) were in the 31–40 years age group. About three quarters 2237 (71.4%) had tertiary education, 2174 (69.4%) were married and 580 (18.5%) were nurses. Majority of the participants 1938 (61.9%) had worked for more than 5 years (Table 1).

Knowledge on transmission of hepatitis B infection

Table 2 shows that less than half of the participants knew that hepatitis B could be transmitted by needle prick, sharing of sharp objects, and sexual intercourse, while about 70% knew that blood transfusion was a mode of transmission. Only 3% believed it could be transmitted by shaking of hands and 16.3% did not know any mode of transmission.

Participants in the study flow chart and their uptake of hepatitis B vaccination

Table 3 shows the participants in each stage of the study. A total of 297 (9.5%) doctors, 716 (22.9%) nurses/pharmacists/lab workers, and 2119 (67.7%) administrative staff were involved in the study. Participants who knew their HBsAg status were 893 (28.5%). Twenty one, 21 (2.4%) were HBsAg positive, while 872 (97.6%) were HBsAg negative. Among the 872 participants who were HBsAg negative, 445 (51.0%) have received at least one dose of hepatitis B vaccine while 427 (49.0%) have not received any dose of hepatitis B vaccine.

Reasons for non-uptake of hepatitis B vaccine by the participants

The reasons for non-uptake of hepatitis B vaccination by the 427 HBsAg negative participants included: cost of

Table 1 Socio-demographic characteristics of the respondents ($N = 3132$)

Socio-demographic characteristics	Doctors ($N = 297$)		Nurses/Pharmacists/Lab Workers ($N = 716$)		Admin staff ($N = 2119$)		Total $N = 3132$	
	N	%	N	%	N	%	N	%
Sex								
Male	185	62.3	277	38.7	489	23.1	951	30.4
Female	112	37.7	439	61.3	1630	76.9	2181	69.6
Age – group (Years)								
< 20	0	0	0	0	12	0.6	12	0.4
20–30	94	31.7	84	11.7	414	19.5	592	18.9
31–40	112	37.7	196	27.4	843	39.8	1151	36.7
41–50	66	22.2	298	41.6	558	26.3	922	29.5
51–60	21	7.1	138	19.3	273	12.9	432	13.8
> 60	4	1.3	0	0	19	0.9	23	0.7
Education Level								
Primary	0	0	0	0	269	12.7	269	8.6
Secondary	0	0	23	3.2	603	28.5	626	20.0
Tertiary	297	100	693	96.8	1247	58.8	2237	71.4
Marital status								
Married	198	66.7	510	71.2	1466	69.2	2174	69.4
Single	97	32.6	201	28.1	571	26.9	869	27.7
Separated	0	0	0	0	11	0.5	11	0.4
Widowed	2	0.7	5	0.7	71	3.4	78	2.5
Duration of work (Years of experience)								
< 1 Year	38	12.8	19	2.7	206	9.7	263	8.3
1–5 Years	152	51.2	101	14.1	678	32.0	931	29.8
> 5–10 Years	50	16.8	380	53.1	410	19.3	840	26.8
> 10 Years	57	19.2	216	30.1	825	39.0	1098	35.1

the vaccine (46/427, 10.8%), didn't know where to receive the vaccine (203/427, 47.5%), didn't believe they could be infected (28/427, 6.6%), and other reasons including the long vaccination schedule of the vaccine and lack of time (150/427, 35.1%). Details are as shown in Table 4.

Factors associated with uptake of hepatitis B vaccination among participants that were hepatitis B negative

Table 5 shows factors associated with uptake of hepatitis B vaccination by the participants. After adjusting for age, sex, marital status, level of education, and professional categories, the Odds for uptake of hepatitis B vaccination were higher among single/separated/widowed participants compared to those that were married (AOR = 1.38, 95% CI = 1.01–1.92, $P = 0.050$). The Odds for uptake of hepatitis B vaccination were 22% lower among nurses compared to doctors (AOR = 0.78, 95% CI = 0.54–0.98, $P = 0.037$), while the Odds for the uptake of hepatitis B vaccination increased with increasing age (AOR = 1.30, 95% CI = 1.08–1.59, $P < 0.001$). The Odds for uptake of hepatitis B vaccination also increased with increasing duration of work in the hospital (AOR = 1.19, 95% CI = 1.09–1.32, $P = 0.032$). It was about 2.1 higher among participants who had secondary education compared with those that had primary education (AOR = 2.06, 95% CI = 0.75–5.61, $P = 0.159$), and about twice higher among those that had tertiary education than others that had less education (AOR = 1.96, 95 CI = 0.76–5.07, $P = 0.164$).

Discussion

This study showed that the uptake of hepatitis B vaccination among HCWs in Enugu, Nigeria was poor. This is similar to the study conducted in Pakistan [15], but differs from other studies from India and Ethiopia [16, 17]. The authors found that 28.5% of the participants knew their hepatitis B status, and that 2.4% were hepatitis B positive, while 97.6% were hepatitis B negative. The observed low knowledge of hepatitis B status (28.5%) in this study could be due to absence of pre-employment screening for hepatitis B as well as lack of policy concerning hepatitis B screening in the facility. It also

Table 2 Knowledge on transmission of hepatitis B ($N = 3132$)

Transmitted by:	Doctors ($N = 297$)		Nurses/Pharmacists/Lab Workers ($N = 716$)		Admin staff ($N = 2119$)		Total $N = 3132$)	
	N	%	*N*	%	*N*	%	*N*	%
Shaking of hands								
Yes	11	3.7	24	3.4	49	2.3	84	2.7
No	286	96.3	692	96.6	2070	97.7	3048	97.3
Needle prick								
Yes	280	94.3	293	40.9	749	35.3	1322	42.2
No	17	5.7	423	59.1	1370	64.7	1810	57.8
Blood transfusion								
Yes	284	95.6	614	85.8	1282	60.5	2180	69.6
No	13	4.4	102	14.2	837	39.5	952	30.4
Heat								
Yes	12	4.0	57	8.0	140	6.6	209	6.7
No	285	96.0	659	92.0	1979	93.4	2923	93.3
Sexual intercourse								
Yes	249	83.8	524	73.2	759	0.4	1532	48.9
No	48	16.2	192	26.8	1360	99.6	1597	41.9
Drinking contaminated water								
Yes	49	16.5	105	14.7	232	10.9	386	12.3
No	248	83.5	611	85.3	1887	89.1	2746	87.7
Contamination from surfaces								
Yes	81	27.3	89	12.4	402	18.9	572	18.3
No	216	72.7	627	87.6	1717	81.1	2560	81.7
Sharing of sharp objects								
Yes	258	86.9	204	28.5	1027	48.5	1489	47.5
No	39	13.1	512	71.5	1092	51.5	1643	52.5
Don't know								
Yes	0	0	26	3.6	486	22.9	512	16.3
No	297	100	690	96.4	1633	77.1	2620	83.7

suggests that the facility has not been regularly conducting free or subsidized screening for its HCWs. While it is expected that all individuals who are hepatitis B negative should take the vaccination, while those who are hepatitis B positive receive treatment, the study found that only 51% of participants who are hepatitis B negative have received hepatitis B vaccination.

The overall uptake of hepatitis B vaccination among HCWs in this study was 14.2%. This is similar to what was observed in previous studies [18, 19]. However, it is lower than 22.4% reported in the similar study in 2006 [20], and also among HCWs in a teaching hospital in Ile-Ife, South-West Nigeria which revealed that 65% of the health workers have been vaccinated against hepatitis B virus [4]. The observed uptake in this study is also lower than 54.8% reported among theatre and laboratory workers at a teaching hospital in Imo state, Nigeria [21]. These differences could be due to the fact that the current study involved a larger population, and also administrative staff which were not involved in previous studies. This study also revealed that only 28.5% of the participants had prior knowledge of their hepatitis B status. This poor result could be due to the cost of screening for hepatitis B surface antigen and its poor accessibility in Nigeria. Regular free or subsidized screening programmes might bring improvement in this regard.

It was observed that a higher proportion of administrative staff have not received hepatitis B vaccination compared to nurses, doctors, pharmacists and laboratory technologists. This higher uptake of hepatitis B vaccination among the clinical than administrative staff could be as a result of their pre-employment training and education which might have included the importance and safety of

Table 3 Participants in the study flow chart ($N = 3132$)

Variable:	Doctors (N = 297)		Nurses/Pharmacists/Lab workers (N = 716)		Admin staff (N = 2119)		Total (N = 3132)	
	N	%	N	%	N	%	N	%
Participants who knew their HBsAg status:								
Yes	162	54.6	282	39.4	449	21.2	893	28.5
No	135	45.4	434	60.6	1670	78.8	2239	71.5
Total participants	297	100.0	716	100.0	2119	100.0	3132	100.0
HBsAg of participants who knew their status:								
HBsAg Positive	1	0.6	6	2.1	14	3.3	21	2.4
HBsAg Negative	161	99.4	276	97.9	435	96.7	872	97.6
Total who knew their status	162	100.0	282	100.0	449	100.0	893	100.0
Participants who were HBsAg negative, and took/ did not take any dose of hepatitis B vaccine:								
Took at least a dose	98	60.9	155	56.2	192	44.1	445	51.0
Did not take any dose	63	39.1	121	43.8	243	55.9	427	49.0
Total who were HBsAg negative	161	100.0	276	100.0	435	100.0	872	100.0
Doses of vaccine taken by the participants:								
Participants who were HBsAg negative, and took one dose	8	8.2	26	16.8	122	63.5	156	35.1
Participants who were HBsAg negative, and took two doses	16	16.4	44	28.4	11	5.8	71	16.0
Participants who were HBsAg negative, and took three doses	74	75.4	85	54.8	59	30.7	218	48.9
Total who took at least a dose	98	100.0	155	100.0	192	100.0	445	100.0

vaccination to health. The management of health facilities should pay attention to administrative cadre of staff for improved uptake of hepatitis B vaccination among its HCWs. Similarly, the duration of HCWs that had worked in the facility also influenced the uptake of hepatitis B vaccination. Higher proportion of those who had worked for more than 5 years in the facility received hepatitis B vaccination than those who had worked for less. This result could be due to lack of policy concerning hepatitis B vaccination of workers in the hospital. Also higher proportion of participants older than 30 years of age received hepatitis B vaccination than those below 30 years old. This higher uptake of hepatitis B vaccination among older HCWs who are also more likely to have worked for longer

Table 4 Reasons for non–uptake of Hepatitis B vaccine by the Participants ($N = 427$)

Reasons:	Doctors (N = 63)		Nurses/Pharmacists/Lab Workers (N = 121)		Admin staff (N = 243)		Total (N = 427)	
	N	%	N	%	N	%	N	%
Cost								
Yes	4	6.3	7	5.8	35	14.4	46	10.8
No	59	93.7	114	95.2	208	85.6	381	89.2
Don't know where to take the vaccine								
Yes	34	54.0	35	28.9	134	55.1	203	47.5
No	29	46.0	86	71.1	109	45.9	224	52.5
Don't believe I could be infected								
Yes	1	1.6	3	2.5	24	9.8	28	6.6
No	62	98.4	118	97.5	219	90.2	399	93.4
Others e.g. long vaccination schedule and lack of time								
Yes	3	4.8	19	15.7	128	52.7	150	35.1
No	60	95.2	102	84.3	115	47.3	277	64.9

Table 5 Factors associated with Uptake of Hepatitis B Vaccination among participants that had Hepatitis B Negative (*N* = 872)

Variable:	Uptake of Hepatitis B Vaccination (*N* = 872)				Chi-square (X^2)	*P* value	AOR (95% CI)	*P* value
	Yes	%	No	%				
Sex								
Male	124	27.9	135	31.6	0.558	0.455	1.00	
Female	321	72.1	292	68.4			0.93 (0.69–1.24)	0.305
Age group (Years)								
< 30	60	13.5	80	18.7	14.048	0.003	1.00	
31–40	187	42.0	191	44.7			1.30 (1.08–1.59)	< 0.001
41–50	126	28.3	117	27.4			1.38 (1.09–1.65)	< 0.001
51–60	72 16.2		39	9.2			1.41 (1.12–1.73)	0.032
Marital status								
Married	327	73.5	293	68.6	1.981	0.576	1.00	
Single/Separated/Widowed	118	26.5	134	31.4			1.38 (1.01–1.92)	0.050
Education level								
Primary	8	1.8	13	3.0	1.825	0.768	1.00	
Secondary	58	13.0	56	13.2			2.06 (0.75–5.61)	0.159
Tertiary	379	85.2	358	83.8			1.96 (0.76–5.07)	0.164
Professional Categories								
Doctors	98	22.0	63	14.7	11.108	0.049	1.00	
Nurses/Pharmacists/Lab workers	155	34.8	121	28.4			0.78 (0.54–0.98)	0.037
Admin staff	192	43.2	243	56.9			0.23 (2.67–5.69)	0.241
Duration of work in the hospital								
< 1 Year	33	7.4	124	29.0	18.742	< 0.001	1.00	
1–5 Years	109	24.5	95	22.3			1.19 (1.09–1.32)	0.032
> 5–10 Years	128	28.8	93	21.8			1.26 (1.08–1.45)	0.043
> 10 Years	175	39.3	115	26.9			1.28 (1.12–1.49)	0.042

AOR Adjusted Odds Ratio, *95% CI* 95% Confidence Interval, *Reference category* 1, X^2 = Chi-square

duration might be due to their previous observations. It is possible they might have observed their colleagues suffer fulminant hepatitis and/or liver cancer as a result of possible non-uptake of hepatitis B vaccination. The reason for this higher uptake among this category of HCWs may also be due to previous hepatitis B vaccination related encouragements from colleagues. Such encouragement could lead to increase in awareness and knowledge of importance of screening and uptake of hepatitis B vaccination for those who are hepatitis B negative, and treatment for those who are hepatitis B positive. Formulation of policies to make screening for hepatitis B surface antigen and uptake of hepatitis B vaccination compulsory and at free or subsidized cost for all HCWs may bring improvement in uptake of hepatitis B vaccine.

This study found that 48.9% of those who were vaccinated had full coverage of the three doses of the vaccine, while 16 and 35.1% took two or one dose respectively. This is similar to the study conducted in Tanzania, and India among HCWs where 48.8 and 50% received three doses of the vaccine respectively [22, 23]. It is also similar to the study conducted among doctors and nurses in Lagos, Nigeria where 48.5% completed three doses of hepatitis B vaccination [24]. It is however lower than results documented in the study conducted among doctors and nurses in Iran which reported that 86.2% completed the recommended three doses of vaccine [25]. This difference might be due to the fact that the present study involved all health workers including administrative staff compared to study from Iran where only doctors and nurses were included. Thus, the differences in this study compared with other studies could be due to the inclusion of administrative staff, and the larger sample size. Interestingly, those who received three doses of vaccine in the current study is higher than the findings in other studies conducted in Nigeria, Sweden, Pakistan, and South Africa which reported 16.3, 29.7, 39.8, 37.2, and 19.9% respectively [20, 21, 26–28]. However, it is lower than the findings in a study done in Ethiopia where 61.2% of those vaccinated had received all 3 doses of the vaccine [17].

Our study revealed that age, staff category and duration of work in the facility significantly influenced uptake of hepatitis B vaccination, but no factor significantly influenced full vaccination status. However, after adjusting for confounders, the odds for full hepatitis B vaccination were higher among female participants than males (AOR = 1.17, 95%CI = 0.76–1.78, $P = 0.265$), tertiary education compared to primary education (AOR = 2.94, 95% CI = 0.64–12.43, $P = 0.328$), and among participants with longer duration of work (AOR = 1.23, 95%CI = 0.96–1.59, $P = 0.106$). These observations are similar to findings from some other studies which reported that sex, years of occupational practice, and educational status significantly influenced vaccination pattern [4, 20, 21].

The findings in the current study showed that 10.8% of the participants did not receive hepatitis B vaccination because of cost of vaccination, 47.5% did not know where to take the vaccination, 6.6% believed they could not be infected, while 51.1% gave other reasons such as long vaccination schedule, and lack of time. These findings are similar to a study conducted to find reasons for non-uptake of vaccine which reported inadequate vaccine information as a factor [11] and unavailability of vaccine and high cost of vaccine as major determinants [29]. The prevalence of HBV markers which includes individuals with HBsAg, anti-HBc, and anti-HBs who do not need hepatitis B vaccination is 72.5% in Nigeria [30]. Recommendations from American College of Physicians and the Centers for Disease Control and Prevention is that screening for HBV should include testing to three HBV screening sero-markers so that persons can be classified into the appropriate hepatitis B category and properly recommended to receive vaccination, counselling, and linkage to care and treatment [31]. However in Nigeria, accessibility and cost of hepatitis B serological tests for HBV markers is a great challenge. The authors' opinion is that all HCWs should be screened for only HBsAg, and those that are negative should receive hepatitis B vaccination to reduce the cost and other challenges.

Conclusions

This study revealed that uptake of hepatitis B vaccination as well as number of doses received was low among HCWs in Enugu, Nigeria. Age, staff category, and duration of work in the hospital, were independently associated with hepatitis B vaccination. It is therefore recommended that Management of health facilities in Nigeria should provide hepatitis B surface antigen screening facilities and hepatitis B vaccination sites for easy accessibility, and also subsidize the cost of screening for hepatitis B surface antigen and hepatitis B vaccination for all HCWs. They should also formulate policies that make screening for hepatitis B surface antigen and uptake of hepatitis B vaccination for hepatitis B negative HCWs compulsory and at free or subsidized cost. If possible, the Management should also frequently organize free screening for HBV for all its HCWs. This would increase the proportion of HCWs that know their hepatitis B status, as well as stimulate those that are hepatitis B negative and positive to receive the required vaccination and treatment respectively.

Abbreviations

Anti-HBc: Antibody to hepatitis B core antigen; Anti-HBs: Antibody to hepatitis B surface antigen; AOR: Adjusted Odds Ratio; CI: Confidence interval; COR: Crude Odds Ratio; HBsAg: Hepatitis B surface antigen; HBV: Hepatitis B Virus; HCWS: Health Care Workers; OR: Odds Ratio; SPSS: Statistical Package for Social Sciences; UNTH: University of Nigeria Teaching Hospital

Acknowledgements

We thank the management of University of Nigeria Teaching Hospital, Enugu. All the participants are acknowledged. We equally thank Ms. Ngozi and Ms. Ndidi who assisted in data collection and data entry.

Funding

There was no external funding received for this study. It was completely funded by the authors.

Authors' contributions

All authors participated in and approved the study design and data collection tool. BIO participated in the designing, coordination, drafting and arranging the manuscript to the publishable level. IUN and MAI participated in data analysis and critical revision of the work for intellectual content. OO, ODO, ANC, OLC, and EOU participated in the critical revision of the paper. BIO, NT, and IUN conceived the study and designed the work and also participated in data collection and manuscript preparation. OVE, BIO, OO, ODO, ANC, OLC, and EOU participated in data acquisition, data analysis and interpretation of findings. EOU was responsible for language and technical editing/copyediting of the manuscript. All the authors read and approved the final manuscript.

Consent for publication

Not applicable

Competing interests

The authors declare that they have no competing interests.

Author details

[1]Department of Community Medicine, College of Medicine, University of Nigeria, Enugu Campus, Nigeria. [2]Department of Medicine, College of Medicine, University of Nigeria, Enugu Campus, Nigeria. [3]Department of Chemical Pathology, College of Medicine, University of Nigeria, Enugu Campus, Nigeria. [4]Department of Haematology, College of Medicine, University of Nigeria, Enugu Campus, Nigeria. [5]Department of Dermatology, College of Medicine, University of Nigeria, Enugu Campus, Nigeria.

[6]Department of Obstetrics and Gynaecology, College of Medicine , University of Nigeria, Enugu Campus, Nigeria.

References

1. Erhabor O, Ejele OA, Nwauche CA. Epidemiology and management of occupational exposure to blood borne viral infections in a resource poor setting: the case for availability of post exposure prophylaxis. Nig J Clin Pract. 2007;10(2):100–4.
2. Bello AC. Prevalence of hepatitis B virus markers in surgeons in Lagos, Nigeria. East Afr Med J. 2000;77(5):283–5.
3. Chang MH, Hepatitis B. Virus infection. Semin Fetal Med. 2007;12:160–7.
4. Fatusi AO, Fatusi OA, Esimai AO, Onayade AA, Ojo OS. Acceptance of hepatitits B vaccine by workers in a Nigerian Teaching Hospital. East Afr Med J. 2000;77:608–12.
5. WHO. Global policy report on the prevention and control of viral hepatitis in WHO member states. World Health organisation; 2013.
6. Ceters for Disease Control and Prevention. Protection against Viral hepatitis. Morb Mortal Wkly Rep. 1990;39:1.
7. Bojuwoye BJ. The burden of viral hepatitis in Africa. West Afr J Med. 1997;16:198–202.
8. Dannetum E, Tegnell A, Torner A, Giesecke J. Coverage of hepatitis B vaccination in Swedish health care workers. J Hosp Infect. 2006;63(2):201–4.
9. WHO. Hepatitis B: Key facts. World Health Organization 2016. Available: http://www.who.int/mediacentre/factsheets/fs204/en/. Accessed 27 Nov 2017.
10. Bonani P, Bonnaccorsi G. Vaccination against hepatitis B in health care workers. Vaccione. 2001;19:2389–94.
11. Bridget M, Saad BO, Beatrice M, Trish A. Protecting health workers from nosocomial hepatitis B infections: a review of strategies and challenges for implementation of hepatitis B vaccination among health workrers in sub-Saharan Africa. J Epidemiol Glob Health. 2017;6:229–41.
12. Runner SC, Bare B. Brunner and Suddarth's textbook of medical surgical nursing. 10th ed; 2003.
13. Ogunbodede EO. Occupational hazard and safety in dental practice. Nigeria J Med. 1996;5:11–3.
14. Trinkoff AM, Le R, Geiger-Brown J, Lipscomb J. Work schedule, needle use, and needle stick injuries among registered nurses. Infect Control Hosp Epidemiol. 2007;28:156–64.
15. Kumar A, Khuwaja AK, Khuwaja AM. Knowledge practice gaps about needle stick injuries among healthcare workers at tertiary care hospitals of Pakistan. J Ayub Med Coll Abbottabad. 2012;24(3–4):50–2.
16. Sukriti Pati NT, Sethi A, Agrawal K, et al. Low levels of awareness, coverage, and the need for boosters among health care workers in tertiary care hospitals in India. J Gastroenterol Hepatol. 2008;23(11):1710–5.
17. Gedefaw A, Muluken A. Hepatitis B vaccine knowledge and vaccination status among health care workers of Bahir Dar City Administration, Northwest Ethiopia: a cross sectional study. BMC Infect Dis. 2015;15:30–5.
18. Ademowo CA, Ajuwon A. The immunization status and level of knowledge about hepatitis B virus infection among Nigerian surgeons. West Afr J Med. 1997;16:93–6.
19. Sofola OO, Uti OG. Hepatitis B virus infection and prevention in the dental clinic: knowledge and factors determining vaccine uptake in a Nigerian dental teaching teaching hospital. Nig Q J Hosp Med. 2008;18:145-8.
20. Ibekwe RC, Ibeziakor N. Hepatitis B vaccination status among health workers in Enugu, Nigeria. Nigeria J Clin Pract. 2006;9(1):7–10.
21. Okwara EC, Enwere OZ, Diwe CK, Azike JE, Chuwulebe AE. Theatre and laboratory workers awareness of and safety practices against hepatitis B & C infection in a suburban University Teaching Hospital in Nigeria. Pan Afr Med J. 2012;2(1):45-8.
22. Mueller A, Stoetter L, Kalluvya S, Stich A, Majinge C, Weissbrich B, Kasang C. Prevalence of hepatitis B virus infection among health care workers in a tertiary hospital in Tanzania. BM Infect Dis. 2015;15:386.
23. Singhal V, Bora D, Singh S. Prevalence of hepatitis B virus infection in healtg care workers of a tertiary care centre in India and their vaccination status. J Vaccines Vaccine. 2012;2:118.
24. Abiola AO, Agunbiade AB, Badmos KB, Lesi AO, Lawal AO, Alli QO. Prevalence of HBsAG, knowledge, and vaccination practice against viral hepatitis B infection among doctors and nurses in a secondary health facility in Lagos state, South-Western Nigeria. Pan Afr Med J. 2016;26:158–62.
25. Hashemi SH, Mamani M, Torabian S. Hepatitis B vaccination coverage and sharp injuries among health care workers in Hamadan, Iran. Avicenna J Clin Microbiol Inf. 2014;31(2):56-9.
26. Dannetun E, Tegnell A, Torner A, Giesecke J. Coverage of hepatitis B vaccination in Swedish health care workers. J Hosp Infect. 2006;63(2):202–6.
27. Mengal HU, Howteerrakul N, Suwannapong N, Rajatanun T. Factors relating to acceptance of hepatitis B virus vaccination by nursing students in a tertiary hospital, Pakistan. J Health Popul Nutr. 2008;26(1):46–53.
28. Burnett RJ, Francois G, Mphahlele MJ, et al. Hepatitis B vaccination coverage in health care workers in Gauteng Province, South Africa. Vaccine. 2001;29(25):4293–9.
29. Ogunlade LO. Perspectives on hepatitis B vaccination among Health Care Workers in Nigeria. Int J Trop Dis Health. 2016;18(3):1–11.
30. Kiire CF. The epidemiology and prophylaxis of hepatitis B in sub-Saharan Africa: a view from tropical and subtropical Africa. Gut. 1996;38(2):s5–s12.
31. Abara WE, Qaseem A, Schillie S, McMahon BJ, Harris AM, High Value Care Task Force of the American College of P, et al. Hepatitis B vaccination, screening and linkage to care: best practice advice from the American College of Physicians and the Centers for Disease Control and Prevention. Ann Intern Med. 2017;167(11):794–804.

Permissions

All chapters in this book were first published in ID, by BioMed Central; hereby published with permission under the Creative Commons Attribution License or equivalent. Every chapter published in this book has been scrutinized by our experts. Their significance has been extensively debated. The topics covered herein carry significant findings which will fuel the growth of the discipline. They may even be implemented as practical applications or may be referred to as a beginning point for another development.

The contributors of this book come from diverse backgrounds, making this book a truly international effort. This book will bring forth new frontiers with its revolutionizing research information and detailed analysis of the nascent developments around the world.

We would like to thank all the contributing authors for lending their expertise to make the book truly unique. They have played a crucial role in the development of this book. Without their invaluable contributions this book wouldn't have been possible. They have made vital efforts to compile up to date information on the varied aspects of this subject to make this book a valuable addition to the collection of many professionals and students.

This book was conceptualized with the vision of imparting up-to-date information and advanced data in this field. To ensure the same, a matchless editorial board was set up. Every individual on the board went through rigorous rounds of assessment to prove their worth. After which they invested a large part of their time researching and compiling the most relevant data for our readers.

The editorial board has been involved in producing this book since its inception. They have spent rigorous hours researching and exploring the diverse topics which have resulted in the successful publishing of this book. They have passed on their knowledge of decades through this book. To expedite this challenging task, the publisher supported the team at every step. A small team of assistant editors was also appointed to further simplify the editing procedure and attain best results for the readers.

Apart from the editorial board, the designing team has also invested a significant amount of their time in understanding the subject and creating the most relevant covers. They scrutinized every image to scout for the most suitable representation of the subject and create an appropriate cover for the book.

The publishing team has been an ardent support to the editorial, designing and production team. Their endless efforts to recruit the best for this project, has resulted in the accomplishment of this book. They are a veteran in the field of academics and their pool of knowledge is as vast as their experience in printing. Their expertise and guidance has proved useful at every step. Their uncompromising quality standards have made this book an exceptional effort. Their encouragement from time to time has been an inspiration for everyone.

The publisher and the editorial board hope that this book will prove to be a valuable piece of knowledge for researchers, students, practitioners and scholars across the globe.

List of Contributors

Arianne B. van Gageldonk-Lafeber, Wim van der Hoek, Sofie H. Mooi, Catharina B. M. Maassen, Barry Rockx and Johan H. J. Reimerink
National Institute for Public Health and the Environment (RIVM), Bilthoven, The Netherlands

Dick J. J. Heederik and Lidwien A. M. Smit
Institute for Risk Assessment Sciences, IRAS, Utrecht University, Utrecht, The Netherlands

Floor Borlée
Institute for Risk Assessment Sciences, IRAS, Utrecht University, Utrecht, The Netherlands
Netherlands Institute for Health Services Research (NIVEL), Utrecht, The Netherlands

C. Joris Yzermans
Netherlands Institute for Health Services Research (NIVEL), Utrecht, The Netherlands

Qinfen Xie and Hainv Gao
Shulan (Hangzhou) Hospital, Zhejiang University International Hospital, Hangzhou 310012, China

Ping Chen
Shulan (Hangzhou) Hospital, Zhejiang University International Hospital, Hangzhou 310012, China
State Key Laboratory for Diagnosis and Treatment of Infectious Diseases, Collaborative Innovation Center for Diagnosis and Treatment of Infectious Diseases, The First Affiliated Hospital, College of Medicine, Zhejiang University, 79 Qing-Chun Road, Hangzhou 310003, China

Jie Wu, Bing Ruan and Lanjuan Li
State Key Laboratory for Diagnosis and Treatment of Infectious Diseases, Collaborative Innovation Center for Diagnosis and Treatment of Infectious Diseases, The First Affiliated Hospital, College of Medicine, Zhejiang University, 79 Qing-Chun Road, Hangzhou 310003, China

Ting Chen and Jiawei Wu
College of Medicine, Zhejiang University, Hangzhou 310058, China

Zhiqin Zhang
Xianju Hospital of Traditional Chinese Medicine, Zhenjiang, Xianju 317300, China

Huseyin Yilmaz, Nuri Turan, Utku Y. Cizmecigil, Aysun Yilmaz and Ozge Aydin
Department of Virology, Veterinary Faculty, University of Istanbul, Avcilar, Istanbul, Turkey

Asiye Karakullukcu, Taner T. Kirazoglu and Bekir Kocazeybek
Department of Microbiology, Cerrahpasa Faculty of Medicine, University of Istanbul, Cerrahpasa, Istanbul, Turkey

Ayse A. Ozkul
Department of Child Health and Diseases, Faculty of Medicine, University of Izmir, Karsiyaka, Izmir, Turkey

Alper Gunduz
Division of Infectious Diseases and Clinical Microbiology, Sisli Hamidiye Etfal Training and Research Hospital, Istanbul, Turkey

Mahmut Mete
Department of Microbiology, Faculty of Medicine, University of Dicle, Diyarbakir, Turkey

Fadile Y. Zeyrek
Department of Microbiology, Faculty of Medicine, University of Harran, Urfa, Turkey

Juergen A. Richt
Department of Diagnostic Medicine and Pathobiology, College of Veterinary Medicine, Kansas State University, Manhattan, USA

Purusotam Raj Shedain
Department of Community Medicine and Public Health, Institute of Medicine/Ministry of Health, RamshahPath, Kathmandu, Nepal

Madhu Dixit Devkota
Department of Community Medicine and Public Health, Institute of Medicine, Tribhuvan University, Kathmandu, Nepal

Megha Raj Banjara
Central Department of Microbiology, Tribhuvan University (TU), Kirtipur, Kathmandu, Nepal

Huang Ling
Department of Preventive Medicine, Medical College of CTGU/Department of Community Medicine and Public Health, Institute of Medicine, Kathmandu, Nepal

Subash Dhital
National Public Health Laboratory, Department of Health Services, Teku, Kathmandu, Nepal

Dotto Aaron, Tumaini J. Nagu and Ewaldo Komba
School of Medicine, Muhimbili University of Health and Allied Sciences, Dar es Salaam, Tanzania

John Rwegasha
Muhimbili National Hospital, Dar es Salaam, Tanzania

Geofrey Amanya, Collins Atuheire, Hellen Nansumba, Stephen Akena Abwoye, Denis Nixon Opio and Edrisa Kibuuka
Clinical Epidemiology Unit, School of Medicine, Kampala, Uganda

Immaculate Nabukenya
Epidemiology and surveillance Division, Ministry Of Health, Kampala, Uganda

Samuel Kizito, Joan Kalyango and Charles Karamagi
Makerere University College of Health Sciences, Kampala, Uganda

Mei-Jun Chen and Yan-Ting Li
Center of Clinical Laboratory, Zhongshan Hospital, Medical College of Xiamen University, 201-209 Hubin South Road, Siming District, Xiamen City 361004, Fujian Province, People's Republic of China

Yong Lin, Zheng-Xiang Gao and Fan Liu
Center of Clinical Laboratory, Zhongshan Hospital, Medical College of Xiamen University, 201-209 Hubin South Road, Siming District, Xiamen City 361004, Fujian Province, People's Republic of China
Institute of Infectious Disease, Medical College of Xiamen University, Xiamen, Fujian Province, China

Xu Shen and Qi-Feng Zhao
Center of Clinical Laboratory, Zhongshan Hospital, Medical College of Xiamen University, 201-209 Hubin South Road, Siming District, Xiamen City 361004, Fujian Province, People's Republic of China
School of Public Health, Fujian Medical University, Fuzhou, Fujian Province, China

Shu-Lian Li and Hui-Ling Lin
Xiamen Huli District Maternity and Child Care Hospital, Xiamen, Fujian Province, China

Jian-Jun Niu
Center of Clinical Laboratory, Zhongshan Hospital, Medical College of Xiamen University, 201-209 Hubin South Road, Siming District, Xiamen City 361004, Fujian Province, People's Republic of China
Fujian Provincial Key Laboratory of Chronic Liver Disease and Hepatocellular Carcinoma, Xiamen, Fujian Province, China

Ling Li and Guojin Ou
Institute of Blood Transfusion, Chinese Academy of Medical Sciences and Peking Union Medical College, Chengdu, Sichuan, China

Tingting Han
No. 1 People's Hospital of Anqing, Anqing, Anhui, China

Liang Zang
Dalian Blood Center, Dalian, Liaoning, China

Libin Niu
Changzhi Blood Center, Changzhi, Shanxi, China

Weifang Cheng
Anhui Blood Center, Hefei, Anhui, China

Hongkeng Lin
Fujian Blood Center, Fuzhou, Fujian, China

Ka Yi Li
Cooper Medical School of Rowan University, Camden, USA

Ruan Cao
Mianyang Blood Center, Mianyang, Sichuan, China

Binghai Zhao
Nanchong Blood Center, Nanchong, Sichuan, China

Yuqiang Liu
Kaifeng Blood Center, Kaifeng, Henan, China

Xiao Liu
No. 1 People's Hospital of Deyang, Deyang, Sichuan, China

Yingjie Qi
Anhui Provincial Infection Hospital, Hefei, Anhui, China

Yanhua Li
Department of Pathology, New York University School of Medicine, NYU Langone Health, New York, USA

Zhong Liu
Institute of Blood Transfusion, Chinese Academy of Medical Sciences and Peking Union Medical College, Chengdu, Sichuan, China
26 Huacai Rd, Longtan Industry Zone, Chenghua District, Chengdu, Sichuan, People's Republic of China

Xiaoqin Zheng, Liang Yu, Qiaomai Xu, Silan Gu and Lingling Tang
Zhejiang University First Affiliated Hospital State Key Laboratory for Diagnosis and Treatment of Infectious Diseases, Hangzhou, Zhejiang, China

C. Cerva, G. Maffongelli and L. Sarmati
Clinical Infectious Disease, Department of Systems Medicine, Tor Vergata University, Rome, Italy

V. Svicher, R. Salpini, L. Colagrossi and A. Battisti
Department of Experimental Medicine and Surgery, Tor Vergata University, Rome, Italy

B. Mariotti, R. Cerretti and L. Cudillo
Department of Hematology, Stem Cell Transplant Unit, Tor Vergata University, Rome, Italy

Frederick Dun-Dery and Martin Nyaaba Adokiya
Department of Community Health, School of Allied Health Sciences, University for Development Studies (UDS), Tamale, Ghana

Juventus B. Ziem
Department Clinical Microbiology, School of Medicine and Health Sciences, UDS, Tamale, Ghana
Clinical Laboratory Department, Tamale Teaching Hospital, Tamale, Ghana

Williams Walana
Department Clinical Microbiology, School of Medicine and Health Sciences, UDS, Tamale, Ghana

Ernestina Yirkyio
Clinical Laboratory Department, Tamale Teaching Hospital, Tamale, Ghana

Li Zhang and Aiqiang Xu
Academy of Preventive Medicine, Shandong University, Jinan, China
Shandong Provincial Key Laboratory of Infectious Disease Control and Prevention, Shandong Center for Disease Control and Prevention, Jinan, China

Jingjing Lv, Jiaye Liu, Bingyu Yan and Yi Feng
Shandong Provincial Key Laboratory of Infectious Disease Control and Prevention, Shandong Center for Disease Control and Prevention, Jinan, China

Zechun Jiang
Rushan Center for Disease Control and Prevention, Weihai, China

Li Li, Guomin Zhang and Fuzhen Wang
Chinese Center for Disease Control and Prevention, Beijing, China

Hong Zhao, Jiyuan Zhou and Linlin Yan
Department of Infectious Disease, Center for Liver Disease, Peking University First Hospital, No. 8, Xishiku Street, Xicheng District, Beijing 100034, China

Yongqiong Deng
Department of Infectious Disease, Center for Liver Disease, Peking University First Hospital, No. 8, Xishiku Street, Xicheng District, Beijing 100034, China
The Department of dermatology, The Affiliated Hospital of Southwest Medical University, Luzhou, Sichuan, China

Guiqiang Wang
Department of Infectious Disease, Center for Liver Disease, Peking University First Hospital, No. 8, Xishiku Street, Xicheng District, Beijing 100034, China
The Collaborative Innovation Center for Diagnosis and Treatment of Infectious Diseases, Zhejiang University, Zhejiang, Hangzhou, China
The coordination innovation centerMinistry of education, Beijing, China

Nan-Yu Chen, Shian-Sen Shie and Ting-Shu Wu
Division of Infectious Diseases, Department of Internal Medicine, Chang Gung Memorial Hospital, Chang Gung University College of Medicine, 5 Fuhsing Street, Kueishan, Taoyuan 333, Taiwan

Zhuo-Hao Liu
Department of Neurosurgery, Chang Gung Memorial Hospital, Chang Gung Medical College and University, 5 FuSing Street, Kueishan, Taoyuan, Taiwan

Tsung-Hsing Chen
Division of Gastroenterology and Hepatology, Department of Internal Medicine, Chang Gung Memorial Hospital, Chang Gung Medical College and University, 5 FuSing Street, Kueishan, Taoyuan, Taiwan

Ralf Reintjes
Faculty Life Sciences, Department of Health Sciences, Hamburg University of Applied Sciences, Ulmenliet 20, 21033 Hamburg, Germany

Amena A. Ahmad
Faculty Life Sciences, Department of Health Sciences, Hamburg University of Applied Sciences, Ulmenliet 20, 21033 Hamburg, Germany
Department of Internal Medicine, University Medical Center Hamburg-Eppendorf, Martinistr. 52, 20246 Hamburg, Germany

Abby M. Falla
Department of Public Health, Erasmus MC, University Medical Center Rotterdam, Wytemaweg 80, 3015 Rotterdam, CN, Netherlands
Division of Infectious Disease Control, Municipal Public Health Service Rotterdam-Rijnmond, Schiedamsedijk 95, 3011 Rotterdam, EN, Netherlands

Erika Duffell and Teymur Noori
European Centre for Disease Prevention and Control, Granits väg 8, 171 65 Solna, Stockholm, Sweden

Angela Bechini
Department of Health Sciences, University of Florence, Viale G.B. Morgagni, 48, 50134 Florence, Italy

Irene K. Veldhuijzen
Division of Infectious Disease Control, Municipal Public Health Service Rotterdam-Rijnmond, Schiedamsedijk 95, 3011 Rotterdam, EN, Netherlands
Center for Infectious Disease Control, National Institute for Public Health and the Environment, Antonie van Leeuwenhoeklaan 9, 3721 Bilthoven, MA, Netherlands

Roberto Bruni, Stefania Taffon, Angela Costantino, Paola Chionne, Elisabetta Madonna and Anna Rita Ciccaglione
National Reference Laboratory for HAV, Viral Hepatitis Unit, Department of Infectious Diseases, Istituto Superiore di Sanità, Rome, Italy

Michele Equestre
Department of Neurosciences, Istituto Superiore di Sanità, Rome, Italy

Eleonora Cella, Alessandra Lo Presti and Massimo Ciccozzi
Epidemiology Unit, Department of Infectious Diseases, Istituto Superiore di Sanità, Rome, Italy

Elitsa Golkocheva-Markova, Diljana Bankova and Pavel Teoharov
Department of Virology, National Center of Infectious and Parasitic Diseases, Sofia, Bulgaria

Rachel Shirazi, Daniela Ram, Aviya Rakovsky, Efrat Bucris, Yael Gozlan and Yaniv Lustig
Central Virology Laboratory, Ministry of Health, Chaim Sheba Medical Center, Tel - Hashomer, 52621 Ramat Gan, Israel

Pninit Shaked-Mishan
Microbiology Laboratory, Carmel Medical Center, Haifa, Israel

Orit Picard
Gastroenterology Laboratory, Sheba Medical Center, Ramat Gan, Israel

Yonat Shemer-Avni
Laboratory of Clinical Virology, Soroka University Medical Center, Beer Sheva, Israel

Haim Ben-Zvi
Microbiology Laboratory, Rabin Medical Center, Petach Tikva, Israel

Ora Halutz
Microbiology Laboratory, Sorasky Medical Center, Tel Aviv, Israel

Yoav Lurie
Liver Unit, Shaare Zedek Medical Center, Jerusalem, Israel

Ella Veizman
Liver Unit, Rambam Medical Center, Haifa, Israel

Matthias Carlebach
Liver Unit, Bnai Zion Medical Center, Haifa, Israel

Marius Braun and Michal Cohen-Naftaly
Liver Institute, Rabin Medical Center, Petah-Tikva, Israel

Amir Shlomai
Liver Institute, Rabin Medical Center, Petah-Tikva, Israel
The Sackler School of Medicine, Tel Aviv University, Tel Aviv, Israel

Ella H. Sklan
The Sackler School of Medicine, Tel Aviv University, Tel Aviv, Israel

Rifaat Safadi
Liver Unit, Hadassah Hebrew University Hospital, Jerusalem, Israel

Orna Mor and Ella Mendelson
Central Virology Laboratory, Ministry of Health, Chaim Sheba Medical Center, Tel - Hashomer, 52621 Ramat Gan, Israel
School of Public Health, Sackler School of Medicine, Tel Aviv University, Tel Aviv, Israel

Ziv Ben-Ari
The Sackler School of Medicine, Tel Aviv University, Tel Aviv, Israel
Liver Disease Center, Sheba Medical Center, Ramat Gan, Israel

Elizabeth M. Temu and Mercy L. Nkwama
Internal Medicine Department, Kilimanjaro Christian Medical Center, Moshi, United Republic of Tanzania

Flora G. Ruhangisa, Jeremia J. Pyuza, Kajiru G. Kilonzo and Furaha S. Lyamuya
Internal Medicine Department, Kilimanjaro Christian Medical Center, Moshi, United Republic of Tanzania
Institute of Public Health, Community Health Department, Kilimanjaro Christian Medical University College, Moshi, Tanzania

Innocent B. Mboya and Venance P. Maro
Institute of Public Health, Community Health Department, Kilimanjaro Christian Medical University College, Moshi, Tanzania

Daniel W. Gunda
CUHAS, Mwanza, Tanzania

Elichilia R. Shao
Internal Medicine Department, Kilimanjaro Christian Medical Center, Moshi, United Republic of Tanzania
Institute of Public Health, Community Health Department, Kilimanjaro Christian Medical University College, Moshi, Tanzania
Better Human Health Foundation, Moshi, Tanzania
Imagedoctors International, Arusha, Tanzania

Sofie H. Mooij, Anna D. Tulen, Wilfrid van Pelt, Eelco Franz and Agnetha Hofhuis
Epidemiology and surveillance unit, Centre for Infectious Disease Control Netherlands, National Institute for Public Health and the Environment (RIVM), Antonie van Leeuwenhoeklaan 9, 3721 MA Bilthoven, the Netherlands

Boris M. Hogema, Hans L. Zaaijer and Michel Molier
Sanquin Research, Department of Blood-borne Infections, Amsterdam, the Netherlands

Simone Vollmer, Andrea Irwin and Prince Alfani
Médecins sans Frontières, Operational Center Amsterdam (OCA), Quartier Aeroport, A1, Rue 1039, Porte 405, BP30, N'Djamena, Chad

Larissa Vernier
Médecins sans Frontières, Operational Center Amsterdam (OCA), Quartier Aeroport, A1, Rue 1039, Porte 405, BP30, N'Djamena, Chad
Médecins sans Frontières, Operational Center Amsterdam (OCA), Plantage Middenlaan 14, 1018DD Amsterdam, the Netherlands

Annick Lenglet, Sibylle Sang and Charity Kamau
Médecins sans Frontières, Operational Center Amsterdam (OCA), Plantage Middenlaan 14, 1018DD Amsterdam, the Netherlands

Boris M. Hogema
Sanquin Diagnostic Services, Department of Virology, Plesmanlaan 125, 1066 CX Amsterdam, The Netherlands

Ali M. Moussa
Ministry of Health, BP440 N'Djamena, Chad

Cono Ariti
Medical Statistics, London School of Hygiene and Tropical Medicine, Keppel Street, London WC1E7HT, UK

Livia Melo Villar, Elisabeth Lampe, Helena Medina Cruz and Leticia de Paula Scalioni
Laboratory of Viral Hepatitis, Oswaldo Cruz Institute, FIOCRUZ, Helio and Peggy Pereira Pavillion - Ground Floor - Room B09, FIOCRUZ Av. Brasil, 4365 - Manguinhos –, Rio de Janeiro, RJ 210360-040, Brazil

Flavio Augusto Pádua Milagres
Federal University of Tocantins, Tocantins, Brazil

Renata Gracie, Monica de Avelar Figueiredo Mafra Magalhães and Anselmo Rocha Romão
Laboratory of Information in Health, Institute of Communication and technological and scientific information in Health (ICICT), FIOCRUZ, Rio de Janeiro, Brazil

Vanessa Salete de Paula
Molecular Virology Laboratory, Oswaldo Cruz Institute, FIOCRUZ, Rio de Janeiro, Brazil

Wail A. Hayajneh
Department of Pediatrics, Faculty of Medicine, Jordan University of Science and Technology, Irbid 22110, Jordan

Vincent J. Daniels, Muhammet Nabi Kanıbir, Matthew Pilsbury, Morgan Marks, Michelle G. Goveia, Elamin H. Elbasha, Erik Dasbach and Camilo J. Acosta
Merck & Co., Inc., Kenilworth, NJ, USA

Cerise K. James
Agile-1 for Merck & Co., Inc., Kenilworth, NJ, USA

Wenhai Yu
Institute of Medical Biology, Chinese Academy of Medical Sciences and Peking Union Medical College, 935 Jiaoling Road, Kunming, China

Chenchen Yang, Xianhui Hao, Tianwu Ma and Fen Huang
Medical School, Kunming University of Science and Technology, 727 Jingming Road, Kunming, China

Yu-Ling Qin, Bo Li, Yue-Su Zhou, Xin Zhang, Lei Li, Bing Song, Peng Liu, Yue Yuan and Tian-Jun Jiang
Beijing 302 Hospital, Beijing, China

Zhong-Peng Zhao, Jun Jiao, Jing Li, Yi Sun, Ya-Jun Song and Jia-Fu Jiang
Beijing Institute of Microbiology and Epidemiology, Beijing, China

Stephen Sevalie and Joseph E. Kanu
No. 34 Military Hospital, Wilberforce, Freetown, Sierra Leone

Foday Sahr
No. 34 Military Hospital, Wilberforce, Freetown, Sierra Leone
College of Medicine and Allied Health Sciences, Freetown, Sierra Leone

Gloria Carmona and Laura Ruiz
Public Health Agency of Catalonia (ASPCAT), Roc Boronat 81-95, 08005 Barcelona, Spain

Sergi Hernández
Public Health Agency of Catalonia (ASPCAT), Roc Boronat 81-95, 08005 Barcelona, Spain
Departament de Medicina, Universitat de Barcelona, Barcelona, Spain

Marta Vilaró and Àngela Domínguez
Departament de Medicina, Universitat de Barcelona, Barcelona, Spain
CIBER Epidemiología y Salud Pública (CIBERESP), Barcelona, Spain

Pilar Ciruela, Mireia Jané and Lluis Giralt
Public Health Agency of Catalonia (ASPCAT), Roc Boronat 81-95, 08005 Barcelona, Spain
CIBER Epidemiología y Salud Pública (CIBERESP), Barcelona, Spain

I. B. Omotowo, V. E. Okoli and A. C. Ndu
Department of Community Medicine, College of Medicine, University of Nigeria, Enugu Campus, Nigeria

U. N. Ijoma, O. Obienu and D. O. Onodugo
Department of Medicine, College of Medicine, University of Nigeria, Enugu Campus, Nigeria

I. A. Meka
Department of Chemical Pathology, College of Medicine, University of Nigeria, Enugu Campus, Nigeria

T. Nwagha
Department of Haematology, College of Medicine, University of Nigeria, Enugu Campus, Nigeria

L. C. Onyekonwu
Department of Dermatology, College of Medicine, University of Nigeria, Enugu Campus, Nigeria

E. O. Ugwu
Department of Obstetrics and Gynaecology, College of Medicine, University of Nigeria, Enugu Campus, Nigeria

Index

www.ingramcontent.com/pod-product-compliance
Lightning Source LLC
LaVergne TN
LVHW080918210926
848485LV00004B/674